THE HOME
HEALTH CARE
SOLUTION

THE HOME HEALTH CARE SOLUTION

Janet Zhun Nassif

A COMPLETE CONSUMER GUIDE

Harper & Row, Publishers
*New York, Cambridge, Philadelphia, San Francisco,
London, Mexico City, São Paulo, Singapore, Sydney*

For Fred Nassif,
my caregiver and friend

The author welcomes the reader's comments about this book. Please address your comments to: Janet Zhun Nassif, % Dept. 382, Harper & Row, Publishers, 10 East 53rd Street, New York, N.Y. 10022.

FIRST EDITION

Library of Congress Cataloging-in-Publication Data

Nassif, Janet Zhun.
  The home health care solution.

  Includes index.
  1. Home care services.   2. Consumer education.
3. Home care services—United States.   I. Title.
RA645.3.N37   1985   362.1′4   85-42582
ISBN 0-06-015471-3   85 86 87 88 89 MPC 10 9 8 7 6 5 4 3 2 1
ISBN 0-06-096012-4 (pbk.)   85 86 87 88 89 MPC 10 9 8 7 6 5 4 3 2 1

CONTENTS

V   HOW TO GET THE BEST CARE

VI   ALTERNATIVES TO HOME CARE

VII   RESOURCE GUIDE TO HOME CARE

ACKNOWLEDGMENTS

In conducting research for this book I expected to find widespread consumer problems in the home care industry much like those that consumers face with the traditional health care system. Instead, I found that the biggest problem was that countless consumers endured needless days of hospitalization or confinement in nursing homes unaware that sound help was available no farther away than their own front door. This problem had struck painfully close to home when my husband's aunt, Mary Hitti, whom I deeply cared for, was forced to live her last days in a nursing home in Brooklyn because no one—neither concerned family nor the professionals from whom help was sought—really understood the home care alternative.

The Home Health Care Solution evolved as an answer to this serious large-scale problem. It's true that in the course of writing this book I discovered some poor practices and shoddy operators. But by and large the people I met were committed to high quality home care, open in their answers to my many questions, and eager to help me so I could help consumers. A large measure of thanks and credit for the book belongs to them.

I would like to acknowledge all those professionals whose names appear in this book but particularly: Florence Moore, long-time home care advocate, formerly of the National HomeCaring Council, who first recognized the need for consumer education and inspired me to write this book—her suggestions and advice put me on the right track and opened many doors to the movers and shakers in the home care network; Elsie I. Griffith, Visiting Nurse Service of New York (VNSNY), who gave me her time so graciously despite her whirlwind schedule and who put the resources of her agency at my disposal; Peter Rogatz, MD, VNSNY, who provided moral support as well as an intelligent interview; Marilyn Dean, RN, Medical Personnel Pool, who is proof that profits and top-notch patient care are not incompatible—her review of portions of the manuscript and her insightful comments enriched this book; Allyson Faist, RN, HNS, who gave, and linked me with, information unavailable in any book; Anne Harvey, American Association of Retired Persons (AARP), who cut through the red tape to help; Nancy Gorshe, National Association of Area Agencies on Aging, who did more than what she was asked to; and Margaret O'Brien, RN, who said she would follow up and did.

Many other professionals, not identified by name in this book, helped shape it through personal interviews, by supplying valuable research material, by reviewing the manuscript, or by arranging cheerfully for me to get to the right people. I am grateful for their participation, and I am sure they will recognize their contributions. They include: William D. Cabin, National Association for Home Care, a consummate professional and a nice guy to boot, who did all of the above for me, often, and more—he remains one of the most reliable men I know; Mary VanMeer, Association for Medical and Health Alternatives, a busy and caring person who believed in the project and was willing to work to make it work.

I also wish to thank Joel Reaser, AARP; Sandra Fisher, Administration on Aging, DHHS; Mike Noble, American Dental Association; Helen Maule, RN, American Red Cross; Dan Lerman, American Hospital Association; Vickie Taylor, ACSW, Bearden Professional Associates, Knoxville, TN; Barbara Berger Opotowsky and Nanci Florin, Better Business Bureau, NY; Clara Simmons, Center for Human Services, Cleveland; Arthur F. Kohrman, MD, Children's Hospital and Research Center, Chicago; Grace Theado, RN, Community Home Health Services, Joliet, IL; Janice Treml, Community Nursing Service, Salt Lake City; George West, RRT, Continuing Care Associates, Canton, MA; Dennis Kodner, Elderplan, Brooklyn, NY; Carol Grigsby, RN, Madeline Kerman Millman, and Shirley Turner, RN, Empire Blue Cross Blue Shield, NY; David Heiden, Glasrock Home Health Care; Arthur Forest, Jim Barnett, and Judith Thomas, HCFA; Camilla Fleming, HRA, NY; Bob Braun, Jim Jolley, and Marie Foster, HRS, FL; Ginny Posid, RN, Home Health Care, Anchorage, AK; Robert M. Allen, Home Health Care Medical Directors Association; Donald D. Jones, Health Insurance Association of America; Jocelyn Griffo, *Home Health Journal;* Paula Fogelberg, MSW, Home Health Services of Tennessee; the staff, Hospice Care, Pinellas Park, FL; Judith Walden, RN, Hospital Home Health Care, Albuquerque; Anne Weiss, Humboldt Senior Resource Center, Eureka, CA; Gregory Wallis, RT, Linde HomeCare Medical Systems; Carol Raphael, Medical Assistance Program, NYC; Diane Justice, NASUA; former Senator Frank E. Moss, NAHC; Jim Warren, National Kidney Foundation; the staff, National Shared Housing Resources Center; Nancy Barhydt and Madeline Penachio, NY Department of Health; Richard McGowan, Judy Holtz, and Raisa Otero-Cesario, Office of Inspector General, DHHS; Ellen Harnett, the Pride Institute; Rita Gorman, Metropolitan Life Insurance Company; Carol Gordon and Amy Hanover, Quality Care; Jere Rowland and Florence C. Scharf, Staff Builders; David Forsee, Travenol Management Services; Eileen Ales, Sandy Calvert, and Sara Craig, Upjohn Healthcare Services; Cynthia Vitters and Joe Fleckenstein, Veterans Administration; Astrida Berzs, RCSW, VNA Home Healthcare, Portland; Martha J. de Ulibarri, VNA of the Denver area; Martha Bergman, Susan Leuris, RN, Edward Mullaney, and Edward Sikula, VNSNY.

Few authors get into print without the benefit of an enthusiastic editor or agent, conscientious secretarial help, and steadfast support from caring family and friends. I am lucky to have had it all. My special thanks to Janet Goldstein, my editor at Harper & Row, who recognized immediately the need for this book and whose warm and professional manner, easygoing editorial style, and perceptive suggestions were a writer's dream and greatly improved this manuscript; Edy Ginis Selman—agent, friend, marketing strategist, health care seer—one exceptional person who can, and does, always read between the lines; Arthur Marcus, Marcia Lewicki, Vicki Vogel, and Irene Cunningham, who helped bring the written word into print with their careful deciphering of my scrawl and their very professional typing skills. My deep appreciation is offered to Virginia Brown, Nancy Crosby, Phil Crosby, Kyoko Eustach, Jean and Don McKerrow, Micheline Nakis and Erik Pitsokis, Mary Jane and Ed Nassif, Pat and Bob Neale, Donna and Will Rogers, Carol and Jim Ross, Mary Ellen Zhun Russell, Mimi Untermeyer, and Henry Untermeyer, who continued to dispense their own special brand of home care while I worked "underground" on this book, keeping their hearts and homes open to me though I could not reciprocate their many kindnesses; to Ellen and Peter Zhun, who have always been more than just parents; to Janet Antoinette and Victoria Grace Russell, who gave up "our" playtime together without complaint; and to Fred Nassif, who gave up our playtime too and who was always my first-line editor and chief morale booster.

Finally I would like to extend my gratitude to the many consumers who shared their experiences, concerns, and questions with me. My heartfelt thanks to those named in the book, to those who wished to remain anonymous, and also to Juanita Biddle, Ruth Haywood, Ruby Levine, Eugene Mechler, Margie Menges, Gladys Marie Smith-Wesp . . . but, most of all, Aunt Mary Hitti.

I

INTRODUCING
HOME CARE

—1—

There's No Place Like Home

Robert W. sat waiting in his hospital bed for his physical therapist to arrive. At age 59, he had been felled by a stroke that left him partially paralyzed on one side. He felt refreshed now that he had bathed, groomed himself, and dressed with an aide's assistance. The aide had also taken his temperature and pulse and carefully noted these vital signs on his patient record. His nurse had stopped by earlier that morning to listen to his heart and lungs. She also checked Robert for any reaction to the new blood pressure drug his doctor had ordered.

Always an independent man, Robert recalled how he felt after he was admitted to the hospital following his stroke. "Once I knew I was going to survive, I wasn't sure that I wanted to. I felt so helpless."

Robert feels better now. His recovery is slow, but he is starting to walk again. He is even thinking ahead to the time when he can return to work. The careful nursing care and regular therapy sessions he receives are working their wonders. "With the good care that I get," Robert remarks, "I'm getting better quicker than I ever expected to."

Nothing is particularly remarkable about Robert's case except one thing. He is recovering at home, not in the hospital. The nurse, therapist, and aide are home care personnel, not hospital workers.

Robert is just one of millions of Americans who have found the home health care solution. Instead of languishing in a hospital or a nursing home, they are cared for at home, where they want to be.

That's where Martha R., age 36, wanted to be when she

became terminally ill with stomach cancer. Surrounded by her loving family—her husband, two children, and family dog—she spent her last days without pain at home, thanks to a community hospice program. Despite her serious illness, she was very much a part of everyday family life, and she continued her duties as a mother. Both her husband and her children cherish the memory of their last days together.

For another mother, Patricia C., age 26, home care was prompted by a joyful event, the birth of her second child. Instead of remaining hospitalized for several days, she went home within 24 hours where her 3-year-old son was waiting anxiously for his mommy and his new baby brother. A specially trained nurse visited twice to monitor Mrs. C.'s health and the baby's. A part-time homemaker helped her with household chores, which eased her hospital-to-home transition.

Bachelor Peter Q., age 35, found the home care solution when a car accident left him with multiple broken bones mending in a neck-to-knee body cast. His choice? Transfer to a nursing home for six weeks or more, or go home with help. It didn't take him long to make the home care decision.

"'Til death do us part' was the vow that we made," Mr. G. said, as he recalled his feelings when his wife of 62 years started to fail. "A nursing home—never." With home care help, Mr. and Mrs. G. were able to remain home together until Mrs. G. died peacefully at home a year later.

When it comes to needing care, regardless of age or situation, people are rediscovering that there's still no place like home. Home care—the oldest form of health care—is enjoying a revival.

For many older Americans, the concept of home care has a familiar ring. Before the advent of our modern health care system, most people began life at home and ended it there too. When they were downed by illness, injury, old age, and infirmity, they were cared for in their own homes by family, friends, and the family physician.

Change began with the discovery of diagnostic tools like X rays and wonder drugs like penicillin. Medicine, which up to then had been largely a homespun, bedside art, moved almost overnight into the realm of science and technology. Health care became more organized and specialized, and the growth spurt of hospitals started. Soon hospitals, with their technological wonders, became the patient's mecca for medical miracles.

At the same time, advances in technology slowly altered American social structure and values. Families became more mobile. The extended family disappeared. Many older people were left living alone, with relatives far away. Women, the traditional caregivers, joined the work force in great numbers. The result was the birth of nursing homes to fill the void. In the public's mind, nursing homes gradually became an accepted institution for senior care.

As so often happens, the pendulum is now swinging the other way. Just a few years ago, hospitals and nursing homes had the market cornered on health care, while home care was health care's "best kept secret."

Not so any longer. The message is getting out loud and clear to those who have a stake in health care—doctors and other health professionals, government officials, employers, insurers—and most important to you, the consumer.

The home care boom has just begun. It won't be kept under wraps any longer.

HOME CARE AND YOU

If you are an older American, are disabled, or are in failing health, you may be already keenly interested in home care. That's important, because home care can be the key to maintaining your most prized possession—your independence. If you're younger and in good health, you may think, "So what—home care has nothing to do with me." Yet reality says otherwise.

It's a fact. Sometime during your lifetime, you, a family member, or someone you know and care about will almost certainly need home care. If you require hospitalization at any age, you can cut short your hospital stay. Home care brings the same personnel who provide hospital care to your door so you can recover in the comfort and privacy of your own home.

Are you in your forties? With our increasing life span, the chances are four out of five you will have responsibility for an elderly, ailing parent or relative for a long period of time, perhaps even into your own "golden years." Maybe that day has already arrived. If so, you are one of some 22 million Americans whose parents are now struggling with problems that impair their daily life. In such cases, home care presents a sound solution you would be wise to explore now.

If you are a woman, take special note of home care. Statistics show you will probably have to care for two sets of aged parents, yours and your husband's. Also, as a woman you are more likely to spend your last days in a nursing home unless you discover a different solution.

In the pages ahead, you will learn the ins and outs of the home care solution. Though home care is the best thing that's happened to health care in some time, it's becoming big business. "Inevitably whenever an area begins to attract billions of dollars, it will attract the sharks and the entrepreneurs," cautions National Association for Home Care (NAHC) president Val Halamandaris. "We're starting to see some signs of that in home care."

Home care headlines about unscrupulous business practices, slipshod care, and sometimes outright abuse are now surfacing sporadically. In more than one instance, consumers have been ripped off by the personnel paid to provide tender loving care. Mix money and medicine, and you have the prescription for serious potential consumer problems.

However, you needn't let the dark side of home care worry you: You will get the best of what home care has to offer if you become home-care-wise. This book will help you do just that. If you happen to be in the helping professions, whether you are a doctor, nurse, hospital discharge planner, social worker, community service worker, volunteer, or employee assistance manager, you will also find practical advice that can help you better assist those you serve.

WHAT IS HOME CARE?

Although health professionals usually understand the phrase "home care," the phrase misleads some consumers and mystifies others. Home care suffers from an image problem. The title of this book deliberately includes the word "health" so you will not mistake its message.

From the outset, let's set the record straight. *Home care* means *people care at home.* It is diagnosis, treatment, monitoring, rehabilitation, and supportive care provided at home, rather than in an impersonal hospital, nursing home, or other institution.

Home care is the preferred term, not *home health care,* because it is far more than just health care. At its best, home care is holistic, providing in-home health, social, and other human services that can help you as a whole person, not just as a "patient."

Home care also means services to families to help them cope with the problems of caring for loved ones. Home care means more than just providing services "for" people. It means teaching people needed skills so they can manage on their own, with less stress and more satisfaction.

In this era of great specialization, think of home care as the "quality of life" specialty.

THE HOME CARE SOLUTION

Earlier you met several consumers, each with different problems. Like them, you can turn to home care as a solution to varied personal situations.

You can substitute home care for inpatient care whenever possible, and as soon as possible. One insurer conservatively estimates that 7 percent of all hospitalized patients on any given day could be treated at home. Many patients remain hospitalized for injections, monitoring, and therapy, all services which are readily available in the home.

In some cases, home care can help you avoid hospitalization

altogether, as Mr. N., 45, a self-employed businessman, learned. When Mr. N. accidentally injured his back, his doctor advised a week's hospitalization, traction, and follow-up physical therapy. Not one to agree easily to anything, he explored his other options. That same day, he was in a hospital bed at home, in traction, with a home care agency providing care according to his doctor's orders.

Mr. N.'s experience counters one mistaken, widely held notion about home care: Home care is not just for the elderly. It can be a boon to people of all ages, including children and families. In fact, one out of every four people currently receiving home care is under age 65. The number of younger consumers is expected to grow as more people learn about home care availability and benefits, and many heretofore hospital-only treatments become more routine at home. For example, for infants born with a jaundice condition, home bilirubin phototherapy is now available. This treatment, which requires controlled exposure to ultraviolet light, normally keeps an otherwise healthy newborn hospitalized for three extra days, as well as mom. Now mother and child can begin their bonding process at home without needless delay.

Though home care among the younger population is on the upswing, older Americans represent the largest group of home care consumers. The positive impact of this care on their lives cannot be overstated. With a sound plan for home care services, the vast majority can maintain independent living at home and avoid nursing home placement . . . despite even overwhelming odds.

Such is the case with Mrs. P., an elderly Italian Brooklynite who receives home care through the Metropolitan Jewish Geriatric Center of New York. That Mrs. P. can remain at home is a wonder. At age 82, she lives alone, though she suffers from severe arthritis, heart disease, is partially blind in both eyes, and is hard of hearing. But she's at home, assisted by an aide four hours a day, four times a week. A nurse visits Mrs. P. every two weeks and monitors her health. When needed, the program's doctor provides medical care. The social worker helps her with financial matters.

Because of her health problems Mrs. P. loses her balance

easily, so as a security measure, the agency has installed an in-home emergency response system that will bring help promptly should Mrs. P. fall at any time of the day or night.

Twice a week, the agency has arranged transportation services so that Mrs. P. can participate in the center's adult day care program. Mrs. P. looks forward to these outings with great anticipation. She gets to visit and chat with friends, easing her loneliness; and she participates in the center's exercise program, which helps keep her mobile.

Of her home care program, Mrs. P. says: "Without it, I could not manage to take care of myself at home alone. I would probably be in a nursing home."

Mrs. P. is right. On a disability scale used to rate people who require nursing home care, Mrs. P. is a shoo-in candidate. So is Mr. Jacob G., another elderly person served by Metropolitan.

Most observers would have automatically assumed that a nursing home was the best place for this 98-year-old gentleman when his existing health problems—circulatory disease, hardening of the arteries, and congestive heart failure—were complicated by a recently broken hip. Yet with an aide five days a week, a nurse to check his progress, and regular physical therapy, he stayed at home, close to the neighborhood temple he loves. His hip has healed well, and he walks with only a slight limp, assisted by a cane. With the help provided by the agency, Mr. G. safely manages three flights of stairs each morning to attend temple, where he still serves as a cantor.

Both these seniors are receiving care through an innovative long-term home care program aptly called the Nursing Home Without Walls. Designed to show that even the elderly with multiple problems can live safely at home with proper care and at a cost 25 to 50 percent *less* than comparable nursing home care, this program has rescued thousands of elderly in New York State from almost certain nursing home placement. Similar programs are scattered in other states throughout the country.

Some Intangible Benefits

When it comes to personal satisfaction and contentment, home care wins hands down over institutional care. Universally, surveys of home care users of all ages report a high measure of consumer satisfaction. If you have ever been hospitalized, you understand why.

When you enter a hospital—even a good hospital—suddenly you become "the patient." Like joining the army, this depersonalization process begins with induction (patient admissions). You are given a tag (a patient identification bracelet), and your clothes are exchanged for a hospital uniform (an all-too-revealing gown). No matter how independent you have been before, your daily routine must revolve around the hospital's schedule. Dependence and your sick role are encouraged at every turn. You're no longer permitted to walk to X ray if you need one; you're wheelchaired. Visitors may come only during specified hours. No children. No pets. No privacy. No phone calls after hours. If this isn't demoralizing enough, the food is usually as institutional as the surroundings.

Home care is a human solution to institutional treatment. At home, you can arrange for care according to a schedule that meets your life style and needs. You can enjoy meals with taste appeal and eat when you want to. Visitors can come and go at times convenient for you and for them, and everyone you want to see is welcome. It's a comfort just to have familiar belongings around you.

Most people eat better, sleep better, and feel better in their own homes, so it is not surprising that better health is another home care dividend. Yes, home care is a healthful solution. Contrary to some opinions, it's definitely *not* second-rate care. The American Medical Association endorses home care, as does the American Hospital Association, among other organizations.

A U.S. Department of Health and Human Services (DHHS) study on home health services stated: "The quality is typically quite high, primarily because of the service ethic and professionalism of the nurses. The fact that as home health nurses they function in a much more independent manner than is customary for nurses (especially compared with hospital settings) seems to bring out the best in them."

It also brings out the best in patients. The happy feeling of being cared for at home seems, indeed, to be healing. Repeated studies have found that on the average, people recover faster at home. Among the chronically ill, home care is associated with improved or maintained mental function and social activity. More than one research study has also credited home care for the lower death rates among the elderly receiving this service. Examining the data on home care, a U.S. General Accounting Office study "found evidence that individuals who receive expanded home care services live longer than others who use currently available health services."

A government imprimatur is reassuring, but you have only to speak to consumers to appreciate the health benefits home care can bring. Colonel McKaig saw a dramatic change in his wife, who at age 82 began to decline rapidly, physically and mentally. "The doctor said there was nothing that could be done. When Shirley [a home health aide employed by Upjohn Health Care Services] walked in, I knew we had a professional and someone who knew what it was all about. She would bathe her, change linen, and was psychologically sympathetic. My wife had a friend. Shirley didn't do anything you would call 'therapeutic,' but my wife improved markedly. Her alertness improved. She became a different person."

Since coming home for care, 3½-year-old Don Broom, a multiply handicapped child who is on a life support ventilator, has started to thrive. He now talks and sits up, reports his father, and receives constant love and care. "That's something we couldn't give Don when he was 24 miles away at the hospital," his father, Frederico Broom, explains.

The scientific reasons behind the health payoffs of home care are undergoing study. One researcher suggested that for the chronically ill, the answer may be the "ounce of prevention" principle. He noted that through regular home care, any developing problems were detected earlier and treated sooner. Without care, key symptoms were often ignored until more serious and harder-to-treat illnesses were apparent. The plain fact that home care keeps people out of hospitals or nursing homes itself may promote health. Though hospitals are designed to restore health, inherent problems exist within the system that work against this mission.

For starters, it's highly stressful. Two well-recognized stressors—life change and lack of personal control over situations—are inescapable realities of institutional care. Stress, we are learning now, can help precipitate or worsen health problems. So just going to a hospital for some consumers, particularly for the elderly, may be enough to send a person in declining health into a tailspin.

Hospitals are repositories of infection. Most hospitals employ a special nurse epidemiologist whose sole role is to prevent, track down, and correct outbreaks of infection. With constant personnel changes, hospital patients risk medication mistakes or other human errors. No one can deny that hospitals deserve credit for accomplishing life-saving miracles; but unless absolutely necessary, they can be "hazardous to your health." Public health analysts have found that during strikes, when patients are kept out of hospitals, community death rates actually go down.

Nursing homes suffer from institutional problems akin to those of hospitals. In most nursing homes, care is highly regimented, even to the point of scheduled toileting. The use of "chemical restraints"—deliberately overmedicating patients to keep them "trouble-free" for staff—is widespread despite regulations against such practices.

One nursing home resident told a government survey worker: "I hated to give up my belongings. I worked all my life and valued my independence. I cried for the first one-and-one-half years I was here."

About 25 percent of the elderly who move to nursing homes die within the first year of residence. This percentage is far higher than can be explained by illness alone. When life is no longer worth living, it seems that people just give up.

New inroads into the dynamics of health and illness underscore that medical care is not the only mainstay of health. Our social ties and support may be even more critical to our well-being. On this point, home care rates high, as it keeps people close to family, friends, and the community—in other words, within the social support network. Researchers theorize that social support acts as a buffer against stress, thereby preventing or minimizing the negative effects of stress on well-being.

The Financial Benefit

Perhaps the most tangible benefit of home care is that it can help you save money.

Many Americans are vulnerable to the high costs of care. A Robert Wood Johnson study conducted by Louis Harris and Associates found that one out of ten families randomly surveyed had at least one member with a serious illness and one-quarter of these families said the illness caused major financial problems.

While health insurance helps shoulder health care costs, unless you have 100 percent coverage, even a short-term hospital stay can put a serious dent in your budget. In 1983, a *U.S. News & World Report* article on soaring hospital costs cited the case of a man who underwent two-hour knee surgery at a public hospital in the Northeast. Imagine his shock at seeing his bill. After just two and a half days of care, it totaled a hefty $12,046.

Now consider the home care solution. As a rule, home care costs considerably less than care in institutions, where you are charged a day rate based on *all* the general services the facility must provide in order to operate. In hospitals, this includes nursing care, therapy, X-ray and laboratory units, food service, laundry, and medical equipment. Also built into the cost equation is the high cost of administration, plus the cost of the building itself. Usually, added to the day rate are individual costs for each extra item provided beyond room, board, nursing, and general medical care. Thus you are charged, for example, for an X ray, each laboratory test, and even an aspirin.

Upon receipt of the hospital bill, patients are stunned to

find that the cost of certain extras is often astronomical. Colonel McKaig, who kept accurate records of all his wife's medical expenses, found he was charged $2.40 for each absorbent bed pad, which cost him 30 cents at his local drugstore. A common drug, Lasix, cost $1.50 per pill in the hospital. He was accustomed to paying $3.95 for 100, about 4 cents apiece.

Reported examples of hospital overcharges include a $19.75 to $148 spread for a complete blood count, a common lab test that costs the hospital about $6 to run; a $12 to $142 range for an intravenous solution that wholesales for 94 cents. With such overcharges, the cost of a simple two-day nonsurgical hospital stay can quickly top $1,000.

With home care, you are charged only for the professional health or personal services you need. Home care agencies have lower administrative costs, and you can obtain your own drugs and supplies, which usually mean an additional cost savings. The time factor also alters home care costs, usually in your favor. Institutions must provide round-the-clock care. Home care is seldom provided 24 hours a day, and fewer hours means lower cost. Your family also saves on the transportation costs of hospital visiting.

The cost of home care provided over a period of a few weeks can come close to what you might pay for a *single day* of hospital care. A 1984 study by the U.S. House of Representatives Select Committee on Aging assisted by the National Association for Home Care reports that in 1982, the average home care client received 9.6 visits for a *total* home care cost of $364.32. For Medicare patients, hospital stays averaged 10.5 days, at an average cost of $350 per *day*.

By exchanging your home for the hospital room, you automatically save daily. In 1982, a semi-private hospital room, before extras, averaged $178.49 a day. If you consider that hospital charges account for nearly two-thirds of the average total medical bill, the opportunity to save through home care can be substantial. The Hospital Home Health Care Agency of California reports that in 1982 the average day in a California hospital topped $700, while an average home care day for its patients was a mere $70. In cases of catastrophic illness or accident, the savings are dramatic. Aetna Life and Casualty Company, through a program that encourages home care, reports of savings of $78,000 per patient over conventional care.

For anyone who must pay for some health care costs out of pocket, home care will generally save money. Let's consider the potential savings home care can mean to Medicare recipients. Those eligible for Medicare hospital or nursing home care generally qualify for home care too, which Medicare fully covers. Medicare will even allow the use of home care to avoid hospitalization.

Medicare data for 1982 placed the average annual cost per beneficiary for hospital care at $3,675, for nursing home care at $1,710, and for home health care at $819. In the case of hospital and nursing home bills, these patients often paid better than 50 percent or more of the bill out of pocket. The $819 home care bill was completely covered by Medicare; beneficiaries did not have to pay a penny.

Small wonder that in its Medicare booklet the American Association of Retired Persons stresses that home care visits "frequently enable people to manage a good part of recovery at home and greatly reduce the risk of heavy expenses for long-term care."

If you are on Medicare or privately insured through your employer or other plan, home care represents an opportunity to save not just money, but your benefit days should serious illness or injury later strike. You won't be charged a hospital or nursing home day when you substitute home care instead. Many insurers and employers themselves now encourage home care.

If you are considering a nursing home for long-term care, home care can offer ample savings. Even the cheapest homes cost over $1,400 per month, which is seldom covered by insurance. Colonel McKaig's monthly home care bills for his wife averaged $700—not cheap, and not insured either, but still far less than a nursing home, which was his only alternative.

These are but a few examples of the financial benefits you

can derive by choosing the home care solution. It makes good consumer sense to get well at home, or to continue to live independently at home and keep your money in the bank.

HURDLES TO HOME CARE

Despite its benefits, the home care option remains seriously underused. According to Val Halamandaris, NAHC president, "Consumers still don't know that home care exists."

The Information Gap

Part of the problem is that the professionals consumers rely on for help often don't know about home care either, or know far too little. Several studies found that social service personnel did not suggest home care as an alternative to those applying or admitted to nursing homes. Yet experts reckon that close to one-third of all current nursing home residents could be cared for at home if home care and other community services were provided.

For consumers who are hospitalized or about to be, physicians are often a major stumbling block. While growing numbers of physicians advocate home care, far too many still think office, hospital, or nursing home when they think of patient care.

That's not surprising if you consider that of 127 U.S. medical schools, only 15 require future MDs to take courses in geriatric care. Few medical and osteopathic schools ever take the student out of an institution to see and experience patient care at home. For the fledgling physician, the hospital is where the action is.

Peter Rogatz, MD, whose varied career includes hospitals, medical education, and the health insurance industry, and who now serves as vice-president for medical affairs, Visiting Nurse Service of New York, sees other issues as well. "Many physicians are afraid of losing control of their patients. They may perceive the nurse as a competitor, or may think if the patient finds out he or she can manage at home with a visit from a nurse every couple of days, that patient may not come and see me so often." Dr. Rogatz points out this block is overcome when the Visiting Nurse Service, as does any professional home care agency, makes it clear that the doctor's orders are meticulously followed.

"My doctor didn't suggest home care," said Mrs. R., "until I told him my Medicare coverage was running out. Until then, my husband had been either hospitalized or cared for in a nursing home." Many doctors don't prescribe home care because they think it is an expensive add-on cost to patients. Often physicians plan treatment according to what kind of insurance coverage you have. Like consumers, by and large they are unaware that insurance now often covers home care. Therefore doctors automatically gear treatment to hospital care.

"We realize now that when it is left for doctors to initiate home care," said Katherine Daley of Connecticut General Life Insurance Co. in *Business Week,* "they don't." This insurer stations a nurse in the hospital to review patient records and spot likely home care candidates.

Whatever your doctor's reason, if he or she does not discuss home care as an option, Dr. Rogatz suggests you ask your doctor directly, "Isn't there some way I can get this care at home?" Don't debate the issue, but become informed enough to discuss it. Often a little prodding on your part will make the difference.

These information gaps mean that many consumers and families are missing out on the home care solution. They are in hospitals and nursing homes needlessly or are struggling at home, unaware that home care is available to assist them. Recent studies estimate that there are some 5 million consumers who could benefit from home care services, but are not receiving them.

Now that you are home-care-aware, help spread the good news. Don't hestitate to put your neighbors, friends, or relatives in need in the know. Share the message with professionals too.

The Financial Gap

The costs of care prevent some consumers from seeking and obtaining needed health services of any kind, home care included. In situations where loved ones require long-term care, many families experience financial hardship. The cost of caring for a severely disabled person, without drugs or doctors' fees, may exceed $5,000 per year.

Much of the problem can be traced to the way health care is financed in our country. Medicare and most private insurance are geared toward help for acute, not chronic, care. This leaves many people trapped in what Senator John Heinz, chairman of the U.S. Senate Special Committee on Aging, refers to as "no care zones." Heinz says these Americans are "caught between a rock and a hard place. They have just enough income to disqualify them for Medicaid, but neither the money nor the insurance to cover their long-term bills."

The answer to the problem lies partly in political solutions. As a nation, we must be willing to redirect our priorities toward prevention and away from institutional care.

For anyone caught in the financial gap, there are no easy solutions. But many organizations can help. Later chapters will provide advice and cost-saving tips.

IS HOME CARE FOR YOU?

The home care solution is waiting for you, but first you have to recognize whether or not you have a problem that it can help. As you have seen, you can't always rely on professionals for guidance. In health care, it always helps to understand one's own needs, whether for the short or the long term.

The questions below will give you some insight into whether home care may benefit you or someone you care about. If the answer is "yes" to any of these questions, consider or suggest home care.

If you are at home:
  • Are you ill, disabled, elderly, and frail—living alone, or

with someone whose health is also impaired?

- Are physical or emotional problems making it hard for you to manage daily tasks like bathing, dressing, getting in and out of bed, shopping, cooking, housekeeping, child care?
- Has someone—physician, relative, friend—suggested that you give up living at home, or move in with your children, because of needed care?
- Are you scheduled for, or considering, outpatient or same-day surgery or a 24-hour maternity center, and worried about aftercare?
- Are you recently discharged from hospital or nursing home, but not fully recovered and finding it hard to follow your doctor's recommendations for care, such as taking medicine or doing prescribed exercises?
- Are you having trouble coping with poor health or performing medical self-care tasks such as giving yourself injections or ostomy care, or checking blood sugar?
- Do you have a chronic condition that requires frequent or ongoing monitoring, such as heart or kidney disease, breathing difficulties, diabetes, muscle-nerve problems?
- Are you terminally ill and afraid or depressed? In constant pain? Worried about your family? Wanting to remain at home?

If you are a hospital or nursing home patient:

- Are you past the acute phase of your illness, but still need regular or periodic monitoring, nursing care, therapy, or other health services?
- Are you receiving ongoing institutional care mainly because you need rehabilitation? Intravenous (IV) antibiotic therapy? Artificial feeding? Ventilator support for breathing? Or because your condition is terminal?
- Are you receiving institutional care *mainly* because you live alone and need help with daily tasks that a spouse or other family member cannot provide? Because you need part-time nursing supervision?
- Are you ready for discharge but concerned about your ability to care for yourself, your home, or your family?

If you are a caregiver for an ill or disabled child, spouse, parent, or relative:

- Are you unsure of your caregiving skills or feel that they could be improved with professional assistance?
- Has your loved one experienced lack of expected or hoped for progress? Does he or she seem to be declining?
- Do you often miss work in order to provide care?
- Do your responsibilities prevent you from getting a regular break for relief or taking a vacation?
- Are you often angry, anxious, frustrated, or exhausted because of your caregiving responsibilities?
- Does the family member under care have a condition that requires regular health monitoring?
- Are family relationships seriously strained or breaking down because of caregiving pressures?

In situations such as these, a sound home care program that includes one or more services may work well for you. Of course, home care is not the only or even the best solution for every individual situation. When someone needs extensive care, treatment, and supervision round-the-clock for months or indefinitely, a hospital, nursing home, or rehabilitation facility may be more appropriate. However, it is important to keep in mind that few absolutes dictate when institutional care is a must. Each person, each family, each situation is unique and should be evaluated carefully on an individual basis. When home care is appropriate, many people who have serious and often multiple problems can live at home where they want to, and ideally should, be. They are at home even though involved health professionals, concerned family members, or others believed "it couldn't be done."

—2—

The Home Care Revolution

Although history buffs trace the first organized home care program back to the Boston Dispensary in 1796, home care was not officially launched into the mainstream of American health care until 1965. That year brought the passage of Medicare, Title XVIII, and Medicaid, Title XIX, of the Social Security Act. This was the beginning of large-scale reimbursement for home care services. The seeds of the home care revolution were sown.

Around the time of this landmark legislation, only 250 agencies existed that would fit today's Medicare agency mold. By 1984 their numbers had swelled to more than 5,000, with the greatest growth spurt occurring in the last five years. In 1982 alone, these agencies made over 28.1 million home care visits to Medicare recipients. Each year the number of consumers served continues to increase.

Why the home care revolution now? If you follow the news regularly, the reasons for the turnabout from institutional to home care begin to surface.

HEALTH CARE COSTS

Over the last twenty years, health care costs have risen rapidly and are still rising. In 1965, costs hovered at $41.7 billion. By 1985, HCFA predicts the figure will reach a staggering $456 billion—more than a tenfold increase.

You might argue that the cost of everything has gone up with inflation. True enough, but the rate hike for health care has regularly outpaced the consumer price index (CPI) by a wide margin. For example, in 1982 the CPI rose 6.1 percent over 1981, while health care costs saw a full 11.6 percent increase. Hospitals, with a 15.7 percent jump, were the big offenders. In 1976, the American Hospital Association reported that average daily cost per hospital day was approximately $152; by 1982, the day cost had risen a whopping 115 percent to $327.40.

Recent data point to a more moderate trend in rising health costs as hospitals tighten administrative controls and reduce personnel costs. Even so, HCFA experts say that by the year 2000 the national price tag for health will exceed a monumental $1 trillion. These out-of-kilter costs have created a national health care crisis affecting everyone from the individual consumer to the giants of industry.

If You Are on Medicare

It's frightening but true: Medicare, the national health insurance payment program for the elderly, is slated for bankruptcy in the 1990s unless serious measures are taken to save it.

In 1983, as part of its belt tightening, Medicare changed its payment rules for hospitals. Under the old system, hospitals literally received a blank check for treating Medicare patients. The longer a patient stayed, the more services rendered, the bigger the bill. Medicare paid, with few questions asked. Hospital administrators understandably liked the system.

Those days are gone forever. Now a flat payment system is in effect, akin to a restaurant's fixed-price menu. With a system called DRGs (diagnostic related groups), hospitals get paid a preset price for the patient's total care. This predetermined price is based mostly on the admitting diagnosis, one of 467 possible diagnostic categories. The government pays not a penny more than the DRG fee schedule allows, no matter how many tests are ordered or how long the patient is hospitalized.

While this may sound bad for hospitals, it can be a boon. The government allows hospitals that can provide care at a cost *below* the established DRG fee to pocket the difference. Now, at last, hospitals have an incentive to scrutinize plans for treatment according to what is most cost-effective. The system also encourages hospitals to discharge Medicare patients as soon as they can. Critics charge this means "sicker and quicker" than even before.

For Medicare patients, no longer is home care just a possible option; it's becoming a short-term necessity as hospitals deliberately discharge recovering patients earlier than before. But if you haven't reached those golden years, don't breathe a sigh of relief. As Medicare goes, the private sector is sure to follow. It's happening already.

If You Are Privately Insured

If you are a typical working American under age 65, your employer foots the lion's share of the health care costs for you and your family through private health insurance programs. The more employees use health services and the more costly these services are, the higher your employer's insurance costs. In 1984, employers spent an estimated $17 billion on health insurance premiums, a figure higher than corporate dividend outlays. In some cases these out-of-sight insurance costs cut seriously into profitability and may even threaten a company's existence.

Big business is feeling the pinch. Take Chrysler Corporation, for example. Its annual health insurance tab alone runs about $373 million. This is not bad news just for Chrysler; it's bad for consumers too. These hefty insurance costs translate into a $600 higher sticker price per car.

Employers are no longer accepting ever-mounting insurance costs as an inevitable part of doing business. They are fighting back, and the name of the game is "cost containment."

One prime cost containment strategy is to make you as an employee more aware of health care costs so you will select and use health services more prudently. Many businesses are requiring employees to pay more for health care than ever before, a definite attention grabber. The days of $50 and $100 deductibles are fast disappearing in exchange for deductibles in the $200 to $600 range. Companies are demanding that employees split the bill through new or higher co-payment systems. Such tactics can be effective. A Rand Corporation study found that the fully insured spent up to 60 percent more on health care than those partially insured.

Some companies use both the carrot and the stick approach to reducing health costs. They offer employees incentives to use cheaper care, or penalize them for use under certain conditions. Full payment may be made for outpatient same-day surgery such as a hernia repair, but only 50 to 80 percent coverage will be offered for the repair as an inpatient operation. In nonemergency surgical cases, coverage may be reduced unless a second opinion confirming the need for surgery has been obtained.

Cost savings from such measures can be dramatic. At a Phoenix hospital, for example, the costs for a D&C, a gynecologic surgery, were four times as high as those costs at Surgicenter, a Phoenix same-day surgical facility. The renowned Massachusetts General Hospital now performs about 200 different operations on an outpatient basis. Outpatient costs range up to 75 percent less than the same operations performed with normal two-day hospitalization.

Businesses are also forming health groups or coalitions—over 100 nationally—in order to learn the health care ropes, share effective cost-containment strategies, and exert collective influence on the system. These coalitions are making headway too. The Denver Colorado Coalition for Health, for example, obtained discount hospital rates when its members agreed by contract to use the services of Presbyterian/St. Luke's Medical Center's six-hospital system.

As costs have risen, insurers have not sat idly by just collecting higher premiums. Pressured by unions and employers, and fearful of losing their policyholders, they too have joined the fray to streamline costs. Insurers like Connecticut General, Prudential, Transamerica Occidental, and Equitable have started innovative hospital preadmission review or certification programs. Since hospital costs account for up to 65 percent of all employee health expenses, reducing hospitalization can mean substantial savings to both insurers and employers.

Under these programs, prior to hospitalization your doctor

submits information on your symptoms, diagnosis, and proposed plan of treatment and length of hospital stay. The insurer's reviewer, a specially trained nurse or physician's assistant, then scans the treatment plan for its appropriateness according to preset medical guidelines. Plans outside these guidelines are referred to a physician for closer review and discussion with your doctor. Adjustments may be made, or some alternative measures such as home care may be recommended. Hospital stays that are deemed not medically necessary are paid for by the insurer at lower rates or sometimes not at all.

Insurers have also been keeping a close watch on the Medicare DRG system. They have noted that DRGs have significantly slowed increases in treatment costs for Medicare patients. What is good for keeping costs down for Medicare patients, insurers believe, can be good for holding down costs for everyone. Speaking for the industry, Daniel Thomas, assistant director, Consumer and Professional Relations Division of The Health Insurance Association of America, emphatically states: "Reimbursement reform of the DRG nature is what must be done to address the cost problems of the entire system."

The insurance industry is pushing such legislation at the national and state levels. In the CIGNA Corporation's booklet "Your Guide to Cost Containment," designed for employers, CIGNA states its intention to develop a "DRG-based reimbursement option for all group policyholders."

For consumers, this message should be clear. It's only a matter of time before private insurers will pay hospitals by the head, by the diagnosis for *all* patients, not just for seniors. As a patient you will no longer be able to entreat your doctor to allow you to stay hospitalized just "one day longer" until you feel completely recovered and ready for home once again. If you do, you may get the okay, but the stay will be at your expense, not your insurer's or employer's. In the new employer-insurer health care scheme, home care is a more important option to you than ever before.

AN OLDER AMERICA

The reason for the home care revolution can also be seen in the changing face of America. Though the media still portrays a youth-crazed culture, the truth is that the American population is getting older.

This population trend, which has been called the "graying of America," will continue well into the twenty-first century. A 1983 Census Bureau report noted that in the past twenty years the number of people age 65 and over has grown twice as fast as the rest of the population. Today about one out of every six persons is aged 65 or older, compared to one out of sixteen at the turn of the century. By 1990 the ratio will drop to one out of five and decrease again to one out of three by 2025.

Within this generation, increasing life expectancy has made the so-called old-old, those over 85, the most rapidly growing age group. While some 2 million Americans fall into this age category now, by the mid-twenty-first century they will number about 16 million, more than twice the current population of New Jersey.

The health of older Americans is far better than most younger Americans imagine. A 1979 National Health Interview Survey found that 95 percent of all seniors aged 65 to 74 can enjoy life independently without help at home. As a group, however, increasing age does eventually take its health toll. By the time people reach age 85 or older, about one out of three require some kind of personal assistance, and about 20 percent receive nursing home care.

All this has budget implications for older citizens and the entire country. Despite Medicare, older Americans continue to spend more of their own money each year on health care. HCFA reports that their annual health tab equals a hefty 20 percent of their average yearly income. Nationally, about one-third of all health costs go for senior care. Yet older Americans today represent only about 11 percent of the population. The reality of an ever-expanding older population intensifies Medicare's financial straits. As America grays, rising federal outlays—and taxes—are inevitable.

Nursing homes can no longer be a solution. In 1982, the Department of Health and Human Services reported to Congress: "There is considerable evidence that the current supply of nursing home beds is not sufficient to meet the demand for care." Particularly hard pressed are the elderly poor, whose nursing home costs are paid for through Medicaid. Nursing homes that operate on a for-profit basis control a large part of this industry. To ensure greater profits, many are seeking to fill limited space with higher-paying customers. Some homes are turning in their Medicaid authorizations, thereby forcing their Medicaid patients out. A 1984 Senate Special Committee on Aging investigation found that many nursing homes illegally required families to make cash payments or sign private contracts as a condition of admission for potential Medicaid clients.

Reliance on nursing homes as an answer raises both cost and "quality of life" issues. Nursing home care doesn't come cheap. Annual costs range from $15,000 to $50,000 per person. Most people who enter homes as paying patients eventually deplete their assets and end up Medicaid paupers. Medicaid, like Medicare, is financed by tax dollars.

Older people universally agree that nursing homes are no place to live. Investigations by consumer groups such as the National Citizens' Coalition for Nursing Home Reform (NCCNHR) confirm this. Elma Holder, NCCNHR founder, reports that during 1984 and 1985 NCCNHR interviewed nursing home residents nationwide about their living conditions. Residents universally agreed that patient care suffered because homes lacked enough staff to provide top-rate care and that the available caregiving staff was generally poorly trained. Foremost among the complaints was lack of freedom to make even the most basic life-style decisions, such as when to rise in the morning. Ms. Holder cited many homes for "failing to provide any therapy, recreation, and real patient attention." Not all nursing homes, of course, fall short, but few can substitute satisfactorily for the home.

THE CONSUMER TIDE

The groundswell of health care consumerism has also helped pave the way for the home care renaissance. There's no doubt that consumers are taking greater interest in and more control over their health than ever before. Joggers, health food stores, and fitness centers bear witness. The neighborhood pharmacy now routinely stocks home pregnancy tests, blood pressure cuffs, and any number of self-care and home care products.

On TV or radio you'll get the latest update on health together with news, sports, and weather. Health even has its own forum on Lifetime, a major cable television network, and in publications like *Prevention Magazine.*

All this, plus organized consumer groups, are divesting health care of its mystique and making waves in the system. The old doctor-patient relationship is fast disappearing in exchange for a true health partnership, with the doctor no longer an absolute authority, but a valued competent technical advisor.

Consumers, taking a hard look at institutional care, don't always like what they see. They are demanding—and getting—the changes they want as hospitals feel the sting of competition and dwindling revenues. For example, home-style birthing centers, almost unknown a decade ago, have become standard at many medical centers in response to consumer pressure.

As consumers seek alternatives to traditional care, home care emerges as the most appealing. A survey of 1,000 consumers conducted by the National Research Corporation found home care ranked number one on their priority list of alternative health services needed in their communities.

This consumer trend is no mere flash in the pan. Long-standing organizations, such as the American Association of Retired Persons (AARP), have become consumer health activists. In its "Healthy Us" campaign, AARP urges members to "make smart consumer choices" and "investigate health care alternatives" including home care and hospices. New consumer health groups are springing up to educate consumers about such options. The People's Medical Society (PMS) board chairman, Robert Rodale, asserts: "Our goal, as organized lay people, is going to be to show everyone why medicine must undergo a vast transformation."

THE IMPACT ON HOME CARE

As cost containment, consumerism, and concern about aging America sweep the nation, the home care revolution builds.

Many states now mandate that insurers offer home care benefits in employee health insurance programs. However, many insurers and employers do not need legislative prescriptions to put into practice what they believe makes good health and economic sense.

Transamerica Occidental Life's Patient Care consultant Bevlyn Mathews says her company "firmly believes that home health care and home hospice care are cost effective." As proof of her company's commitment, she points out that Transamerica has "revamped its home care benefit to encourage its use. Now home health care and hospice care are reimbursed 100 percent and are not subject to deductible allowances."

Insurers are also testing new ground for covered home care benefits. Empire Blue Cross and Blue Shield (formerly Blue Cross and Blue Shield of Greater New York) is among the insurers experimenting with a home care option for low-risk mothers after childbirth. In its program, instead of a three-day hospital stay, mothers leaving within 24 hours receive follow-up care at home by a nurse practitioner and even a homemaker for a short spell of initial home relief.

Home care's cost-saving potential has definitely caught the employer's eye. In 1981, the State of Colorado, one of the largest employers in the state, grossed a $163,000 savings in the first year it added home care to its employee benefit package. With its home care coverage, Kodak Corporation reports it nets about $160,000 in savings each year.

Business coalitions are educating employers about such results. The Midwest Business Group on Health, for example, surveyed 86 employers in its eight-state region on their home care coverage. Forty-nine employers, over half, had or planned home care benefits, and another 20 percent were considering it.

Industry Expansion

These trends have not gone unnoticed by home care agencies, would-be home care entrepreneurs, and the health industry at large. The financial community is also following home care with great interest, as private marketing research firms like Cleveland-based Predicasts forecasts that "Home health care is expected to be the most dynamic segment within the health care field in the 1980's."

The arrival of high-technology treatment in the home has sparked wildfire interest. In *Modern Healthcare,* John Arlotta, vice-president, Travacare, of Travenol Laboratories, Morton Grove, IL, reports: "In the TPN [one high-tech treatment] market alone you're talking about 2,200 patients currently getting therapy. That's about $60–$80 million in terms of business."

Everyone who can is getting into the home care market; those already there are generally expanding their operations. Traditional suppliers of temporary office personnel such as Kelly and Manpower are now in the home care business. Major corporations like Avon and Union Carbide own medical equipment companies or other home care subsidiaries. Doctors who once disavowed house calls will now gladly come to your door. Even pharmacists have branched into home practice.

The number of Medicare-certified agencies is increasing rapidly, HCFA reports, at a rate close to 100 a month in 1984. The most dramatic increases have occurred in states without certificate of need (CON) regulations. CON laws control the numbers and growth of publicly funded health services such as hospitals or home care agencies according to demonstrated need. In Texas, for example, where CON laws don't operate, the number of certified agencies leaped from 80 in 1980 to 443 in 1984.

Just how big is the industry picture? No one knows for

sure. There is no single, reliable source for these data. In Florida, for example, where demand for services is high, HCFA counted 149 Medicare-certified agencies in 1984. The Florida Association of Home Health Agencies reckons another 400 to 600 agencies are doing business. In 1983, certified agencies in New York State numbered 131, while 446 non-certified agencies had also set up shop.

The majority of hospitals, which once had little or no interest in home care, are seeing it as a new opportunity as revenues decline due to empty beds and ever-shortening patient stays. Now, instead of losing patients when they are wheeled through the discharge door, many hospitals are holding on by offering home care services. HCFA reports a 48 percent boost in hospital home care agencies between November 1983 and November 1984. With the DRG system in place, hospitals with their own home care agencies can "double-dip"—push Medicare patients out soon enough to pocket a DRG surplus; then get a second Medicare payment when these patients use their home care services. High-tech care patients are particularly lucrative.

For-profit investor-owned hospital chains have been quick to cash in on the profit possibilities. Some, like National Medical Enterprises, Inc., operate hospitals, nursing homes, home care agencies, and medical equipment outlets, so that patients and their dollars need never leave their cash-flow system.

The wholesale hospital move into home care worries many long-time community home care agencies. In the past, these agencies depended on hospitals for patient referrals. The added competition could threaten their existence. The community nonprofit sector is taking a long hard look inward and changing to meet the times. They are adopting basic marketing and management strategies that heretofore were often foreign ground. In some cases they work directly with hospitals in joint home care ventures.

Groups like visiting nurse organizations are banding together to meet the competition head on. Arthur Rice, executive director of the newly formed American Affiliation of Visiting Nurse Associations and Services, explains: "The organizations, seeing an erosion of their market share and the changes in the industry, decided they needed a vehicle to assist them in developing marketing programs and additional revenues." Already the affiliation has paid off. In 1984, contracts were signed with American ContinueCare, Travenol, and Health-dyne, all high-tech companies, to provide national IV (intravenous) therapy service.

Competition and the Consumer

There's no doubt that home care has become highly competitive and that competition is here to stay. Agencies are working hard to make themselves known to doctors, social workers, hospital discharge planners, and anyone else who can ultimately help them reach their objective—serving consumers.

For you, this wildfire industry growth and rapid change present both risks and opportunities. In some respects it is the best of times and the worst of times for home care consumers.

The increasing competition has helped bring home care into less populated areas. It is also making consumers more aware that home care provides an option to hospitals and nursing homes. With such industry growth, never before have consumers had so many choices in home care. But choices without consumer know-how can be bewildering. Not all agencies that offer home care can deliver what they promise. And of those that can, some do a much better job than others.

Home care has some inherent risks because it involves more responsibility not only for consumers, but for agencies too. Once you bring care inside the home and close the door, the best or worst can happen. But the flipside to this picture shows the tremendous opportunities available to the consumer who is willing to become involved and exert normal consumer pressure. The competition in home care is fierce, and agencies want to please. They aim to build and maintain solid reputations that can only work in your favor—if you know what to do and what to look for.

II

BUILDING
CONSUMER SAVVY

—3—

A Consumer Primer

If you look in the Yellow Pages in most urban and suburban areas, you will find lots of home care listings, often pages and pages, and *plenty* of advertising. Among the most popular catch phrases are variations on the "caring" theme. "We care," "The secret of our care is caring," "Caring . . . the best medicine." Such messages all sound very reassuring . . . they are designed to!

Advertising is all right provided an agency makes good on its claims. But it's not solid consumer information. Ads won't help you sort out which agencies give good, fair, or poor care. To make these distinctions takes basic consumer savvy, which you can acquire. Your education process begins when you become more familiar with the world of home care—the available services, how home care works, who provides it, and the basic terms used in the field.

WHAT SERVICES ARE AVAILABLE?

"When you talk about hospital care," says Elsie Griffith, board chairman of the National Association for Home Care, "people know what you mean. They can visualize their community hospital and the services it provides. They have a frame of reference. That's not true for home care." This worries Ms. Griffith because, as she points out, "lack of awareness prevents people from taking full advantage of what home care has to offer."

Indeed home care, as provided by a network of agencies across the country, has much more to offer you than the standard health services.

Health Services

Skilled nursing has become the best known home care service thanks to the century-old tradition of the visiting nurse organizations. If you need dressings changed, drugs administered, close monitoring for serious changes in health or other complications, you need skilled nursing care. Teaching newly discharged hospital patients and their families how to perform skilled nursing procedures so they can do it themselves also falls under the heading of skilled nursing. Simple tasks such as taking a temperature or pulse rate are considered "basic," not skilled, nursing.

Personal care is a mainstay for many patients during recovery periods, for the frail elderly, or for the partially or totally disabled. As the term suggests, personal care includes help with daily activities related to maintaining personal health and hygiene, dignity, and self-respect. Assistance with bathing, toileting, grooming, dressing, eating, and moving about are personal care services.

Therapy of many types adds to the spectrum of health services. All types aim to restore, maintain, or enhance the abilities of those under care. Physical therapy focuses on physical movement. Speech therapy aids communication problems. Respiratory therapy concerns breathing difficulties. Occupational therapy helps people overcome problems of daily living at home or work that can occur when normal abilities are limited. These may include how to manage personal care, household tasks like cooking or childcare, and job duties like typing or phone work.

Nutrition services help meet special dietary needs related to illness and also improve on normal diets to promote wellness.

Diagnostic aids and *high-tech treatments,* common to hospitals, are becoming commonplace in home care. Blood or other samples may be taken in the home for later lab analysis; some lab tests can be done on the spot. Portable X-ray units can be brought to the home, as well as electrocardiographic (EKG) equipment. Chemotherapy, intravenous (IV) therapy, and other "high-tech" treatments once considered too sophisticated for home care are now available.

Medical and dental care round out the roster of major home health services. Yes, doctors are making house calls again, sometimes in cooperation with home care agencies. Dentists too provide some in-home services through special programs for the homebound.

Medical Equipment and Supplies

If needed, it's possible to transform the home into a mini medical unit. Hospital beds, walkers, wheelchairs, and oxygen equipment are among the items routinely available for home use. In addition, advancing technology is bringing an array of other devices into the home, including life support systems and cardiac monitors. Emergency response systems that act as electronic home companions link ill or frail persons living alone with immediate backup support when needed.

Homemaking Services

If you think about the many tasks essential to running a home, the day-to-day household chores like light housekeeping, laundry, food shopping, planning and preparing meals, and paying bills, you have a partial picture of what *homemaking services* involve. Beyond these, many other homemaking services are available, depending on the individual situation.

Childcare may be provided as a homemaking service when a caregiving parent is ill, absent, or otherwise unable to assume the normal parental role. Teaching others home management skills such as budgeting or shopping or child-rearing techniques is also a homemaking service.

Social Services

Once you have reviewed the array of home care services, you'll have an appreciation for the role of *social services,* sometimes called *medical social services.* One key function is to help coordinate the home care agency's many services with other beneficial community programs. Indeed, helping consumers negotiate the maze of available services and pulling

them together into a comprehensive personalized plan is
emerging into a distinct subspecialty service called *case management* (see Chapter 17). In addition, social services help
people cope with the many individual problems that illness
and disability may bring to home life.

Hospice Services

Hospice services provide health care, and social, emotional,
and spiritual support to the terminally ill and their families
during the last months of life. Hospice services, however, do
not stop with death, but continue afterward to help families
during the grieving period. (For a full discussion, see Chapter
18.)

Support Services

The services already described form the backbone of home
care. In addition to these basic services, many other services
that help support independent living or home care goals may
be available.

Respite care brings temporary relief to family members
who care for ill, disabled, or failing loved ones. For many
families, respite care makes the difference between continuing
care and finally, very reluctantly, giving up and turning to
institutional care. Said one husband of a stroke patient,
"Before they came [home care agency staff], I was nearly sick
with worry. I carried her to the doctor. She was agitated if I
would leave her at all. Now I can get some relief. I can even
tend my garden."

Respite can be provided through a variety of arrangements:
at home by allowing family caregivers to take a break from
the stress and pressures of ongoing care, or it can be arranged
on a residential basis in a hospital, nursing home, or sometimes
a private home for a temporary period ranging from a few
days to a few weeks. Such relief can allow caregivers the
chance to go out of town on business or take vacations
knowing their loved ones are in good hands. Adult day care
and foster care can also provide respite for family caregivers.

Many respite projects underway serve families whose loved ones are developmentally disabled or are Alzheimer's or senility (dementia) patients.

Chore services help with heavy-duty household tasks that go beyond the scope of homemaking. This includes floor or window washing, yard work, and minor home maintenance and repair. Without such services, many adults cannot continue to live safely in their homes.

Home-delivered meal services, often called Meals-on-Wheels, bring free or low-cost nutritionally sound meals to those who cannot prepare food themselves (usually an elderly person). Often a hot noonday meal may be delivered, together with a cold meal for the evening. Sometimes a frozen, easily reheatable meal may be left for later.

Besides good nutrition, such meal programs provide personal contact and a sense of security for the homebound, especially if they are living alone. Meal services also have a preventive role. "Food is a therapeutic way to help the elderly stay well," asserts one visiting nurse. "If left to their own devices, they will often forget to eat. Many of them don't have the energy to prepare meals."

Friendly visiting or companionship services are just that. A welcome scheduled visit and friendship can help break the loneliness and depression experienced by many homebound people. For many people, this socialization prevents decline, and maintains and improves mental alertness and interest in life.

Telephone reassurance services help ensure personal safety by linking the homebound via the phone with a daily prescheduled call. Should someone fail to answer, a backup plan goes into effect, and the caller sees that a personal in-home check is made. Beyond safety, these calls also bring friendly, daily visits via the phone.

Transportation and escort services are a vital home support. In one government survey, home care consumers and their families most often cited this need. Transportation services usually work together with escort services that provide physical support, encouragement, and protection to help the otherwise homebound chance a trip into the community. Mini-vans, private cars, or public transit systems may be used to transport the frail or disabled to medical appointments, shopping, or recreational or social events.

Adult protective services help the adult who can no longer adequately manage personal finances or legal affairs. Usually the adult lives alone. These services go beyond simple bill paying, providing for people with small stocks and assets the kind of financial management or conservatorship that banks provide. For example, they will transfer funds usually held by seniors in low-yielding passbook accounts into higher-interest-bearing funds.

HOW HOME CARE WORKS

You may be familiar with the services. But if you are like most consumers, you will have had no real experience with home care until you need it. Let's take a step-by-step look at how home care works, with a professional home care agency. To make the process clearer, we will follow Robert, the stroke patient described in Chapter 1, through each step of his home care experience, from start to finish.

The Decision

You may decide yourself that you want home care; or a family member, a friend, or your doctor or other health professional may suggest it. In Robert's case, he was anxious to leave the hospital as soon as possible and pressured his doctor to "Get me out of here!" The doctor mentioned home care, and Robert agreed eagerly to try.

If you are undecided about home care, discuss this option with your doctor, your family, hospital discharge planners, or other appropriate professionals. Home care personnel can also help to advise you.

The Doctor's Prescription

When you need home care for medical reasons, as in Robert's situation, your doctor normally writes an order for home care just as he or she would prescribe a drug or other treatment. Robert's prescription read: "Skilled nursing and physical therapy." In nonmedical cases, such as help for failing elderly persons who do not need skilled care or therapy, a doctor's okay is not necessary.

Agency Selection

You should choose an agency that meets your needs for service and operates with the highest professional standards. Robert's doctor mentioned the hospital's own home care program and advised his family to check with the hospital discharge planner or social worker for other recommendations. The family also contacted a friend who had used home care before. The family then talked with each suggested agency and selected the one they felt was right for them.

Agency Assessment

The agency you choose conducts what professionals call an *assessment*. This is a detailed evaluation of your situation which confirms the need for services ordered and identifies any other beneficial services. The assessment helps determine how much daily or weekly help is required to promote recovery or help maintain independence.

Because Robert was hospitalized, the agency nurse conducted this initial assessment in the hospital. Normally, the first assessment takes place in your own home.

The Care Plan

After an assessment, the agency tailors a home care plan just for you and reviews it with you. Before making the plan final, the agency advises your doctor of its assessment results and presents the plan for your doctor's approval. The plan outlines key details, including the treatment goals, the specific services, the level of care that will be provided, and any medical equipment and supplies that may be needed.

The levels of care may range from intensive care for medically unstable but not life-threatening conditions, to intermediate care for stable conditions like Robert's that require skilled services and home support for recovery, to maintenance care that helps a frail, disabled, or chronically ill person remain at home.

After Robert's assessment, the agency nurse recommended an aide's assistance to help him with personal care and basic daytime nursing since his wife worked. Robert's doctor, who was unaware of the family situation, agreed that an aide's help was essential to enable Robert to go home. The doctor's original order was revised and the needed medical equipment (in this case, a hospital bed) was added.

Basic Paperwork

The agency usually asks you to sign one or more forms in order to initiate home care. These may include: a consent agreement, release of medical information forms, a service contract or letter outlining services to be provided, costs and payment obligations, and financial or insurance disclosure authorizations.

Robert signed the agency's standard service agreement and a form that allowed his insurance carrier to pay the agency directly. The agency had already contacted his insurance carrier to confirm Robert's home care coverage.

Services and Supervision

The agency then selects and assigns appropriate personnel and provides or helps arrange for needed medical equipment and supplies, if you wish. Provisions are made for any additional services you need that the agency does not render. Supervision of personnel begins the first day home care personnel come into your home.

After meeting his nurse and aide, Robert and his wife felt reassured about his decision to leave the hospital early. Both the nurse and the aide were experienced and clearly knew what to do. The nurse answered Robert's questions and began to teach him basic self-care. The aide helped reinforce what the nurse had taught and encouraged Robert as he tried to do certain tasks himself. The agency supervisor called Robert on the aide's first work day to see if he had any questions or problems. A few days later, the supervisor visited Robert to double-check the suitability of the care plan and to observe Robert's condition and care firsthand.

Ongoing Care

The agency continues to provide ongoing care and regular, in-home supervisory visits. When more than one type of health worker provides service, home care becomes a team effort. Those involved confer on an informal or formal basis to discuss your progress and changing needs. Your doctor is informed through telephone and written progress reports, and updates the care plan as needed in consultation with the agency.

As Robert's home care progressed, the agency nurse and physical therapist continued to teach him and his family health care skills. Aide visits were cut back as his condition improved. After a team conference, physical therapy was also decreased. But occupational therapy was added on his doctor's orders to improve Robert's ability to manage basic tasks at home. The supervisor visited Robert regularly and phoned him in between to ensure that the agency's standards for care were being maintained.

Payment

The agency bills you and/or your insurance company for services on a regular basis. The agency maintains all responsibility for personnel payroll, insurance, and social security. Personnel timeslips are provided for your review. If you are on Medicare and qualify for home care according to Medicare guidelines, the agency bills the government directly. There is no cost to you for Medicare-qualifying home care expenses.

In Robert's case, his insurance company paid 80 percent of his bill; the agency billed him for the remaining 20 percent. Of course, not every insurer covers home care; nor does every available home care service qualify for insurance payments. (See Chapter 10.)

The Finish

In most situations, home care is of short duration, a few weeks or months. Once the treatment goals as outlined in the care plan have been reached, services and insurance coverage usually end. The decision to conclude services for health reasons is based primarily on your progress and your doctor's judgment. As a consumer, however, the option is always yours to end services earlier or extend them if you wish, although insurance would no longer pay.

Robert's home care program was concluded after he was well enough to get about with the assistance of a walker. By then his blood pressure had stabilized, and drugs and diet controlled his condition. Through the agency teaching, he was able to follow up with the prescribed exercise himself. His family provided the extra support he still needed to manage at home.

Looking back at his experience, Robert credits home care for his faster-than-average recovery. Most of all, he is thankful that he could get well at home.

Your personal experience with home care may vary somewhat from the steps outlined above. For example, should you need certain supportive services like friendly visiting, payment may not be an issue. Such services are usually available free in the community. In nonmedical cases, supervision, though important, may be less frequent, depending on the type of service provided.

WHO PROVIDES HOME CARE?

Without a doubt, families, often aided by friends and good neighbors, provide more home care to loved ones than anyone else. Some families also rely on individuals they hire directly from the community for help with childcare, home nursing, homemaking, or chore work. This is grassroots home care, which may be the only kind of help available in some rural areas.

In most areas, however, you'll find many agencies and organizations that make up the world of home care. These groups may be broadly divided into home health or home support agencies.

Unlike the home health agencies, support-type agencies do not provide skilled nursing or therapy of any kind. They do offer homemaking, basic home nursing, personal care, social services, and other support activities such as companionship that make independent living possible.

The home care agencies and organizations include:

- Visiting nurse organizations
- Community service organizations, including those serving senior citizens, families, and the disabled
- Agencies based in hospitals, nursing homes, or rehabilitation centers
- Commercial firms varying from large nationally known chains to smaller private agencies
- Homemaker–home health aide services
- Government agencies like the Veterans Administration (VA) hospitals or county health departments
- Hospice organizations

The home care agencies represented by these groups number in the thousands. But no matter whether they are large or small, well-established or newcomers, expensive or cheap, home care agencies come in two brands: the professional agencies and the others.

The Professional Home Care Agency

Professional agencies provide top-notch care that results in the home care success stories described earlier. With quality-minded agencies, these successes are not just here and there examples. They happen every day. What's their secret?

The pros work hard at what they do. They don't cut corners in care to cut costs. They hire carefully and are quick to fire employees who can't pass muster. They spot any rejects fast because they supervise all their employees. They properly assess your situation to work out a plan that's right for you, keeping good care and its cost to you in mind.

The pros aren't in business just to supply personnel; they are dedicated to preserving the quality of life at home. Not only do professional agencies do their jobs well, but they do a good job consistently. They have a track record you can depend on.

The "Other" Agencies

Among these agencies you will find certain subgroups.

The "earnest entrepreneurs" aspire to make the professional grade. Some may be nurse-owned or started by other people with a background in the helping professions. These agencies understand what quality home care means and strive to provide it, but they fall short on the necessary business and management expertise. This lack can cause consumer troubles, such as insurance payment problems and frequent employee changes. Poor care is seldom an issue.

The "get-rich-quick" entrepreneurs see home care mostly as a golden financial opportunity. They may have only one office or many home care branches. They try to project a professional image, but often don't practice what they preach. They go through the motions of assessment, developing a care plan, employee screening, and supervision in order to avoid obvious problems that, if publicized, could hurt their business. But these entrepreneurs focus on *their* profit first, *your* care second. With these, you may get marginal to good care, and sometimes serious problems. Your experience largely depends on your luck with the personnel they assign to you and the extent of agency supervision.

The "mom and pop" operations may be run by well-intentioned people or the care-nots. Though some have been in business many years and advertise that they provide home care, they do not understand the professional concept of home care at all. With these agencies, you order the personnel you want. They handle payroll, provide personnel, and sometimes supply *loose* supervision. With them, expect get-by care, and sometimes very poor service or serious problems.

The "nurses registries" or "health employment agencies" provide personnel for you to hire, and little else. This amounts to do-it-yourself home care, described in Chapter 8, and often brings plenty of problems.

The "fly-by-night" operations are the sharks of the home care industry. They masquerade as professional home care agencies in their ads, while they are seldom more than a card file and telephone outfit. They hire personnel wholesale through employment ads without any reference checks or proof of adequate experience or training. Once hired, employees seldom see these employers face-to-face again. Employees are sent out by phone, paid by mail, and never supervised on the job.

These agencies provide a body and a bill for their services, nothing more. As you might suspect, whenever an agency brings unskilled strangers off the street into your home, the worst can and often does happen. These agencies are mostly responsible for the hard luck or home care horror stories that sometimes hit the headlines. These agencies are a small group, but their shoddy, dangerous care unfortunately gives all home care agencies a bad name. Obviously you will want to avoid these agencies at all cost.

Rest assured that if you do your consumer homework, these frauds are not hard to spot. Nor will you have much trouble sifting through the other agencies to get to the pros, who are in the majority.

To help you wade through the maze of agencies and

advertising appeals, let's look at the basic terms used in the field and what they mean to you as a consumer. How to select a pro agency is covered in Chapter 6.

THE BASIC TERMS

Whenever you hunt for health services of any kind, you will often encounter unfamiliar jargon. In health care-ese, for example, a professional, an institution, an organization, or an agency that offers health services becomes a "provider." The consumer becomes a "case," "patient," "client," "customer," "recipient," "beneficiary," or "bennie," depending on the provider's own vocabulary.

Let's translate other basic terms into consumer language.

Bonding—Agencies and Employees

The words "bonding" and "bonded" often appear prominently in advertising. Though people often associate bonding with safety in care or protection against theft or property damage, John Gay, a bonding agent for the Mutual Insurance Agency, admits: "It's more or less an advertising gimmick."

To bond its employees, an agency normally pays a preset fee based on the dollar size of the bond, much the same way anyone buying insurance pays a varying premium according to the size of the policy. Any security check of bonded employees is rare. In fact, most bonds are purchased as "blanket" bonds that cover employees in general and do not cite individuals by name.

What happens in case of theft or property damage by a "bonded" employee? Normally the consumer can collect for losses only if the employee is convicted of theft, or if the consumer sues in court for property damages and wins. Financial settlements are not paid directly by the agency; the money comes from the bonding company. Bonding really acts as a kind of insurance that protects the agency against financial claims involving its employees.

In some states, agencies themselves must be bonded in

order to obtain an operating license. In these cases, financial claims made against the agency itself—for example, government losses due to Medicare fraud—would be recovered through the bond.

As a consumer, you must realize that bonding has little practical value. It does not help you avoid problems in any way and usually helps you recover losses only after successful court action.

The Licensed Agency

A *license* is a legal permission usually granted by a public authority. It gives a person, an organization, or a business entity that meets certain requirements the right to engage in an occupation or activity. A license is a regulatory device which in theory is supposed to protect the public interest. States license health institutions such as hospitals, nursing homes, and laboratory facilities which have met state minimum standards.

You might suppose, as a public safeguard, that every state would have special licensing laws for home care agencies as they do for other health institutions. However, many states— 19 as of December 1984—do not specifically license home care agencies at all. In those states, agencies may be "licensed," but the license is a standard operating or occupational license, the kind needed by any business to set up shop. Among states with specific licensing for home care agencies, laws vary from weak to strict. So don't look to licensing for all the answers.

Because of quirks in some state licensing laws, sometimes fine agencies cannot be licensed. For example, states may license only home health agencies, so a good homemaker– home health aide agency, because it isn't considered a home *health* agency, cannot qualify. One state may license only agencies that are eligible to receive public funds. Thus an agency that serves only the privately paying or insured public cannot become licensed.

From a consumer viewpoint, this means don't count on the label "licensed" as a guarantee of quality. The state department of health usually licenses home care agencies. Check with this department if you want specific up-to-date information on licensing requirements in your state.

The Certified Agency

While the definition of a licensed agency varies among states, the term *certified* has uniform meaning nationwide. A certified agency is one authorized to receive payment for Medicare home health services, and in some states for Medicaid/Medi-Cal or other publicly funded home services.

The state health department certifies and monitors qualified agencies on behalf of the federal government. However, to become certified in any state, an agency must meet certain minimum federal standards for patient care and financial management. So a Medicare-certified agency in Texas meets the same federal standards as one in Tennessee.

The basic standards require that the agency provide a written and detailed plan of care prescribed by the doctor as well as written progress reports to the doctor at least every 60 days. An experienced registered nurse (RN) must make the initial assessment visit and supervise all care, including in-home visits at least every two weeks. All personnel must be trained and qualified, and aides must be closely supervised.

As you can see from these basic standards, certification implies a measure of quality. However, it is not foolproof. Quality depends on how strictly each state monitors and enforces these federal standards.

The Accredited Agency

"Consumers have a better chance of a good home care experience when they receive services from an accredited agency," asserts Stephen Holzemer, RN, who oversees the National League for Nursing's accreditation program. The reason? "An accredited agency has gone that extra mile," he explains. "It has undergone a voluntary step-by-step process that shows it is meeting above-average patient-care and operating standards, and that it is also responsive to the community's needs for service."

The value of accreditation is often hotly debated among health professionals. But consumers can be sure of one important fact: An accredited agency has been carefully evaluated and judged satisfactory against tough professional standards set by nongovernmental organizations that work to promote excellence in home care.

Four organizations accredit home care services:

- The National League for Nursing (NLN) accredits non-hospital community home health agencies. Each level of its review process involves consumer representation.
- The Joint Commission on the Accreditation of Hospitals (JCAH) accredits hospitals after a careful review of all their operations. When hospitals operate home care departments or hospices, they must meet specific standards in these areas to become JCAH-accredited.
- The National HomeCaring Council (NHC) accredits or approves homemaker–home health aide agencies or services within multiservice community organizations or home health agencies. NHC standards emphasize careful screening, training, and supervision of aides.
- The Council on Accreditation of Services for Families and Children (COA) also accredits homemaker–home health aide services with standards parallel to those of NHC. Most of its accredited home care services exist within family or children's social service agencies or agencies that provide mental health services.

Accreditation can be very useful to consumers because, as David Shover, COA executive director, explains: "Home care is often needed at a time of crisis, when people are desperate for services and don't have the luxury of carefully checking an agency out. Accreditation gives the consumer a benchmark of quality to use instead of relying on the Yellow Pages."

Accreditation serves as a "Good Housekeeping Seal of Approval" that you will want to look for. However, it has one major drawback. At present, too few agencies seek accreditation. Finding an accredited agency in many locales is like looking for a needle in a haystack. For example, as of April 1, 1985, only 120 agencies nationwide were NLN-accredited; NHC boasts 131 accredited services.

All accrediting groups are stepping up efforts to promote accreditation among professional agencies as well as consumers. "Consumers can help," states Florence Moore, NHC executive director, "by demanding accreditation when possible." But perhaps the most effective means to boost accreditation is to link it to key funding sources.

COA is exploring with the United Way the use of accreditation to identify agencies worthy of United Way's financial support. NLN has already made progress in this respect. Mr. Holzemer reports that Philadelphia Blue Cross, an important health insurer, requires home care agencies to bear the NLN stamp for full reimbursement.

By all means, look for accredited agencies. And expect to find more in the future.

Proprietary Versus Nonprofit Agencies

The labels *nonprofit* and *proprietary* (profit-making) have special meaning in the minds of many consumers. Nonprofits may translate into "community service," "quality care," or "fairly priced"; profit-making may be interpreted as "anything for a buck," "cut-rate quality," or "making money on sickness."

What's the truth? Neither generalization is accurate. Essentially, the terms proprietary and nonprofit reveal only the extent of an agency's tax obligation. An agency's reputation must depend on its standards and quality of care, not its income tax status.

Among nonprofit agencies, you should know that nonprofits may be either *voluntary* or *private* agencies. Voluntaries are community service-oriented agencies with boards of directors comprised of a broad spectrum of community leaders. Private nonprofit agencies, as this term suggests, are run by one individual or family or a small board of people who are often really business partners. In such cases, the agency has usually been formed as nonprofit in order to take advantage of certain tax and state licensing laws.

You may view the profit motive in health somewhat suspiciously. Yet, like it or not, the profit element is well entrenched in our health care system. One-third of all community hospitals are now owned by for-profit groups. In home care, the number of profit-making agencies has been steadily increasing. In 1982, the federal government, in effect, gave its stamp of approval to the proprietary sector. This was accomplished through a legislative change that now allows Medicare payments to qualified for-profits. In 1984, 30 percent of all certified agencies were for-profits.

Many excellent community nonprofit agencies, like the Visiting Nurse Service of Denver (VNS), work cooperatively with proprietaries. The Denver VNS contracts with Upjohn Health Care for certain personnel services. Many well-respected nonprofits are becoming involved in for-profit enterprises, again proof that the word "proprietary" means little by itself. The Visiting Nurse Service of New York, for instance, has formed its own for-profit subsidiary, called Partners-in-Care, which provides nonskilled services only. VNS chief executive officer Elsie Griffith proudly states: "Since Partners was founded, never once has the Board suggested we cut costs that would affect the quality of care." Profits derived from the Partners company are pumped back into the parent VNS so it can provide even more free community service.

Personnel Terms

If you have had little experience with health care, you may be surprised by the variety of personnel who provide services. Before we look at these caregivers in the next chapter, you should understand three terms: licensed, certified, and registered. These are important professional credentials related to one key issue: consumer protection.

The Licensed Professional

Workers whose jobs may risk public health, safety, or welfare are generally licensed by the state. Teachers, lawyers, stockbrokers, and beauty operators are among the nonhealth personnel that states typically license. In the health field, all states license doctors, including chiropractors, podiatrists, dentists, and optometrists, as well as nurses, physical therapists, and pharmacists. For other health personnel, licensing varies by state.

Generally, to become licensed health professionals must: (1) submit proof of graduation from an approved course of study; and (2) successfully pass a written examination, which may be combined with oral and practical tests. This done, the state issues a license permitting them to work. Usually the State Department of Education, Higher Education, or Department of Health acts as the licensing agency. Often licensing is done jointly with a state specialty board such as a Board of Nursing or a Board of Medicine.

Licensing is supposed to protect the public against poor or dangerous care by screening out incompetent personnel. But it does not assure good care. Licensing only tests initial ability. In many states, licenses are renewed annually just by mailing in a yearly licensing fee. In nonhealth fields, rubber-stamp relicensing may not be harmful. But within the constantly changing world of health care, watch out. Those physicians, for example, who were licensed twenty years ago but have failed to keep up with advances in diagnosis and treatment are ill-equipped to practice good medicine today. In health, the quality of patient care depends on continuing education and work experience, not just a license.

The Certified or Registered Professional

Licensing is a state-run program with varying standards. Programs that certify or register personnel are usually national in scope and sponsored by national organizations representing the health professions. For example, the National Association of Social Workers represents the social work profession much the same way the American Medical Association represents physicians. Among other activities, these health profession organizations, through special boards, councils, or similar bodies, help set national standards for education and professional practice.

Strictly speaking, registration means listing of professionals by name on an official roster of a state agency or organization;

for example, nurses are registered with the state once they become licensed. Practically, however, for most other professionals, certification and registration are equivalent terms.

Certification and registration procedures normally parallel licensing, but are generally viewed as signs of quality for two reasons: (1) The national standards of a professional organization are usually much tougher than those of states. Many organizations require professionals to undergo continuing education and/or periodic reexamination to maintain certification or registration status. (2) Participation is generally optional. Professionals can choose whether or not they will "go" for these credentials, since they can legally work without them. Therefore, these credentials generally indicate high-caliber personnel.

Because certification and registration operate independently of licensing, personnel may be certified or registered as well as licensed.

WHAT IS QUALITY IN HOME CARE?

The most important consumer term has been saved for last. Ellen Winston, NHC consumer advocate, notes that as consumers, "We demand 'quality' in the goods we purchase for our homes. We want clear labeling on products. We want guarantees. Shouldn't we pay equal attention to and demand that same kind of quality when it comes to the care we receive in our homes?"

Granted, it's no simple task for consumers to judge quality in health care, period. Organizations that set standards for care often don't agree on even bare-bones standards. However, among home care experts there is some consensus on what quality means. Certainly it begins with honest, reliable, competent, and caring help at home. But home care becomes *quality* home care when it offers the following:

- *The right mix of personnel and services.* The personnel who assist you are appropriate for the tasks at hand.

Provisions are made so you receive any and all the services that can benefit you.

When the mix is right, for example, you don't receive care from a nurse when the services of an aide would do. You or your family should not struggle alone to cope with the emotional stresses of failing health when social services can help all concerned. When support services can enhance life, like friendly visiting, they are suggested and become part of the overall home care program, if you agree.

- *The right level of care.* You get the "proper balance" of care—not too much so your condition lingers or you grow dependent needlessly on others, nor too little so you are left still struggling at home. You get enough help so you recover as quickly as you can or remain independent in your own home as long as you can. For instance, when the level of care is right, you won't get round-the-clock care when just several hours of help a day will do.

- *Coordination of care.* Even if you have a single condition, you may be cared for by several different doctors, each with varying treatment agendas. Each doctor may discuss treatment with you, but too often they don't talk to each other and coordinate their individual treatments into a single plan of care. "Fragmentation," or the bits and pieces approach, is one of the biggest problems consumers face with our health system today.

In home care you often have several different kinds of health personnel involved—the family doctor, the nurse, the therapist, and the aide. More than one organization may play an ongoing role in assisting you too. For example, a home care agency, an adult day care center, and a Meals-on-Wheels program may all provide help.

Home care clicks when the various personnel and organizations concerned know about one another's involvement. They share information about your condition and progress. They coordinate their services and avoid duplication. In short, they work together to improve the quality of your life.

- *Continuity or continuum of care.* There is an uninterrupted "flow" from one kind of appropriate care system to another as your health and needs change. You might be moved from home care to the hospital to a nursing home and back to home care again. However, such changes should occur only when they are the best solution to your health and care needs. You should never be left midstream at home without proper help until alternative care is arranged. Nor should you be kept lingering in a hospital or nursing home when you could be cared for at home.

—4—

What Services Do You Need?

Before you seek home care, it's smart to have some idea of what help you may need. A 1983 poll conducted by *Better Homes and Gardens* magazine found that almost half of its readers preferred live-in help if a parent became incapable of living alone. How do you feel about it? Though this costly option gets a high consumer rating, it is often far from the best solution.

If you are a newcomer to home care, it's easy to misjudge what services you actually need. If you are sick, you may think "nurse," as in private duty, or "live-in," if abilities start to fail. Yet in professional home care circles, old-fashioned private duty nursing (which insurers sometimes still insist upon) is strictly passé. In hospitals, most patients do not need, nor do they get, eight hours a day of one-to-one nursing care. *Geriatric Nursing* reports that in nursing homes patients received an average of only 12.5 minutes a day of RN care. Likewise, intensive skilled services are seldom needed at home except in unusual cases.

As for live-in help, let's look more closely at this particular option.

THE LIVE-IN

Before an agency will provide a live-in, you must have adequate sleeping accommodations. This doesn't necessarily mean a private room (although it will be harder to get a live-in without one). But it definitely means a bed and some privacy, not a couch in the living room.

If you assume a live-in means 24-hour help, you are

mistaken. Usually a live-in must be guaranteed 8 hours of sleep a day, 1 hour off for each meal, plus 3 hours a day of personal time. Add it up and you get 10 hours of "round-the-clock" care.

Today, with coordinated teamwork available at professional home care agencies, emergency response systems for backup, and a widening range of community services, live-in help is usually an unnecessary security blanket. It also carries a risk of providing more help than needed, which can worsen a situation by fostering dependence. Such dependence could encourage premature institutionalization.

Just as well-meaning adults often fail to credit children with their real strengths and abilities, as people age they become labeled by numbers that carry preconceived notions about what senior citizens can and cannot do. In a *U.S. News & World Report* interview, "If You Have to Care for Your Aging Parents," noted geriatrician Dr. Stanley Cath explains that many elderly people can stay on their own despite "severe physical handicaps such as progressive immobilizing arthritis, prolonged convalescence, paralysis from strokes, and hearing and visual losses . . . provided," says Dr. Cath, "they link up with key supportive services. . . . Regular visits from supportive and reassuring people are often enough to keep older people independent and at home, while some require professional evaluation and medication. . . ." "Older people," Dr. Cath prescribes, "when physically able, should be expected to pitch in and do some of the chores."

Psychologist-researcher B. F. Skinner, active and alert at age 80, also firmly believes in "doing" as a key to maintaining lifelong independence. "Those that help you very often interfere when you feel okay. I walk two miles to work every day. When my younger friends (who don't expect to live as long as I do) drive by in their cars, I always tell them I don't want a lift unless it's very bad weather. If they give you a lift, they deprive you of a chance to do something interesting and helpful. I think it's very important not to help unless help is needed," Dr. Skinner asserts. "That's one of the problems of caring for people in nursing homes. Nursing homes find it easier to do things for old people." Frequently this is counterproductive.

If you must arrange for home care, avoid this common consumer pitfall. Don't self-prescribe or insist upon unnecessary services. For the elderly, this amounts to "killing with kindness"; but at any age, this practice can slow recovery.

Discuss with your doctor *specific* needs for care, and don't jump to conclusions. "A doctor may make an offhand passing remark in the hospital," observes Jean Langevin, RN, "like 'You shouldn't leave your wife home alone.' The husband interprets this as a 'my wife needs 24-hour care,' though this is seldom the doctor's meaning."

Following a doctor's statement that "nothing more could be done at the hospital," one consumer arranged for home care for his elderly mother, not wanting to put her into a nursing home. His mother had suffered a stroke that had left her partially paralyzed and her speech badly impaired. Assuming that the doctor meant no further recovery was possible, the well-intentioned son did not seek an agency that could provide the physical, occupational, and speech therapy his mother needed. Instead, he arranged for three shifts of aides to provide custodial care round-the-clock.

Professional home care agencies will work with you and your doctor on a sound plan of care. However, as a wise consumer, you need a good understanding of who's who in home care to participate fully in this process. Let's look at the personnel who comprise the home care team, and the role each plays in recovery and self-maintenance.

THE HOME CARE TEAM

The bottom line in home care is people. Every agency is only as good as the people it hires. Home care is always a team effort. Even if only one worker provides "hands on" care, behind the scenes there are other personnel involved in the caregiving. The skills of all those in an agency's home care team largely affect the quality of care.

Who's Who at the Agency

The organizational structure of an agency varies by size. A very large agency, whether profit or nonprofit, is usually organized like any corporation, with officers or directors for key operational areas such as patient services, finances, personnel, education development, marketing, or public relations. In smaller agencies, these functions are usually combined, and one person may handle several areas.

As a home care consumer, four operational positions in the agency most directly affect your care. Their job titles and specific duties may vary somewhat by agency. Again, in a small agency these jobs may be combined. When you contact an individual agency, discuss who is responsible for each of these roles.

The Home Care Coordinator

Generally the coordinator processes initial requests for home care, taking key information and answering basic questions. The coordinator can be a nurse, a social worker, or a "clinical" coordinator, but most agencies employ trained, nonprofessional clerical workers in this role.

Coordinators also assign and schedule personnel, usually paraprofessionals. Clerical coordinators also supervise paraprofessionals with respect to general employee performance, *not* patient care. For example, if an aide is repeatedly late for work, this problem goes to the coordinator. If there is a personality clash or you want to change your care schedule, the coordinator would assist. If you have problems with the quality of your care—for example, an aide who doesn't know how to help you transfer from a wheelchair to a bed—you contact the nursing supervisor.

The Nursing Supervisor or Clinical Coordinator

The nursing supervisor is like the head nurse on a hospital floor who usually assigns and schedules professional personnel, and oversees and helps coordinate your "hands on" care. The supervisor may conduct the assessment, develop a care plan, confer with your doctor, and monitor your progress and the quality of care provided by all caregiving personnel, professional and paraprofessional.

The Director of Patient Services

Sometimes known as director of quality assurance or operations, this is the nursing supervisor's supervisor, who is responsible for maintaining the agency's professional standards of patient care. This professional acts like the hospital director of nursing, and may develop procedures and guidelines for patient safety and care, conduct inservice training, and regularly review every aspect of the agency operations that can affect the quality of care you receive.

The Administrator, Manager, or Executive Director

This is where the buck stops at an agency. The administrator, like the head of any company, is responsible for any and all activities of the agency and its administrative and caregiving personnel. The caliber of the administrator reflects the caliber of the agency.

The Nurses

Nurses come in two basic types: the registered nurse, or RN; and the licensed practical nurse or LPN (called licensed vocational nurse, LVN, in the states of California and Texas). Both types provide skilled nursing care. So what's the difference between the two?

Registered nurses have training that covers not only skilled nursing techniques, but emphasizes the psychological and social aspects of illness. Nurses who hold a four-year college nursing degree, a BSN (Bachelor of Science in Nursing), are considered the cream of registered nursing, prepared to assume greater responsibility in the nursing world. During study, they learn how to make independent judgments about a patient's condition and care, perform basic patient physicals, and usually learn community or public health nursing. All this makes them more attuned to the needs and demands of home care practice.

LPNs, on the other hand, complete much shorter training that develops routine nursing ability. Independent skills are not emphasized, since in hospitals or elsewhere LPNs almost always work under direct RN supervision.

The specific skilled tasks nurses may perform are governed by state laws (usually called Nurse Practice Acts) and the employing agency. Generally, both types of nurses may change dressings, administer oxygen, insert and irrigate urinary catheters, give enemas, and assist with rehabilitation. Depending on *demonstrated* ability, an LPN may be allowed other tasks; for example, to give medications or suction and care for a tracheostomy. Otherwise these are strictly RN jobs. LPNs never draw blood or start intravenous fluids, or perform patient assessments.

Within registered nursing, there are a growing number of specialty areas, most of which are officially recognized by special training courses and additional professional credentials. Among these specialties, here are some often found within home care:

- *Nurse practitioners (NPs).* They provide total patient care for the well or chronically ill, uncomplicated patients. In some states, these nurses virtually work like doctors, prescribing drugs, giving immunizations, and making professional judgments on common medical diagnoses. They work with physician backup or collaboratively with doctors, and may specialize in pediatrics, geriatrics, and nurse midwifery, among other areas.
- *Enterostomal or "stoma" therapists (ETs).* These nurses provide direct care to patients with bowel and bladder diversions, such as a colostomy; serious wounds, including draining wounds and pressure sores; and incontinence problems. They teach patients and families self-care skills, and how to use services or medical supplies and devices related to such problems. Because their work is highly specialized, many ETs work as consultants to home care agencies rather than being full-time employees.
- *Critical Care Registered Nurses (CCRNs).* These nurses usually work inside hospital intensive care units. Some now provide assistance to home care agencies involved

in high-tech home care. CCRNs are specialists in the latest technological nursing techniques.

- *Certified Rehabilitative Registered Nurses (CRRNs)*. These nurses mostly work in hospital rehabilitation units or centers and are now moving into home care, since patients needing even intensive rehabilitation can be cared for at home.

If you are the *average* home care patient, either an LPN or an RN may provide satisfactory skilled nursing care. However, whenever a person is acutely ill, or has several different health problems that must be managed at once, an RN's expertise is needed. Likewise, RNs have the professional background needed to perform most high-tech home care. Most agencies assign RNs whenever patients and families need detailed teaching of self-care skills such as catheter care or bowel and bladder training.

The nursing supervisors in all professional home care agencies are registered nurses, most with public or community health experience. In some agencies, RNs may also function like social workers and help identify, obtain, and coordinate any nonnursing services that may be needed.

Therapists and Their Assistants

All therapists are highly skilled rehabilitation specialists. Also working in the field are assistant-level personnel who handle more routine and simple rehabilitation cases, with direction. You can compare the assistants to lesser-trained LPNs, and therapists to more highly skilled RNs.

If you cannot move normally, you may need a physical or occupational therapist's help. *Physical therapists (PTs)* are concerned with helping patients reach their peak ability to function physically. *Occupational therapists (OTs)* are concerned with peak function too, but they focus on improving physical, mental, or social abilities. It's easy to confuse the jobs of these therapists, who often work together and complement each other.

Let's take the case of a woman who has suffered a stroke

and is now partially paralyzed on one side. In this case, the physical therapist will help her perform specific exercises that will strengthen her weakened arm and leg muscles. The PT may fit her for a wheelchair and teach her how to use it. The occupational therapist will help this newly disabled woman learn to change or adapt her normal daily routine so that important daily activities such as cooking and dressing are possible. The OTs work will help strengthen muscles too, but it is mostly geared to helping the woman live as normally as possible at home.

For many ailing or arthritic older Americans who do not otherwise need skilled care, an OT can be a miracle worker. The therapist's trained eye can spot scores of ways one's home and routine can easily be adapted to improve safety, and to conserve time and energy. For example, the therapist might suggest a simple, inexpensive lever system to replace sink faucet knobs. This would eliminate the need to grasp and turn knobs, which often is troubling.

For a kitchen work surface, a heavy plastic called Dicem is available to provide traction and help prevent bowls from slipping during mixing. The therapist may analyze how someone prepares a meal, noting how much excess energy is spent making unnecessary trips. Motion savers would be suggested, including reorganizing the kitchen to save steps. As experts in activities of daily living (ADL), OTs have tricks that can make life easier at home for the most able-bodied. But for someone who wants to maintain and improve their functioning, OTs are too often an underutilized resource.

Physical therapist assistants (PTAs) work under the supervision of PTs and help with simpler exercises and treatment, and routine instruction on use and care of braces, walkers, or wheelchairs. *Occupational therapy assistants (OTAs)* are their counterparts in the occupational therapy field. They may teach basic self-care skills after the therapist's evaluation.

If normal speech is or becomes impaired speech therapy can help. *Speech therapists (STs),* known in professional circles as speech pathologists and audiologists, may opt to work in only one of two areas: in communication disorders caused by *any* problem, such as stroke, brain injury, or diseases; or in audiology, the prevention, diagnosis, and treatment of *hearing-related* speech disorders or basic hearing problems.

Respiratory therapists (RTs) provide services to aid breathing-impaired patients who suffer from heart-lung conditions such as heart failure, asthma, and emphysema. Even patients who cannot breathe without the assistance of a ventilator can now be cared for at home. Therapists may help monitor patients for breathing-related conditions, or take arterial blood samples for tests that measure the effects of oxygen or other therapy. Therapists also test and monitor in-home respiratory equipment for safety and proper function, and teach patients self-care skills. This therapy may also be provided by a *respiratory therapy technician (RTT)*, who handles stable patients needing routine care.

Dietitians

Diet is as important to recovery as any prescribed drug; and for health maintenance, a healthful diet is essential. Dietitians, sometimes called nutritionists, or RDs (registered dietitians), assess a person's dietary needs, evaluate current diets, and plan a nutrition program to promote health.

Because dietitians' services are seldom reimbursed by insurers, the majority of home care agencies do not, unfortunately, have a dietitian as a regular home care team member. Some agencies employ dietitians as needed as home care consultants.

Social Workers

Traditionally, social workers help consumers and their families quickly identify and tap into other needed community services, from Meals-on-Wheels to vocational rehabilitation. In many instances, they provide case management services (see Chapter 17) and deal with the financial side of home care. They explain Medicare or Medicaid coverage, negotiate with private insurance carriers, or find community resources that can help consumers pay for home care or obtain alternative care.

But professional social workers can perform many other valuable services when called upon to do so. They can:

- Counsel patients and help them to cope with the wide variety of nonphysical problems that illness and disability often bring, such as the hardships of dealing with job loss, changing family roles, or depression
- Appraise the patient's in-home social environment and its effect on the recovery process, and suggest measures to help improve overall care as well as the quality of life at home
- Act as patient advocates with caregiving team members and the agency so, for example, clients are provided clear, easy-to-understand self-care instructions or explanations about home care procedures

Professional social workers have completed either a bachelor's college program in social work (BSW) or a graduate-level master of social work (MSW) program. The BSW can handle the traditional social work role, perform basic home evaluation, and assist consumers with less demanding personal problems. The MSWs can "do it all," including helping you through difficult situations that require skilled counseling. MSWs with postgraduate training, known as *clinical social workers,* are qualified to provide psychotherapy. In fact, in many states these clinical social workers can even hang out a shingle and work in private practice just as psychologists and psychiatrists do.

Homemakers and Home Health Aides

If you ever need home care, homemakers and home health aides may become the most important personnel in your life. These team members provide the kind of day-to-day help that can often make the difference between hospitalization, nursing home care, or staying at home.

Most agency brochures list homemakers and home health aides separately, yet their job responsibilities often overlap. Within many agencies, the "homemaker" and the "home health aide" are one and the same person who just switches titles according to the job assignment.

Homemakers may also be called housekeepers, home helpers, or home managers. Home health aides may be called nursing assistants, health aides, home attendants, or personal care workers or aides. The National HomeCaring Council (NHC) prefers the job title and promotes the concept of the homemaker–home health aide, who is trained to manage the full range of household and basic nursing care tasks. Because Medicare and other insurance carriers use the title home health aide, it is well recognized.

What an Aide Can and Cannot Do

At most agencies, home health aides perform three general services on the job: (1) personal care; (2) basic nursing; and (3) incidental homemaking.

An aide may provide only basic, *not* skilled, nursing tasks. For example, an aide can take and record your temperature, pulse, and respiration rate, and make sure you follow simple medical recommendations such as getting more exercise. If you need outside treatment, an aide can accompany you to the doctor's office or hospital clinic. Whether or not the aide can actually drive you there depends on the agency's policy.

An aide can also assist with self-administered drugs, which are drugs you normally take by yourself. What "assist" means depends on the agency's policy and your state laws related to drug administration. For example, if you are a diabetic, you might give yourself daily insulin injections. However, state laws prohibit aides from giving drug injections even if you or a family member normally do this. Injections are considered skilled nursing requiring the services of a nurse.

As minimally trained personnel, aides are not usually permitted by law *physically* to hand you prescription drugs, in the interest of patient safety. Where state laws do not specifically prohibit this practice, agencies often do because of liability worries. Normally, to assist you with drugs, an aide may:

• Arrange drug bottles or medicines by the bedside or

elsewhere so they are convenient for you to use
- Bring you a glass of water or whatever else you may need so you can take your drugs
- Remind you when it is time to take your medicine
- Stand by and watch that you do not mix up medicines and see that you take the right drug in the right dose

Despite these concerns over patient safety, in many states aides are permitted to refill insulin syringes for the patient's own use. If this seems contradictory, realize that this practice has been encouraged by Medicare regulations. As a cost-saving measure, Medicare will not pay a nurse to do this task unless state law specifically bans aides from doing so. Some states concerned about patient safety have passed such legislation as a safeguard for senior consumers.

Also coming under the heading of basic nursing care are more specialized tasks that aides may perform *provided* they have had *advanced* training. Aides may:

- Irrigate a Foley catheter
- Assist with ostomy bag changes
- Assist with self-administered oxygen therapy
- Reinforce and change simple *nonsterile* dressings
- Assist with prescribed skin care
- Assist with simple prescribed exercises and mobility devices (walkers, crutches, etc.)
- Perform simple urine tests for sugar, albumin, etc., and record results
- Apply ice cap collars or binders or supports
- Measure fluid intake and output as ordered by the doctor
- Prepare special diets as prescribed by a physician or dietitian

Some agencies prefer to assign LPNs to perform these duties. However, aides who have received the proper advanced training, and who are experienced and well supervised, can safely perform these tasks. But aides cannot give enemas or douches, change sterile dressings, tube feed, or handle any other skilled nursing tasks.

Under the heading of personal care, sometimes called *custodial care,* an aide assists with normal activities of daily living (or ADL for short). The aide will help you bathe, toilet, dress, groom, get in and out of bed, eat, walk, and so on.

Last, the home health aide's job description includes *some* homemaking. The word is emphasized because Medicare and other insurers will seldom cover an aide's services if they are primarily homemaking. If insurance is not involved, the aide can do more, depending on the agency's own policy. Homemaking covers a wide variety of tasks that keep the home clean and safe, and generally contribute to a person's well-being. Under basic housekeeping, an aide might tidy rooms, dust, vacuum, make and change the bed, wash dishes, and wet or dry mop floors. Aides may also prepare and serve meals, shop for food, and do laundry, including light ironing and mending. Sometimes they help a disabled person pay bills or carry out other essential errands.

What the Homemaker Can and Cannot Do

The homemaker's job includes the homemaking services just described, but these activities form the bulk of the daily work. Notice that the outlined homemaking tasks do not include heavy cleaning. Homemakers never perform heavy "chore" work, no matter how much it is needed in the home.

Personal care is another homemaker-aide overlapping work area. Many agencies assign homemakers when someone needs light help with personal care, but does not need basic nursing. For example, a homemaker might assist an elderly arthritic adult to dress or shampoo hair.

Two unique homemaker responsibilities lie in the area of childcare and teaching home management and parenting. When the mother or other primary caregiver is absent, ill, or disabled, homemakers "mother-substitute," providing partial to complete childcare that differs from run-of-the-mill babysitting. On the teaching side, they instruct in the practical how-to's of home management and parenting:

- Making the home clean, safe, and hazard-free
- Shopping for food or other household goods with quality and economy in mind
- Planning and managing a household budget

- Planning and cooking nutritious, economical meals
- Caring for newborns and children
- Recognizing the needs of children and disciplining them
  properly

Such teaching can benefit very young mothers who have
trouble coping with children and home life, or parents who
have abused or neglected their children. Or it may help a
young retarded or disabled adult learn how to live independently. Likewise, teaching can help the inexperienced elderly adult, usually male, learn to manage the home when the
wife or other primary homemaker becomes ill, disabled, or
dies.

Pastoral Counselors

These professionals become involved in home care usually in
connection with hospice services. They help the very ill and
their families share their concerns about living and dying.
Their focus is nondenominational.

Companions

Job duties for companions, whether paid or volunteer, vary.
As a rule, the companion's main job is being a friend,
someone who will read, talk, listen, and engage the person
needing care in hobbies or stimulating activities, easing loneliness and isolation.

Companions may help with letter writing or phone calls
that keep up the person's interest in daily life. They will
accompany clients on walks or outings to shop, handle
errands, or just relax outdoors.

In addition, they will make a light meal, and at some
agencies they will assist with light personal care. At some
community service agencies, companions may complete application forms for community programs or assist with home
budgeting.

Chore Workers

These personnel are the heavy-duty household workers, some-times called "Handy Andys." If you need floors or walls scrubbed, trash hauled, or windows washed, you require chore services. Chore workers will also perform outdoor yard work and maintenance as well as minor home repairs.

Volunteers

Why are volunteers included among home care personnel? Because many home care services could not operate without this dedicated help. Volunteers, supervised by professionals, help to extend home care to the maximum number of people possible, usually at the lowest cost. Volunteers are usually the mainstays of such programs as Meals-on-Wheels, Friendly Visiting, Telephone Reassurance, and transportation and escort services. Hospice programs also consider volunteer assistants critical. In fact, the federal government requires that Medicare-certified hospices must have volunteer pro-grams.

ASSESS YOUR NEEDS

With this overview of who's who in home care in mind, think about the day-to-day tasks, the individual services, and how much home care you may need. Why not just leave this assessment to the home care pros? You can, of course; but realize that when an agency makes its assessment, it may overlook a helpful service it does not provide.

Take the case of an agency that provides skilled nursing, homemaker, and home health aide services only. Now, sup-pose you need home care as a result of crippling arthritis, but are otherwise well. The agency may advise a homemaker to help with light cleaning, cooking, shopping, and personal care, when in fact you may need a few visits by an occupational therapist who can help you do more yourself than seemed possible. Yet the agency that does not provide occupational therapy probably won't recommend it. All too often agency assessments are geared to the services the agency can supply.

However, just because an agency provides a full range of services is no guarantee that gaps won't occur. For example, at such agencies the social worker's common complaint is, "Why wasn't I involved sooner in home care?" Gaps can occur at any full-service agency, because professionals do not always grasp the full range of each other's roles in care. Doctors, for example, may only see a problem as medical, never recognizing the effects of social factors related to old age, illness, and recovery.

Your assessment won't guarantee that all gaps will be eliminated. Your assessment should not replace the agency's assessment either. But it may help spot potential needs for services which you should discuss more fully with agency professionals.

Reread the range of home care services in Chapter 3 and the personnel descriptions just covered. Use the comprehensive self-assessment checklist on page 386 as an additional guide. With this consumer homework done, you're ready for the next step—hunting for home care.

CONSUMER TIP

If you—or your doctor—are unsure whether or not home care is appropriate, take advantage of a *free* in-home assessment that professional agencies offer. Or if you are not convinced an agency has assessed your home situation properly, or will be sensitive to your needs, get a second opinion. You are under *no* obligation to contract with any agency simply because it conducts an assessment.

—5—

Hunting for Home Care

When you hunt for home care, be prepared for a degree of frustration. If you live in an urban area, your problem may be too many choices; in a rural area, too few. Should you need low-cost care or long-term care, finding help is seldom simple. And if you have to arrange for care for a loved one at long distance, your stress may approach record levels.

There *is* help out there, although searching for it is like looking for undiscovered gold. Finding it takes time, persistence, and patience. But there is far more help waiting than most people realize—if you know where and how to look.

One of the most commonly used, but often least useful, ways to find help is through the telephone directory. In it, you will find home care services under varied listings. In the Yellow Pages, check under Home Care, Home Health Care, Nurses, Nursing Services, Senior Services, Social Services Agencies/Organizations, Homemaker–Home Health Aide Services, and Family Services. In the White Pages, look alphabetically under Meals-on-Wheels, Visiting Nurse, Hospice, or agency names with "Home" or "Home Health" prefixes.

The telephone directory provides mainly a name and a number, so you must phone randomly until you find appropriate help. This chapter describes the many local, state, and national resources that can help you avoid this shotgun approach. You will find the addresses and phone numbers of asterisked (*) resources listed in the Resource Guide, which starts on page 385. You can make the most out of these resources if you do a little advance planning.

BASIC POINTERS

1. *Identify any and all services you may need.* If you haven't done this already, see pages 71–72. The more specific you can make your request, the more likely you will get to the right source(s) of help faster. Remember, if your condition requires *skilled* nursing or therapy, a home health agency is needed. If your situation requires only nonskilled or support services such as respite care, a wide variety of agencies, organizations, or special programs may also be available to meet your needs.

2. *Get recommendations.* "Agencies, like people, have reputations," advises Val Halamandaris, president, National Association for Home Care; "Ask around." Avoid the maze of Yellow Page ads. Get professional references on agencies and community programs from the staffs of the health and social service resources described in this chapter. Seek personal recommendations from those listed on pages 75–76. Ask for more than a name; ask for an explanation as to why an agency or program has been suggested.

3. *Prepare before you phone.* Be ready with pen, paper, and plenty of prepared questions. Have any applicable checklists on hand (see the Resource Guide). If you still don't know what you need or are just plain confused, don't hesitate to holler "Help!" (but be prepared to describe your situation briefly and to the point). When you call, record names and numbers and take notes so you can review your information later, and follow up with further calls if necessary.

4. *Target your phone calls.* Is your situation related to the problems of aging, family troubles, a specific disease or condition? If so, call the resources that work exclusively in that given area first. Sometimes these resources provide direct services. If not, they often serve as an expert referral source for help.

5. *Special situations often require special strategies.* To locate help, try the resources described in this chapter, as follows:

—*In rural areas:* Look beyond your community for services. Often agencies and organizations in neighboring communities will help despite the distance. To locate these quickly, turn to the sections on word of mouth; the hospital and local social security office; then check with publicly funded resources.

—*For low-cost help:* If this is a priority, say so when you call. Look first to United Way, 3A, religious, or other nonprofit community or public agencies for help. Also see Chapter 11. If you are a veteran, see page 170.

—*For help long distance:* If your distant loved one is or was recently hospitalized, try that hospital first. Contact the National Resource Center or appropriate national and state organizations described here for shortcuts to home care in distant communities. Local religious organizations may be able to refer you to out-of-town affiliates. Case management agencies described in Chapter 17 can also help. Always keep a copy of your relative's hometown Yellow Pages on hand in your home as a backup. (Request a copy from your local phone company. There may be a charge.)

LOCAL RESOURCES

Community Referral Services

Many communities operate a telephone "information and referral service" often listed in the phone book by just that title, or I&Rs for short. Other common names for I&Rs are CONTACT, HELP, Help Line, Hot Line, Community Information Service, ACTION, or Action Line. You can often find the phone number for your local I&R on the inside cover flap or on the first page of the telephone directory, where fire and police and other important community numbers are listed. If you can't find an I&R listed in your directory, ask your telephone operator for assistance.

I&Rs do not specialize in health and home care per se; they are an all-purpose community reference point for a wide variety of local services. As such, they can link you with health and mental health care, social services, welfare programs, education, job training, rehabilitation agencies, recreation, and community activities.

If you want to locate local services for the aging, call here. Likewise, contact an I&R for help in locating specific home care support services such as Meals-on-Wheels. If an I&R cannot help you, it can usually direct you to an agency that can.

As an all-around community resource, I&Rs are a good starting point for local assistance.

Word of Mouth

This is one of the oldest and often most reliable methods for finding what you need. "The experiences of friends are very important sources of information," reminds Anne Harvey of the American Association of Retired Persons (AARP). Take the initiative and ask anyone who may be able to help. This includes:

- *Friends or neighbors and acquaintances.* If you do a little digging, you will be surprised to find that many people have had experience with home care.
- *Your doctor.* This is one key resource you shouldn't overlook. Talk to your physician (or call any local physician if you don't have a personal doctor). Often the doctor's nurse, or other staff who work with patients, are home-care-aware and can help too.
- *Local clergy.* Clergy often have extensive experience with home care in the course of their work. Ask for their recommendations on agencies. Many local churches, synagogues, or similar groups provide direct informal home care services to their members or to the community at large.
- *People at work.* If you work, or are a company retiree, ask your union or worker's compensation representative, employee benefits or personnel manager, or others who may help, advise on, or administer health insurance benefits. If you are lucky enough to have an employee

health department, talk to the nurse, social worker, health educator, or counselor there. Many unions now offer special services, such as Friendly Visiting, to their retirees.

- *Your local librarian.* This may seem like an odd suggestion, but the local librarian is often an excellent resource for locating community organizations. Most libraries have a reference section that contains directories of local community services. Libraries often maintain community bulletin boards that display circulars or local programs that may be of assistance to you.
- *City, county, state, or federal elected officials.* These people are all in business to serve. Many officials maintain staffs to help consumers with a variety of problems. So contact the mayor's office, the board of supervisors, or your state or U.S. senator or representative.

Your Local Hospital, Nursing Home, or Rehabilitation Center

Some hospitals operate home health agencies, but even when they don't, they can usually provide home care information. Many hospitals have discharge planning units, which are not to be confused with hospital-based home care services. Sometimes the social service department may handle this job. The discharge planner coordinates follow-up care, including home care, as needed after the patient is released from the hospital.

Since discharge planners often work with several home care agencies, they can recommend or arrange services. Most hospital social service departments can advise you about local social and health programs, including traditional home health agencies or hospices, as well as supportive services.

Even if you are not a hospital patient, contact your local hospital discharge planner or social worker. In some cases, personnel will recommend agencies or services to anyone looking for help. Some hospitals also run health-related I&Rs as a community service. Check with the hospital telephone operator.

Note that discharge planning generally occurs in rehabilitation centers and nursing homes too, so they can also be a source for help. While you may think of nursing homes as the last stop for most people, not all nursing home occupants become permanent residents. To assist those patients who continue their care at home, many nursing homes have discharge planning staff (who may officially work as floor nurses or social workers). Like hospitals, many nursing homes and rehabilitation centers are also starting home health services.

Self-Help Mutual Aid Groups

These support groups, composed of consumers who share a common experience, are caring communities within the community. They focus on mutual concerns, and on sharing feelings, perceptions, and problems. Divorce, Alzheimer's disease, long-term care for elderly parents, ostomies, home care for children, overeating—almost every human condition imaginable has a self-help group somewhere. Frank Riessman, founder of the National Self-Help Clearinghouse, estimates some 500,000 groups exist involving some 15 million Americans. "People want to have control over their own lives," says Riessman. These groups help people do just that. They are an amazing source of self-help ideas and comfort, sharing not just problems, but solutions as well. Some are even organized to provide respite care or other services to group members.

To locate a self-help group, contact local community health agencies or hospitals, which often sponsor groups, or you can contact the National Self-Help Clearinghouse* or its regional members.*

The Social Security Office

According to the Social Security Administration (SSA) Claims Manual, "An essential part of SSA's service to the public is providing information about the programs and services of other public and voluntary agencies." In other words, your local social security office should perform information and referral services. That's the official statement for the record.

What help you will actually get when you call a social security office may be another story. A government survey found that many SSA offices had little information available on community services, and what information they had was often outdated. The survey also noted the social security staff was often indifferent to I&R requests and handled them in a perfunctory manner. That's the bad news. But there is good news too.

Some offices surveyed did an excellent I&R job. Many of these were located in smaller and rural areas. Since you can't predict what your SSA experience will be, and since this is the one single resource that is generally available by phone everywhere in this country, it's worth a call. Most local social security offices can refer you to local physicians and medical equipment dealers who accept Medicare assignment. Other information, such as where to apply for Medicaid, food stamps, or other government programs, should also be readily available. Some SSAs will have much more community service information.

Don't rely on the SSA office for any information on Medicare home care benefits other than a strict reading from the beneficiary booklet. The SSA clerks cannot and should not evaluate your eligibility for Medicare home care. This advice is available only from a Medicare-certified agency, not SSA, or the hospital or nursing home discharge planner.

Publicly Funded Agencies

State, county, or city agencies can sometimes help you locate home care services. However, dealing with the public agencies can often be frustrating. The difficulty often lies first in trying to identify the correct agency and department within the agency; and then in finding a knowledgeable person within that agency.

For starters, regardless of age, try local programs that deal with the aged. Since the elderly are the largest single users of home care services, the staff at senior centers will know what you mean when you ask about home care. Some senior centers sponsor support programs. Also, try the city or county

health department. Don't deal with the operator; talk to a
public health nurse who can explain health department
services. Many provide home care or can refer you to other
appropriate state or local government agencies. The public
department of social services, sometimes known as the department of welfare or public assistance, deals with home
care too, usually in connection with Medicaid/Medi-Cal
reimbursed services. Again, don't rely on the operator. Ask
to talk to a social worker or a supervisor. Some social service
departments assist only Medicaid recipients. Others serve the
public at large. They will provide free information, will help
arrange for certain home care services, or provide case
management for a reasonable fee.

Some state departments of health or local health planning
councils, sometimes called health systems agencies, publish
home care directories that list home care agencies and their
services.

Religious Organizations

Since home care revolves around human needs, many reli-
giously affiliated organizations, large and small, have become
involved in home care to varying degrees. Many organizations
provide free information and referral. Some go further and
provide certain home care services directly, either by running
their own programs or by contracting for services through
local home care agencies. Because these are charitable organizations, the cost of these services is usually based on ability
to pay. Local offices of Catholic Charities, Jewish Family and
Children's Agencies, the Lutheran Council, and the Adventist
Health Network can be found in many cities across the
country. They are among the religious organizations that
assist.

If your own religious persuasion differs or you don't abide
by any religion, don't let this be a stumbling block. Call these
organizations anyway, since they usually assist regardless of
religious belief or affiliation.

Area Agencies on Aging (3As)

Everyone in the 60 and older set should know about the *Area Agencies on Aging (3As)* for many reasons, not home care alone. These agencies sponsor many other worthwhile community activities, including legal, social, and vocational programs; health screenings; and preretirement counseling. They act as an I&R and can help you tap into many other senior-related services such as adult day care.

Nancy Gorshe, associate director of the parent National Association of Area Agencies on Aging, also points out: "The 3As have a major advocacy role. This may mean helping people gain access to needed services or strengthening the work of the nursing home ombudsmen program. We're an advocate for the client not the system."

The Area Agencies on Aging were established through an amendment to the Older Americans Act (OAA), a federal law called Title III. Two major legislative goals are to help older Americans maintain independence and dignity at home and to prevent unnecessary or premature nursing home placement. Given this mandate, the Area Agencies have a natural emphasis on home care services.

The 3As number about 665 and form an "aging network" across the country. They plan, coordinate, and advocate comprehensive services for the 60 and over population in their designated geographic area. Nationwide their programs span almost any nonskilled or supportive home care service you can name. Case management, homemakers, chore services, including home repair, home health aides, transportation and escort services, and shopping assistance are some of the offerings.

The *specific* home care programs you may find available in your community depend on local priorities. One 3A may give priority to homemaker services, while another may focus on nutritional programs.

Here are two examples of the fine work of the 3As:

- A 60-Plus Home Health Maintenance Program in Toledo,

Ohio, provides a nurse at no charge to assess abilities and refer seniors to community services if help is needed; monitor health conditions; teach self-care skills; and counsel seniors on health care options. By providing such preventive services, the goal is to maintain independent living by avoiding complications that would require hospitalization.

- Florida's Community Care for the Elderly (CCE) is administered by the 3A. It aims to help seniors live with dignity in their own homes or homes of concerned relatives or other caregivers and provides adult day care, health maintenance services, respite care, personal care, and an emergency response system, among other services.

Other than information and referral services, agencies seldom operate programs directly. Most sponsor programs awarding contracts to local community organizations or businesses to provide the services. The Area Agency does, however, closely monitor awarded contracts to ensure that services contracted for are in fact delivered. Since 3As regularly evaluate and monitor community enterprises, staff can often advise you about the quality of certain local services, such as home health aide, homemaker, or chore services.

Your designated 3A can sometimes be hard to find. Administratively, they may be located within existing regional planning agencies, economic development commissions, government councils, or city or county governments. Many are incorporated as private nonprofit agencies. In less urban areas, there may be only one or two area agencies per state or region.

To locate an area agency, check your local phone directory, an I&R, or ask local service organizations for seniors such as a branch of the American Association of Retired Persons or a senior center. If you still cannot find a 3A, contact the National Association of Area Agencies on Aging, 600 Maryland Ave SW, Washington, DC 20024, or your state Unit on Aging* for the 3A closest to you.

Area Agency programs may be free, low-cost, or based on ability to pay. Eligibility is based on age, 60 plus, not income; however, locally seniors with the greatest economic or social need may get priority. Social need is also defined locally. For example, it could mean a frail, elderly person who lives alone without any family nearby. Your local 3A may ask you to apply directly, or it may refer you to a local 3A-sponsored program for application.

Even if you are under age 60, contact these agencies for information and advice. Like religious organizations, the Area Agencies on Aging don't discriminate either. Most will try to help you locate home care services even though you don't qualify for their programs.

ACTION Programs

ACTION, an agency for volunteer service, is a federal agency that sponsors certain home care services at the community level. Its Retired Senior Volunteer Program (RSVP) may provide telephone reassurance or friendly visiting services. The Senior Companion Program (SCP) serves frail and infirm elderly to prevent or delay nursing home placement, or make possible discharge from a nursing home.

Senior companions, who are seniors themselves age 60 or older, are low-income volunteers who receive a tax-free stipend, transportation, and certain other fringe benefits. They provide some personal care, grocery shopping, and general companion services. They help arrange for other community services. It's not unusual to have an active 76-year-old senior companion helping a "junior" senior age 70 maintain an independent life style. Senior companion Val Coughlin, Allegheny County, PA, points out: "The wonderful thing about this program is that volunteers like myself know and care, perhaps better than others could ever understand. Because, very simply, we are seniors ourselves." Senior companions help those who are isolated and homebound. The program is free.

To learn if there are RSVP or SCP programs in your area, contact your local I&R or resources for the elderly. You can also contact the national ACTION office at 806 Connecticut Ave SW, Washington, DC 20525, (800) 424-8580, ext. 239.

It will refer you to the appropriate regional office (eight nationwide) that administers and tracks local community programs.

The American Red Cross—Local Chapters

The American Red Cross deals with more than first aid, bloodbanking, and disaster services. At the local level, its activities can run the gamut of services from health screening to home care.

In home care, chapters offer consumer-oriented basic home nursing courses. Some also train home health aides for employment. For years, various chapters have run medical transportation services for the elderly or the disabled. Lately, to help community residents stay independent at home, some chapters have broadened these services to include transportation for shopping or other nonmedical needs.

One innovative home care program has been undertaken by the New York City chapter to serve a pressing local need. With city funding, the chapter hires, specially trains, and supervises home health aides who provide home care directly to AIDS victims. Jeannette Bushey, RN director of the AIDS home attendant program, explains that the Red Cross program was created "because local agencies wouldn't touch these patients." She admits that "it was hard to get workers for the program." But the program is under way. When it is fully in operation, 200 AIDS patients will receive home care.

Don't contact the *national* Red Cross office about local home care services. It provides general leadership and technical assistance, but does not mandate or list local programs. Each chapter operates independently, developing its own programs and eligibility requirements according to community needs. So inquire locally.

United Way

You may have "given at the office" to the United Way, sometimes known as the United Fund or Community Chest. This organization funds many community service programs, including I&Rs and programs for the aging and disabled. Many voluntary nonprofit home care agencies are funded by United Way. If there is a local office in your area, a phone call may be worthwhile. United Way agencies and programs usually provide services at lower costs or based on ability to pay. Most local United Way offices maintain a roster of the groups that they fund.

Community (Voluntary) Health Organizations

When a specific health problem creates the need for home care, call on the appropriate voluntary health organization. Alcoholism, cancer, heart or lung disease, diabetes, mental illness or retardation, multiple sclerosis, blindness, Parkinson's or Alzheimer's disease, and cerebral palsy are among the conditions for which national organizations exist to help those affected and their families. All have local chapters nationwide, with more local units being added each year. In some cases more than one organization may operate for the same problem or some aspect of it. For example, the American Cancer Society (ACS) is the best-known voluntary health organization agency dealing with cancer problems. But organizations such as the Leukemia Society, which is devoted to blood-related cancers, and Cancer Care exist too.

Voluntary health organizations are normally devoted to research, public education, *and* patient services. Most local chapters have staff that can help you locate services and provide advice about care, self-help, and just plain coping with health problems. Some organizations give limited financial help to help pay for treatment and care-related costs, or they may operate free loan services for medical equipment and supplies.

Some chapters provide services too. Many local ACS groups, for instance, sponsor the Road to Recovery program. It provides free volunteer transportation services that take in-home cancer patients to and from treatment. The people served by the program may be too young, too sick, or too old to drive. Often the lengthy daytime regular treatment some cancer therapy requires can make it difficult for families or friends always to drive. Said one grateful patient afterward: "I simply couldn't have driven home that day. I felt so sick from the chemotherapy. I needed that volunteer waiting for me outside the hospital."

The Road program also includes friendly supportive visits from former cancer patients recovered from the same kind of cancer that the current patient suffers. Cancer Care, a tri-state, New York–based social service agency, assists in counseling and planning for home care services, including hospice care. In Massachusetts, the Easter Seal Society has become a certified home health agency and provides a full range of skilled and nonskilled home care services.

These programs are just a hint of what services community health organizations can provide.

If you can't find an appropriate local chapter in your area, or you don't know whether an organization exists related to your problem, you can contact:

> National Health Information Clearinghouse (NHIC)
> PO Box 1133
> Washington, DC 20013
> (800) 336–4797, (703) 522–2590 (VA)

NHIC is a free service of the Office of Disease Prevention and Health Promotion, U.S. Public Health Service. It is a central source of information and referral for any kind of health question, including identification of national and local health organizations and programs. NHIC maintains a library and a computer database of over 2,000 health-related organizations.

You might also consider contacting:

> Association for Medical and Health Alternatives
> PO Box 112
> Clearwater, FL 33517
> (813) 734–9016

AMHA is a nonprofit membership organization that provides members with information on available health treatments (traditional and nontraditional) and health promotion research. Like NHIC, it has a library and a computer database to help locate national and local organizations of assistance to consumers. There is a $30 membership fee.

Neither organization diagnoses conditions or provides medical advice.

NATIONAL AND STATE RESOURCES

The National Resource Center

Do you need to find a Medicare-certified agency in another state? A rehabilitation center? A lab service that will make home visits, or an air ambulance that can fly you home when you are ill out of state? Just one call to The National Resource Center (NRC) may give you the answers to all these questions and more.

NRC is an information and referral service sponsored by Quality Care, Inc., a national for-profit home care firm. Originally developed for health professionals, NRC services are now available free to consumers too.

The center coordinator is an experienced public health nurse who will link you with needed services directly either through Quality Care or another agency, or refer you to another organization that can help, such as the State Unit on Aging. At present the center's data file includes *selected* listings for Medicare-certified home care agencies, visiting or public health nursing services, medical equipment suppliers, air ambulances, lab centers, therapy services and rehabilitation centers, hospices, as well as skilled nursing facilities and major support groups. To use NRC, call 9 to 5 (Eastern Standard Time): (800) 645–3633; in New York, (800) 632–3201.

Other Resources

In addition to NRC and the national organizations already mentioned, the organizations listed below can help give you a quick fix on certain home care services across the country. Where indicated, you may want to contact existing state organizations first, since they may have more specific information on available services in your locale. For a prompt response when you contact these organizations, enclose a self-addressed, stamped, business-size envelope. Contact:

- The National Association for Home Care (NAHC)* for up-to-date listings of state home care associations.* NAHC has compiled the comprehensive *National Home Care Directory,* which, though geared to professionals, you may find helpful and available through reference, hospital, or other professional libraries.
- The National HomeCaring Council* for local home-maker–home health aide services, both NHC-accredited and nonaccredited.
- The National League for Nursing* for its list of NLN-accredited home health agencies.
- The National Hospice Organization (NHO)* for local hospice care of the terminally ill and their families. NHO also publishes a nationwide directory. State organizations* are very active and consumer-oriented. Read more about hospices in Chapter 18.
- Family Service America* for referral to one of its 268 member agencies. Agencies provide family counseling and assist with home care arrangements and referrals to community service programs of all kinds, including services for the elderly. Fees are usually based on income level.
- The state Units on Aging* for all matters related to older Americans in the state. These units can identify key organizations and agencies within a given locale, such as the 3As, which sponsor home care services or other senior-related services like day care and social services. They can direct you to special programs available for long-term care.
- The American Affiliation of Visiting Nurse Associations and Services (AAVNAS)* for the visiting nurse organization nearest you. These long-established multiservice, community-minded home care agencies have a reputation for providing high-quality care scaled according to ability to pay.

- The local offices of national home care firms, mentioned in Chapter 7, for information on their affiliated branches nationwide. Some companies have toll-free 800 numbers.
- The National Association of Meal Programs* for nationwide information on free or low-cost nutritious home-delivered or community group (congregate) meals for senior citizens, age 60 and over, and the homebound.

———6———

Choosing a Home Care Agency

How should you select a home care agency? In a word, *carefully*—as carefully as you would choose a doctor. The care you receive will make an important difference in your health and the quality of your life.

A 1985 AARP study found an amazing 29 percent of the consumers interviewed chose the first agency they called, even if they had time to shop around. Choose a home care agency on the basis of careful evaluation, not merely cost. An Equitable Life Insurance Company survey found that 84 percent of the consumers queried did not consider fees when selecting their doctors. Yet most consumers who question agencies at all are concerned primarily about costs. Jean Langevin, director of a homemaker–home health aide service, notes that in her eighteen years' experience, "No more than 2 percent of all clients we serve ask questions about our agency services when they call. Yet there is a vast difference between the services agencies provide."

She's right. Not all agencies are alike. They vary not just in the *kind* of services they may provide, but in the *quality* of those services too. Remember, there are the pros and the others. If you leave this choice to chance, you are risking second-rate care and needless problems.

This chapter provides questions and answers that can help you evaluate an agency, as well as the fine points to consider in your decision-making process. The key questions have been repeated on page 389 as a checklist so you can record and compare agency responses.

"Don't hesitate to ask lots of questions," urges Medical Personnel Pool administrator Leonard Panar. "A consumer should never feel any question is stupid or trivial." An agency that shows impatience or makes you feel uncomfortable about asking is sending you a subtle but important message about its care.

If you are pressed for time, concentrate your questions on the development of the care plan, personnel qualifications, screening, and supervision.

If the care is for children or someone who lives alone, be extra cautious about agency selection. Problems often occur in these high-risk situations if the agency is not a pro.

THE AGENCY'S RÉSUMÉ

If you know little about an agency other than its name, start as an employer would, with questions that provide background information about the agency itself.

Is the agency a home care agency, or a nurse's registry, or an employment agency?
Many registries or employment agencies list themselves in the Yellow Pages under the same general categories as bona fide home care agencies. Often you cannot identify these registries by name alone. If you want to consider a registry, first read more about them in Chapter 8; then decide.

Can the agency provide professional references?
Any professional agency can supply you with solid references from doctors, hospitals, or community social work personnel. Request specific names; don't settle for the name of a hospital or organization. Don't go any further if an agency cannot provide this information.

Does the agency limit eligibility for service in any way?
Many agencies, particularly community or hospital-based agencies, may service only a certain geographic area. A public agency such as a county health department may limit services to people according to income. Occasionally agencies may

provide care only if there is at least one family caregiver in the home or if insurance coverage is available.

Is the agency accredited, Medicare-certified, or licensed?

The meaning of these terms is discussed in Chapter 3. Remember, licensing and Medicare certification do not imply excellence, so you should continue the evaluation process. These credentials, however, are often important for insurance purposes, so be sure to ask.

What is the background of the agency's top management personnel?

Quality home care needs operational support and guidance from the top. So this question can help you spot the professional agency from the fly-by-nighter. However, ask this question regardless of how long an agency has been in business. The answer may provide a clue about "mom and pop" operations or how patient- versus profit-oriented the agency's approach to home care may be. Management does not mean only the nurse supervisor. It includes the local agency administrator or director of operations, or in the case of small for-profits or private nonprofits, the board of directors.

Be wary when management lacks prior experience in home care or other health or social service fields, or when the board is comprised of people with vested agency interests.

Is the agency fully insured against problems?

Chapter 3 points out that insurance, including bonding, does not protect consumers or indicate that an agency provides quality services and personnel. In fact, many professional agencies do not bond their employees. However, the professionals always carry malpractice and liability insurance.

How long has the agency been in business?

Don't dismiss an agency simply because it is new; but keep in mind that fly-by-night agencies are a growing problem. If the agency has been in business less than a year, consider this: A brand-new legitimate agency, or even a new branch of an established agency, may not have ironed out all its operational standards. When you evaluate the "new" agency, be extra alert to answers about the care plan, supervision, personnel, insurance, and billing. You may find that a new agency is eager to establish a good reputation, has high standards, and will make every effort to satisfy you. Or you may discover that for whatever reasons, the agency seems poorly prepared to handle potential problems and business essentials.

What services does the agency offer?

If the agency offers the services you need, discuss the range of other available services too. Situations can change. Here is a case in point. An out-of-town son called the agency long distance, requesting immediate homemaker and companion services for his elderly father. The son had not visited for some time, and was unaware that his father's home had become a minor disaster area. Weeks of unchanged kitty litter, accumulated garbage, trash and dirt greeted the assessment nurse upon arrival a few hours later. The nurse immediately arranged for heavy-duty cleaning through the agency's affiliated chore service.

If home care is needed for an elderly person, especially one living alone, the availability of social work services is very important. Independent living often becomes possible *if* a well-coordinated agency and community services program is developed. When you consider an agency on the basis of its services, don't reject an otherwise fine agency if it does not provide everything you may need. For example, many home care agencies, even those that are Medicare-certified, often do not directly provide medical equipment and supplies or chore services. If it meets your essential needs, then ask:

Will the agency help you obtain other services, if needed, which it does not provide? If so, how?

This answer often underscores important differences between agencies. In the case cited above, some agencies might simply have notified the son about the household problem and refused the case until the son himself could arrange to have the situation corrected. Instead of receiving home care help, the son would have received an unexpected headache.

You will have to decide yourself whether an agency's response to this question is satisfactory. You may want to ask about help for support or alternative services such as adult day care or Meals-on-Wheels, as a test. Any professional agency should be able to provide you with the names and telephone numbers of local programs that run these services. Many agencies will do far more; they will actually contact and arrange for services in your behalf.

If yours is a borderline nursing home situation, find out what help the agency can provide with placement should the patient's health seriously decline. Don't accept assurances that "someone" will help; ask for the person's name and discuss the nature of the help in detail.

When are the agency's services available? How soon can services begin?

Agencies operate on different work schedules. Some follow a fairly standard work week—daytime hours, no evenings, weekends, or holidays. Others can provide care 24 hours a day, seven days a week, year round. Consider the agency's work schedule from the viewpoint of the care you need, not the cost. For example, hospital discharges often take place on a Friday. Can you wait for home care until Monday? Don't assume that an agency's work schedule indicates its quality of care. A superior agency may only provide daytime services, while an inferior agency may offer round-the-clock care.

Allow as much time as you can to plan for home care, but know that most agencies can provide assessment and/or in-home personnel within 48 to 72 hours, often less. However, if you have a special request—for example, you want an aide who has prior experience with Alzheimer patients, or a male aide, or a live-in—more time may be needed. Advance time may be needed for high-tech care or complex rehabilitation patients. When you discuss "how soon," ask about specific therapies you may need. For example, if you have been receiving daily therapy in the hospital, you should not wait a week for this service at home. If an agency cannot accommodate a *general* request within three business days, go elsewhere.

THE CLIENT ASSESSMENT AND CARE PLAN

The care plan is an important key to sound recovery or to maintaining your independence at home. If an agency doesn't know what a care plan is, or doesn't require one, reject that agency without further question. Agencies generally advertise that they provide assessment as a standard service, but what an agency actually means varies widely. How carefully an agency conducts its assessment and develops its care plan is one good sign of its standards.

Does the agency conduct an in-home assessment prior to developing your care plan and rendering service?
If you call and an agency agrees to "send a worker right over" without further follow-up, don't feel relieved; feel cheated. Except in emergencies, an agency should never write up a care plan and provide care based only on your request for services. Professionally, this would be like a doctor who allows you to diagnose your own illness, prescribe your own treatment, and then simply writes you a prescription and sends you a bill. Only a second-rate agency operates this way.

No matter how carefully you think you have assessed your own situation, an agency has a professional responsibility to conduct its own assessment too. A professional agency will involve you and your family, when appropriate, as it develops your plan of care. A detailed initial telephone assessment won't do. A face-to-face evaluation is a recognized industry-wide standard.

Why can't an agency rely on telephone assessment? "Clients often minimize their need for care when they call," explains administrator Leonard Panar. "Out of pride, they often say that they can do more than they actually can. If I rely on a telephone conversation, I may provide the wrong service or level of care."

An in-home visit allows the agency to assess what problems your home environment may pose. If you are hospitalized, an agency may conduct its firsthand assessment at bedside prior to discharge. However, a briefer follow-up assessment at home is still needed.

If you need home care in a hurry, a careful, detailed telephone assessment is acceptable *if:* (1) Follow-up in-home professional assessment occurs as soon as possible once services begin, ideally within 48 hours. This assessment should verify telephone information, confirm the adequacy of the care plan, and adjust services as needed. (2) The agency consults with your doctor, as advised below.

Does the agency consult with your doctor or other professionals when indicated before developing the care plan?

Agencies routinely contact doctors about the care plan when a doctor's sign-off is needed for Medicare or other insurance. However, whenever you need basic home health aide service or skilled nursing or therapy, regardless of insurance, an agency should always consult with your doctor. A professional agency does this first to ensure safety. The agency will want to make sure your doctor is fully aware of your present medical condition if he or she has not been otherwise alerted. This need for home services may indicate a serious condition or a change in your condition that warrants medical attention. Second, the agency will determine, together with your doctor, whether home care is appropriate for your condition and what combination of skilled services is best.

If you are recently discharged from a hospital, or under ongoing care for any serious condition such as heart disease, or are taking several prescription drugs, for safety's sake a professional agency should still consult with your doctor even if you require only personal care, homemaking, or other nonskilled services. This discussion alerts the agency to any potential problems, whether health- or drug-related, that might occur as it provides care. Also, such consultation may provide the doctor with valuable medical information. For example, if home care was sought for the "sudden" senility of an elderly person, this decline might alert the physician to look for a treatable medical condition or an overmedication problem. Such problems might be missed entirely without the agency's call.

When you discuss this consultation, ask specifically if your doctor will be called. Do not assume that this will happen simply because an agency requests your doctor's name and telephone number.

In addition to contacting your doctor, an agency should, with your consent, also contact other health professionals who may be assisting you—for example, staff at a clinic or adult day care center—in order better to coordinate your care.

Who conducts the assessment and develops the care plan?

A professional assessment means evaluation by a bona fide professional (not an agency clerk or even a trained nonprofessional coordinator). Anything less is second-rate. Any situation that requires skilled or basic nursing requires evaluation by a registered nurse. If the RN has solid experience in public health or community nursing, credit the agency with higher standards. Cases that involve physical therapy should *always* involve a physical therapist in the initial assessment. Other professionals may participate in the assessment as needed.

If you need only nonskilled care (personal care, companionship, etc.), professional assessment may be provided by an RN, a social worker, or a qualified college graduate in a human service field. The professional(s) who assess your situation should develop the specifics of your care plan, following any orders your doctor may have prescribed.

How thorough is the assessment?

Some agencies only do a fast "token" assessment, so be sure to discuss the nature of the actual assessment the agency will provide. A thorough assessment evaluates five areas:

1. *Your ability to perform the normal activities of daily living.* An agency cannot develop a sound care plan without

this information. Therefore, the agency should probe in detail to assess your performance of each basic daily task. This review helps determine what nonskilled services you need and how much help.

Avoid an agency that doesn't determine what you can do for yourself. You will probably end up with a care plan that provides more care than you need. This may not only cost you more, it may hurt rather than help your health.

2. *Your state of health, and what nursing and other assistance are needed.* Regardless of your situation, an agency should assess your physical and mental status. If your case is health-related, a professional agency does not base this assessment solely on consultation with your doctor, a discussion with you or your family, or a review of the hospital record. The RN and/or the therapist should make a personal "hands on" evaluation to assess your condition and determine your skilled care needs. Ask what the RN will do. At a *minimum,* the RN should:

— Review your medical history and diagnosis, confirm current medications, bowel and bladder habits, appetite and dietary needs.
— Check your skin condition.
— Take your vital signs, including pulse and blood pressure.
— Listen to your heart and lungs.

While the RN conducts this evaluation, he or she should also observe your mobility and rate your mental status to note, for example, whether you appear confused, alert, or depressed. Any disabilities such as poor vision or hearing should be noted, as well as your need for special equipment or supplies.

The patient evaluations of some agencies go far beyond this minimum. In its assessment, the Visiting Nurse Service of New York, for example, provides the equivalent of a general office "head to toe" physical that a doctor might perform; in some ways, it's even better. The assessment probes health-related life-style factors such as alcohol, tobacco, or drug use and diet in some detail: the number of meals or snacks eaten, any chewing problems, evaluation of a typical day's diet for nutritional adequacy. When completed, the RN has a thorough understanding of the client's health and skilled care needs, which is the purpose of a personal assessment.

When only nonskilled care is needed, the agency should still assess health status. However, a "hands on" examination is not necessary. In these cases, the assessor should discuss general health, ability to function, medications, and special dietary needs, and observe the client carefully for any obvious difficulties.

3. *Available social support.* Certainly an agency should always have on record the names and telephone numbers of family or friends who should be contacted in case of emergency. Beyond this, an agency assessor should ask about available help from family and friends for the different needs that may affect your care plan.

You may want to rely on help from family and friends for certain tasks rather than on the agency. An agency should discuss this with you in advance and respect your wishes. The presence or absence of social support may affect your home care needs. For example, if you live alone or are socially isolated, the agency may be your only link to the outside world. Certainly a professional agency will make sure there are sound provisions for your safety; it will suggest safety measures if they are needed, such as an emergency response system or a community telephone reassurance program.

4. *Your home environment.* An agency that doesn't consider how your home environment helps or hinders you misses the point of home care entirely. A professional agency will evaluate the home and look for ways it can be adapted so you can live your best there, and for ways to make your home a safer place to be.

5. *Your financial situation.* A professional agency always considers your financial situation as well as your needs for care in the development of its care plan. Any discussion about finances and payment is done discreetly and profes-

sionally. All information is strictly confidential.

Like a good physical that a good doctor will do, a professional assessment takes time. It can't be done in ten minutes. If a nurse whizzes in and out in less than half an hour, you're getting second best.

Do you receive a written, detailed care plan after assessment?
Don't mistake a service agreement or contract, or an employee job description, for a care plan. The service agreement—which you should also receive—generally states the services the agency will provide, its rates, the number of hours of care, and your payment obligations. The job description lists all the work tasks the employee is permitted to perform. The care plan, however, outlines details of your unique care. Most important, it should indicate goals for care, as well as your individual problems and needed services.

Plan formats vary by agency; but in principle, the plan should spell out the general duties of all home care personnel, whether nurses, therapists, or aides. Some agencies use a general master plan that highlights, on a single sheet, each worker's general activities. Then separate plans are drawn up for each team member listing personnel duties in much greater detail. The care plan also lists the supervisor's name and telephone number. A general rule for a care plan is: Make sure that it is customized for you.

THE QUALITY OF SUPERVISION

What kind of supervision does the agency provide?
Check all agencies closely about supervision. Without supervision, you don't have "real" home care; it is as simple as that. Good supervision is a problem preventer and a key to quality care. All caregivers, including volunteer help, should be supervised to some degree. This means ongoing contact between supervisor and worker to discuss and handle problems as they may arise. It also means that someone with greater agency responsibility for patient care—for example,

the nursing supervisor, not the nurse who provides care—visits you *at home* periodically. The purpose? To see firsthand that the nurse, aide, or whoever is assigned is providing proper care. The visit is also an opportunity to note your progress and adjust the care plan as needed. In between visits, supervision takes place through telephone contact between you and the supervisor, and between the supervisor and your caregiving personnel. All home care experts agree, however, that supervision of caregiving personnel by telephone alone is *not* acceptable.

How much supervision is provided?

Once home care begins, supervision should start too. The frequency of ongoing supervision depends on your individual situation.

During recovery or chronic illness use one hard-and-fast rule taken from Medicare standards: If you need the services of a nurse, home health aide, or therapist, an in-home supervisory visit at least once every two weeks is required. Note that *this is a minimum.* More frequent supervision can be required in cases of high-tech care or specialized rehabilitation or when progress is slow and difficult or health appears to be declining.

When only nonskilled care is required, such as personal care or homemaker or companion services, in-home supervision may occur less often. Policies vary among agencies. But remember when comparing agencies that more supervision is better than less. One widely accepted industry standard is a *minimum* visit of once at least every three months. Many agencies exceed this standard for all nonskilled cases, providing biweekly or monthly visits. Some publicly funded home care services provide supervision only at four- to six-month intervals. In any event, weekly contact between supervisor and aide is essential if *only by phone.* Better agencies will contact you weekly to check for satisfaction. Some agencies phone daily to check on proper arrival, departure, or on-the-job alertness.

Remember that these standards are general guidelines. If home care personnel are new and inexperienced, they require more supervision than regular employees. Any situation in which the person receiving care lives alone, and is homebound or bedridden, requires more careful supervision, as does home care for children.

Who provides supervision?

Home health aides and nurses should be supervised only by a registered nurse, preferably one with public health or community nursing experience. Therapists and social workers must be accountable to a responsible person within the agency—if not to the nursing supervisor, then to a manager such as a director of operations or patient services.

If you receive therapy services from assistant-level personnel, a therapist of the appropriate specialty should supervise. The on-the-job performance of nonskilled workers should be supervised by a nurse, social worker, or other professional-level supervisors. A nonprofessional coordinator, however, may monitor adherence to general employee policies such as work schedules.

When is the supervisor available?

The supervisor should always be available to home care personnel, you, and your family during work hours. That's the minimum. At superior agencies, your supervisor or someone equally qualified is always "on call" and available to answer questions, solve problems, and handle emergencies.

PERSONNEL POLICIES

An agency *should* be as careful about its personnel as it is about assessment. One agency administrator put it this way: "Consumers should remember that it is the people you get, not the agency."

You cannot evaluate the agency too carefully on its personnel. Learn the qualifications of anyone who provides care in your home, but pay especially close attention to paraprofessionals—home health aides, homemakers, companions, and so on. Aides may be "certified," meaning they hold a certificate of training. However, unlike RNs or other professional staff, paraprofessionals are not generally licensed by states, nor are they certified by a national organization. Therefore, you must depend almost entirely on the hiring agency's standards to ensure competence.

Experience and Training

Are personnel, particularly paraprofessional personnel, properly trained?

For paraprofessionals, there is no standard definition of training that all experts agree upon. At a minimum, *any* person employed as a home health aide should have completed a formal aide training program, ideally in home health assisting. The National HomeCaring Council (NHC) recommends that training include study in personal care, basic home nursing, first aid, how to work with people, food and nutrition, home safety and management, budgeting, childcare, and family relations. Special instruction in the needs of, and how to work with, the elderly, the disabled, the mentally ill, or the retarded should also be provided.

NHC stresses the importance of this training regardless of whether workers are homemakers or home health aides. Often it is impossible to separate health from homemaking on the job. Consider the homemaker who periodically cleans and shops for an elderly diabetic man. One day he seems out-of-sorts and vaguely confused. The homemaker untrained in basic nursing may overlook these changes, which may signal an insulin problem requiring prompt action.

If an agency trains its own aides, take special notice. Because training adds to an agency's expenses, most agencies do not take on this extra financial responsibility unless they have sound professional standards. By personally training, the agency can control and maintain employee quality. Of course, an agency could run a mill just grinding out "trained" employees, so compare training standards among agencies.

Watch out when agencies state they employ "self-trained" aides. These are workers whose skills were learned solely by caring for sick family members or on the job by working as aides for hire within the community. These workers are often not properly skilled. Be cautious also about nursing-home "trained" or "experienced" aides, since standards here are notoriously low.

Opinions vary on the training needed by other paraprofessionals. All personnel, including chore workers, companions, and volunteers, should at least undergo a careful orientation program.

The NHC recommends, and some states require, formal training for homemakers assigned to any case that involves the care of children or for any worker regardless of job title who provides personal care. Certainly formal training for paraprofessionals can only act as a consumer safeguard.

Does the agency routinely provide continuing education and inservice training for its caregiving personnel?

In the ever-changing world of health, the need for ongoing education and training has been recognized at every level of patient care. According to the standards of the National Association for Home Care (NAHC), a trade association with over 2,400 members, this helps "update knowledge and skills needed to give competent patient care." These training costs are viewed as an essential, not extra, expense of doing business. On this point, over 2,000 agencies can't be wrong. Consider this standard as important as they do.

What experience, if any, does the agency require of personnel?

Experience can be just as important as formal training. Some agencies require that all personnel, professional and paraprofessional, have some appropriate work experience prior to employment.

For aides, NHC advises that prior home care, not nursing home or hospital, experience is what really counts. NHC executive director Florence Moore explains: "In hospitals, or nursing homes, aides are closely supervised and everything you need is at hand. In case something goes wrong, there is immediate professional back-up available. However, in the home, the aide must be able to respond to countless problems without the supervisor's direction. She has to know how to 'make do' with whatever is in the home at that time."

Don't reject an agency that hires well-trained but home-care-inexperienced personnel. Instead, look closely at how the agency screens, assigns, and supervises its personnel.

Screening and Assignment

How are employees screened before hiring?

Standard screening procedures include completion of an application form, submission of references, proof of training, licensing, or other professional credentials, as required, and a personal interview.

Don't place too much confidence in references unless the agency insists on professional references from former *health* employers. Because, as Sharon Hamilton, RN, vice-president of Partners-in-Care, points out: "Almost anyone can get a personal reference from someone." Confirm that the agency carefully checks employer references, state licenses, and so on. But place more importance on the agency's personal interview and the methods that are used to evaluate employee skills.

Quality home care depends on more than employee competence; also needed are common sense, compassion, and the right personality for the job—traits not easy to screen for. Ask how the agency screens personnel through interviewing. For example, Sharon Hamilton instructs her interviewers to ask potential paraprofessionals questions such as these: "What aspects of the job would you find most disturbing?" "What would you do if a client became violent and struck you? Made a sexual advance? Offered you a gift or money?" Ms. Hamilton also advises her interviewers to "trust their instincts" and ask themselves at the interview's end this key question: "Would I want this person to care for my mother?" "If you can't say 'yes' confidently," Ms. Hamilton tells her interviewers, "don't hire that person."

Contemporary Health Care takes a different approach in its hiring interviews. It employs an open discussion about prior work and life experiences in order to identify people-sensitive aides who truly understand the job. By way of example, vice-president Pat Tarantino cited one interview. "She [the applicant] described her work with an elderly woman she had cared for, explaining how she dusted every corner completely as the woman herself had done all her life, though this task wasn't part of the job description. That aide understood the woman's psychological needs, how much it bothered the old woman that she couldn't dust any longer herself. She understood how having someone do it 'her way' made her feel better," said Mr. Tarantino. "We hired that aide."

Kudos to agencies that personally test or assess employee skills, as some do. These professional agencies generally give aides and/or other paraprofessionals written, oral and/or practical tests that cover job essentials. For professionals, agencies generally dispense with tests, since professionals have already undergone state and/or national examination. Instead, professionals are asked to complete a self-assessment skills inventory in order to identify their particular strengths and weaknesses.

How will the agency select and assign personnel for your care?

Don't be concerned about the mechanics here. Look for a professional response showing that the agency matches employees according to the skills you need. If your situation calls for routine care and you are in fairly stable condition, an agency might appropriately assign you a less experienced nurse or aide. A more serious or potentially difficult situation calls for seasoned personnel, often with special experience. An agency which suggests that anyone experienced will do often won't do the best for you.

For example, if you were discharged from the hospital with a serious bedsore, a better agency will assign not just a veteran nurse, but one with specific experience in wound handling. Or if a family needs respite home care for a retarded or otherwise developmentally disabled child, a superior agency will assign an aide experienced with special-needs children, not in just childcare alone.

Will you be assigned the same personnel throughout care, or can you anticipate personnel changes? If so, how often? On what basis are changes made?

It is best to have people who become thoroughly familiar with you, since regulars are more likely to spot problems early and are in a better position to judge your progress. Nurses often care for as many as five patients in a day; aides seldom have more than two or three. So to prevent paraprofessional changes, professional agencies usually consider where you live when they make these assignments. An aide who must travel two hours to get to your home to provide care for four hours may be reluctant to continue your care after a short time. Find out if the agency has aides located within reasonable commuting distance. If not, how can it ensure you regular personnel?

Does the agency consider compatible personalities for ongoing assignments?

In some cases, an aide may care for the same person twenty or more hours per week, so a proper personality mesh can be important to good care. "Some people take a very business-like approach to home care," notes Pat Tarantino. "They want an aide to do the job and then retreat until she is needed again. Other people want talkative aides who become an extension of family." Each situation requires an aide with a different personality.

Can the agency accommodate any special personnel requests?

When you discuss personnel, don't overlook any special needs you may have. For example, most home care personnel are females. If you want a male worker, this is a special request which all agencies cannot satisfy. Or you may need bilingual personnel, or someone experienced in kosher cooking. If you need home care for an elderly parent living alone with a household pet who will also need some care, discuss this special request too. Pet care is considered a special request outside an employee's regular job description.

What specific tasks may personnel perform as part of their regular job duties?

If you check agencies on their job policies, you will find differences that may influence your agency choice. Review your checklist for care and clarify beforehand any "gray" areas pertaining to you. For example, does the agency permit its home health aides, if so trained, to take blood pressure or irrigate colostomy bags? Or do these tasks require the services of a licensed practical nurse? This difference in personnel usually means a difference in cost. Will the nurse make a meal or change a soiled bed? Can aides shop for you or pay bills? If so, how often and under what circumstances? Will the homemaker or companion provide personal care? How much or how little? Can personnel transport you to therapy or medical appointments or to leisure activities such as a beauty parlor? How? By public transportation only, or can you travel by car, yours or the worker's? Is special permission needed in advance? In cases where your auto is involved, most agencies require you to sign a release form in advance absolving the agency from liability should an accident occur.

Realize that answers to some of these questions may hinge more on your insurance than on agency policy. As a general rule, most insurance will not allow aides or nurses regularly to perform "housekeeping" or "custodial" tasks. If your care must be covered solely by insurance, the agency must follow insurer guidelines strictly.

Are all personnel hired and employed directly by the agency?

Many professional agencies employ "independent" contractors. These are professionals—RNs, therapists, and so on—who represent the agency as far as your care is concerned, but who are not bona fide agency employees. These professionals really work for themselves, providing their services to agencies as freelance home consultants. These contractors pay their own social security, taxes, and insurance, while the agency maintains overall employer responsibility for their performance. Generally, there are no problems here. Problems may occur, however, in two cases.

First, be aware that fly-by-night operations that don't care about their clients also don't care about their employees. They typically hire paraprofessionals as independent contractors in order to save the "agency" from paying normal employer expenses. This practice is a sure tipoff to a shoddy agency.

In the second case, many professional agencies "subcontract" for paraprofessional personnel. The agency does not directly hire and employ all the personnel who may be assigned to you. Instead, these so-called "vendor" or "contract" personnel—often home health aides—work for another agency entirely. What's happening here?

Take the case of an agency, perhaps Medicare-certified, that wants to expand its operation but does not have enough personnel. It may subcontract with another agency, perhaps a noncertified proprietary, and in effect "purchase" a given number of hours of aide service each month. Such arrangements are not unusual, and they do not mean automatic problems. You may be surprised to learn, for example, that many hospitals, as a standard policy, regularly use some nonhospital contract staff to provide patient care. If the agency has a vendor agreement, check these points in advance:

- Who provides what supervision? How is supervision coordinated between the two agencies? What happens if problems occur?
- What are the hiring standards of the "subcontract" agency? They should be as high as those of the primary agency. If in doubt, ask for the name of the subcontracting agency and check yourself.

POTENTIAL PROBLEMS

How does the agency try to prevent serious problems or deal with them once they occur?

You are not a pessimist looking for trouble when you raise such questions. Problems can occur even when professional agencies maintain high standards. One clue to quality is how an agency tries to prevent problems and how it handles them should they occur. Discuss any potential problems such as theft, breakage, or substandard care that may worry you. Watch out for any agency person who acts indignant when you raise these legitimate concerns, and who suggests that "such things never happen here." A professional agency representative takes a realistic, matter-of-fact attitude and answers these questions honestly.

For example, at Community Circle of Care (Joliet, Illinois), executive director Beverly Kapinus explains: "I ask each new employee to read an agreement stating the employee will not verbally or physically abuse the client and will uphold the patient's Bill of Rights. The agreement states that failure to do so will mean legal action. The employee is then asked to sign. It's been effective. We haven't had serious problems."

When you discuss problems, don't accept the assurance that "we're bonded" or "we carry insurance." As explained earlier, this in itself means little. Ask about the procedures you must follow in order to collect.

Most professional agencies have specific grievance procedures to handle consumer problems. Check.

YOUR CONSUMER FOLLOW-UP

You can't confirm an agency's every answer in advance. But where you can, don't fail to follow up.

When you contact an agency, don't forget to request its brochures or other available information, such as the annual report. Ask if the agency can provide a rate sheet or will otherwise confirm fees in writing.

Review all material carefully. Look beyond brochure cosmetics. Despite today's competitive marketplace, some very good agencies still have unbelievably dull, institutional brochures. Those that are slick and appealing are nice to look at, but amount to nothing more than good advertising. Check for substance. Does the brochure confirm the key facts you were given? For example, does it confirm that the agency provides stated services, including assessment and supervision, and works with an insurance carrier? Or that it is licensed and Medicare-certified, if applicable?

Some agencies include consumer home care advice and a client Bill of Rights or Code of Ethics as part of their basic promotional material. This is a good step toward consumer education. But whether this information confirms true commitment to top-rated care or is just good public relations, you will know yourself once you have evaluated the agency.

Check with the professional references the agency supplied. Can they confirm the important details concerning supervision, employee standards, and so on?

Contact the local Better Business Bureau for any complaints on file. In high-risk situations, check your local police precinct. One consumer found out *after* a serious theft that there were several similar reports on file for this fly-by-night agency's personnel.

If you want to double-check an agency's claims about personnel qualifications, you can:

- Ask for a copy of the employee job description. Professional agencies have written descriptions that normally include employee qualifications.
- Look through the employment ads of your major newspaper under "Health," "Nurses," "Nurse's Aides," and/or "Home Health Care." Since home care is a growth field, many agencies advertise regularly for nurses and paraprofessionals.
- Call (or ask a friend to call) the agency as if you were a potential job applicant. In most areas aides and nurses are in demand, so it's likely your call will get attention. Ask what qualifications you need to work there.

In any of these cases, see if the qualifications stated match what you have already been told. When I posed as a potential client, some fly-by-nighters and mom-and-pop operations quoted me high standards. Later, as an aide applicant, I found they were either willing to hire me over the phone, or eager to interview me for a job even though they had been told I had no formal training and little related experience.

If round-the-clock services and supervision are important to you, check carefully what a "24-hour" agency means and can provide. Call after hours and test the response yourself.

The New York Metropolitan Better Business Bureau investigated 25 home care agencies that advertised their services in the New York Manhattan Yellow Pages. All the agencies advertised their round-the-clock services with such claims as "call 24 hours, seven days a week," and "immediate response to the needs of your loved ones." Each company was contacted after hours on three separate occasions to request home care services. The results? In more than 10 percent of the cases, no one could be reached at all. And in another 32 percent of the cases, messages were left with answering services, but the calls were never returned.

THE FINE POINTS

During your evaluation, tune into the intangibles of home care. Home care is a very personal kind of industry. Agencies don't have a "product" to sell; they are selling their people and their services.

How the agency treats you when you call, from start to finish, can be very revealing. If you call to discuss home care for an elderly loved one and are immediately put on hold for several minutes, you are off to a poor start with that agency. Likewise, to my way of thinking, an agency makes a poor first impression should you mention an illness like cancer and be bluntly asked "cancer of what"; or, just as bad, should you be fawned over in a patronizing manner. Most people object to such insensitivity from strangers. You don't have to tolerate this in agency personnel. After your talk with the agency nurse or coordinator, answer these questions yourself:

- Did the agency representative put you at ease and make you feel comfortable about asking questions?
- Was he/she knowledgeable? Did he/she instill a sense of confidence about the agency's service?
- Were your questions answered completely? Were you rushed?
- Do you feel you could discuss any problem that might arise with this agency's personnel?

• Do you feel the agency will respond promptly to correct any problems?

If you have time, and especially if home care will be needed for a long period or in a high-risk situation, meet personally with the director of nursing or patient services. After you interview a few agencies this way, you'll see differences and be able to make a sounder selection.

If you are anxious about home care services, or yours is a high-risk situation, insist the agency provide personnel with a proven record *at that agency*. Or ask if you can talk to or meet with the aide who will be assigned in advance. If you prefer, ask to interview personally two or three aides and select your aide yourself.

None of the professional agencies I contacted objected to this, although they stated that they seldom received such requests. However, before you ask, you should be aware of two possible conditions that may be imposed:

1. Because aides are not salaried, but paid hourly for their time, an agency may charge a small fee roughly equal to the aide's hourly wage and transportation costs as compensation.

2. Professional agencies do not permit discrimination in their hiring policies. If an agency suspects you want to interview several aides to circumvent its nondiscrimination policy, it will not honor your request.

Look for any signs during your discussion that the agency takes pride in its employees and treats them with dignity and respect. How agencies treat their employees can affect the employee's attitude toward his/her own job and ultimately the care you receive. Agencies that offer work incentives to paraprofessionals, such as higher-than-minimum hourly wages, periodic salary increases, or certain fringe benefits, usually attract higher-caliber employees. You may also want to ask an agency about its track record on retaining its aides. Since aides have a high turnover rate, this measure is by no means foolproof. But take it as a good sign when agencies retain their aides for long periods.

Other pluses to look for are membership in the state home care association or the National Association for Home Care.

This usually indicates an interest in maintaining professional standards. So does an agency professional advisory committee made up of members (nonemployees) from varying disciplines which usually counsels the agency on care-related issues.

Remember: When you call an agency, you are under *no* obligation to choose that agency or to discuss your situation in detail. For example, you don't have to give your doctor's or the patient's name. An agency will need complete information about any client it serves if it is selected to provide care. But if you choose to make a purely investigative call and make this known, an agency should respect your wishes and answer your questions courteously and completely.

Avoid any agency that uses high-pressure or scare tactics to convince you to use its services. Statements suggesting, for example, that your choice is between home care or a nursing home, or that you don't have much time to look around, are tipoffs. When you look for a home care agency you do not have to tolerate insensitivity, indifference, or unprofessionalism. In most locales home care is competitive, and you can choose among several professional agencies for care.

7

Agency Profiles

In the last chapter, you learned what questions to ask prospective agencies about quality care; Chapter 9 provides questions on cost and payment issues. This chapter profiles some national home care firms, as well as some of their local competitors. These sneak previews, while selective, may serve as a shortcut in your agency selection process. As you review these profiles, read carefully; you will discover differences.

NATIONAL FOR-PROFIT FIRMS

For-profit home care firms are the fastest-growing segment of home care agencies. Between December 1, 1983, and December 1, 1984, Medicare-certified proprietaries increased by 57 percent.

Upjohn and Medical Personnel Pool head the list of the top national for-profit home care chains. National firms are much bigger than locally established agencies, but does this mean they are better? Should you choose a McDonald's (or Burger King or Wendy's) of the home care industry, or should you stick with nonaffiliated local agencies?

There is no clear-cut answer to this question except a qualified "maybe." If you visit any fast food outlet of a given chain across the country, you will find their burgers and fries much the same, as well as their service. Their distinctive quality can be controlled through uniform food purchasing, processing, and serving techniques.

In home care, what you buy cannot easily be standardized, since people, from aides to top agency administrators, are the major ingredient in quality. Despite its national name, any individual office is only as good as its local management and caregiving personnel. Consumers sometimes wrongly assume that because a national firm has many local offices or has grown quickly in an area, this automatically means it provides superior home care. Sometimes a firm may open a branch prematurely, without enough supervising personnel or other staff to provide optimum care. Therefore, your best strategy is to evaluate any office of a national firm as carefully as you would any other agency.

When you consider a national firm, don't assume that it represents big business, and is impersonal or merely profit-oriented. As one administrator earnestly said: "Good care is good business." Many, though by no means all, of the national firms I contacted impressed me with their genuine concern for quality care and professionalism. Some stated surprising flexibility in standard policies in order to accommodate consumers.

What the Nationals Offer

You should find certain standard features among the individual local branches of any particular national firm. These should vary little from state to state and from office to office. Features include uniform:

- Billing, insurance, and office procedures
- Standards for assessment and supervision
- Personnel policies, including standardized job qualifications and duties (local variations will occur to comply with state and city regulations)
- Operating hours

However, the specific services available at offices are not usually standardized. So don't expect, for example, that an Upjohn office in one city necessarily offers the same services in another. Typically national branches offer, at a minimum, skilled nursing, home health aide, companion, and homemaker service with live-in options as standard services. Many firms offer "bed and bath" services that provide a brief morning or evening aide visit for the sole purpose of getting the client into (or out of) bed, bathed, and settled for the night or day. Medicare-certified branches also offer social services and usually most therapies. Some agencies sell or rent durable medical equipment (DME); others will coordinate this service at no cost.

In addition, most firms advertise round-the-clock services seven days a week, so theoretically they should be able to provide services to meet unusual schedules. The largest national firms also have greater purchasing power, which may translate into savings should you need medical equipment or supplies. If you need to arrange for home care at long distance, the local branch of a national firm can usually direct you to its branches in other cities.

Nationals usually provide central quality control. The best firms regularly monitor the performance of their branches.

Profiles

The following profiles are based on questionnaire responses, company literature, and interviews. Note that in follow-ups with local branches in some cities, I found discrepancies. For example, many local offices required service hour minimums, though the national office stated otherwise. Also the BBB investigation described on page 111 cited many well-known national firms for truth-in-advertising failures.

Virtually all agencies run credit checks on their customers, some in advance of care; bill weekly with payment due on receipt; and accept insurance assignment. Free in-home assessment and supervision are built into the service costs of the nationals described here. Note that by law all Medicare cases must be visited in-home biweekly.

> Upjohn Health Care Services
> 2605 E Kilgore Rd
> Kalamazoo, MI 49002–1897
> (616) 342–7000

With 290 offices in 45 states, Upjohn Health Care Services is the largest national home care firm, having entered the home care field in 1969. It is a division of the Upjohn Company, worldwide manufacturer and developer of drugs, founded in 1886. Approximately 105 of Upjohn's offices are Medicare-certified.

Upjohn prides itself on its professionalism and corporate management. "We won't accept a case unless we can do it right." It has a pro-patient philosophy of nursing and a consumer Bill of Rights. Following care, consumers are invited to evaluate their services via a postpaid envelope supplied by the agency.

Services: Standard plus chore services nationwide; therapies, social services, dietitian services at all Medicare-certified offices and some noncertified offices; high-tech services at some offices (cases of children dependent on ventilators for breathing are a specialty); coordinates DME. Offers an economical Independent Living Services program that primarily provides nonskilled personnel.

Personnel: Aides—six months' experience or training course within the last three years; homemakers—no training required; professionals—recent satisfactory work experience and self-assessment of skills required.

Care Plan: In-home RN assessment in all cases except some companion or chore worker cases.

Supervision: In-home visits provided, but frequency varies according to client need, presence of family caregivers.

Payment: No minimums, no credit cards; may require advance payment if credit rating is poor.

Medical Personnel Pool (MPP)
303 SE 17 St
Ft. Lauderdale, FL 33316
(305) 764–2200 (FL); (800) 327–1396

MPP, founded in 1966, is the oldest national home care firm. It has 220 offices in 43 states; 87 offices are Medicare-certified. Owned by H&R Block, Medical Personnel Pool bills itself as an international nursing service providing not only home care services, but supplemental staffing for health facilities in the United States and Canada. It promotes a Code of Ethics that in theory satisfies major consumer concerns about quality in home care. If a local MPP office lives up to this code and its nationally advertised standards, it should rate well in your evaluation.

Following care, customers are sent a postpaid evaluation form (no name necessary) and asked to confidentially rate MPP on: employee courtesy, promptness, professionalism, efficiency, and attitude. Consumers' suggestions are invited.

Services: Standard plus high-tech available nationwide; dietitian and respiratory therapy in most offices. Coordinates DME; case management a specialty. MPP emphasizes wellness and stresses health teaching.

Personnel: All employees must have a year's experience; a standardized skills matching system is used to assign personnel; employees are tested.

Care Plan: In-home RN assessment for all cases.

Supervision: In-home RN visit at least biweekly in all cases.

Payment: Visa, Mastercard, American Express; no minimums.

> Quality Care, Inc.
> 100 N Centre Ave
> Rockville Centre, NY 11570
> (800) 645–3633

Started in 1970, Quality Care (QC) has 165 offices in 43 states; 14 are Medicare-certified.

QC provides clients with a patient policy brochure that clarifies its services. Its treatment plans, assessment forms, and other material are professional, organized, and thorough. As a public service, QC sponsors the National Resource Center, which directs consumers to other available home care resources nationwide (see page 87).

Services: Standard plus high-tech IV and nutrition; chore services; coordinates DME at all offices; respiratory high-tech, therapies, dietitian, social services, and DME sales at some offices. QC specializes in pediatric home care, cancer care, and nervous system diseases/disorders.

Personnel: Aides—aide training plus one year's experience; homemaker—exam, one year's experience; professionals—one year's experience and skills assessment and written tests required.

Care Plan: In-home RN assessment in all cases.

Supervision: In-home visits in all cases, minimum of once every 60 days.

Payment: Generally four hours per week minimum; some branches accept credit cards.

> Beverly Home Health Services
> 23639 Hawthorne Blvd, Suite 202
> Torrance, CA 90505
> (213) 378–9263

Beverly Enterprises, founded in 1963, is best known in health care circles for its nursing homes. In 1982, Beverly Home Health Services was established. It has 138 home care offices in 16 states; 117 are Medicare-certified. In many cities, Beverly offices are known by local community names and are based in Beverly-owned nursing homes.

Beverly maintains a national toll-free consumer advocacy line to take complaints or handle any problems not managed at the local level. It has a patient Bill of Rights.

Services: Standard Medicare services plus DME sales or coordination available at all offices; live-in, all therapies, dietitian, respiratory therapy, and high-tech (including pediatric) care available at selected offices; mental health–psychiatric technician service available at limited offices.

Personnel: Aides—as defined by state law and patient care experience; homemakers—no training required; professionals—one year's recent experience, written test, some skills demonstration.

Care Plan: In-home RN assessment in all cases.

Supervision: In-home visits once every 60 days in all cases; for medical cases, biweekly visit minimum.

Payment: No minimum; no credit cards.

Staff Builders Home Health Care, Inc.
122 W 42 St
New York, NY 10168
(212) 867–2345

Staff Builders Home Health Care, Inc., founded in 1961, entered the home care field in 1971. It has 99 offices in 28 states; 33 are Medicare-certified. Staff Builders' outlines for home care procedures, including high-tech and rehabilitation, employee performance evaluations, equipment inventories, and so on are professional, highly detailed, and extremely well organized. Staff Builders' continuing education program for nurses has been accredited by the American Nurses' Association.

Services: Standard plus all therapies, dietitian, social services; DME coordination and high-tech services available at most offices. Specializes in comprehensive home rehabilitation services; has available COMMUNI-CARE emergency response system.

Personnel: Aides—approved home health training and one year's experience; homemakers—approved homemaker training program or two years' equivalent experience; professionals—one year's recent experience plus CPR, infection control, risk management training; additional training required for certain assignments; skills assessment and written tests required.

Care Plan: In-home RN assessment except in nonmedical cases.

Supervision: Weekly in-home visits in some cases; all seen once a month minimum.

Payment: One visit or four hours per week minimum required; Visa, Mastercard, American Express.

Kimberly Home Health Care
8500 W 110 St, Suite 600
Overland Park, KS 66210
(800) 255–5018

Founded in 1970 as National Medical Consultants, Kimberly Services is owned by Pritchard Services Group of America, a subsidiary of a London-based company. In 1982, Kimberly Home Health Care was established, and it now has 75 offices in 34 states, of which 41 are Medicare-certified. Kimberly has an excellent patient Bill of Rights which it distributes to all clients. Kimberly forms for care are professional and comprehensive.

Note: The 1984 Kimberly service agreement advised clients that employees are not to be left alone in a home with cash, credit cards, or other valuables, and that the client will accept full responsibility for any and all claims, including fire, theft, and property damage. What does this mean to you? Management says this statement is supposed to "provoke discussion" so clients will make their homes secure prior to care. Discuss this clause *very* carefully before signing.

Services: Standard, chore service, all therapies and social services, high-tech available nationwide; no dietitian services; MD service at some offices; coordinates DME; specializes in Alzheimer's and dementia (senile) care, pediatric care, and long-term rehabilitation cases.

Personnel: Aides—recognized training and one year's experience; homemakers—recognized training or extensive life experience; written test for paraprofessionals; professionals—one year's experience.

Care Plan: In-home RN assessment in all cases except some homemaker or chore cases.

Supervision: In-home visits monthly at minimum.

Payment: No minimum; accepts Visa, Mastercard.

Kelly Health Care
999 W Big Beaver Rd
Troy, MI 48084
(313) 362–4444

A subsidiary of Kelly Services, Kelly Health Care was founded in 1976. It maintains 73 offices in 20 states; 40 offices are Medicare-certified.

Kelly distributes a consumer Bill of Rights to all customers which stresses that they have a right to complain or recommend changes in policies.

Services: Standard plus chore, therapies, dietitian, and social services at some offices; does not provide or coordinate DME; high-tech services at some offices.

Personnel: Aides—recognized home health training and one year's recent aide experience; homemakers—no training; professionals—one year's recent experience; skills self-assessment.

Care Plan: In-home RN assessment in all cases, in-home therapist assessment when needed.

Supervision: Monthly visits on average.

Payment: Minimum four hours for one day; no credit cards.

Olsten Health Care Services
1 Merrick Ave
Westbury, NY 11590
(516) 832–8200

The Olsten Corporation was founded in 1950 and entered the home care field in 1971. It has 44 offices in 15 states; 9 are Medicare-certified. Olsten stands by its service. If a customer is not satisfied and notifies Olsten within 24 hours of the time personnel report to the home, there is no charge.

Services: Standard, all therapies, social services, DME, high-tech in all offices; dietitian available in Medicare offices.

Personnel: Aides and homemakers must comply with state and federal standards; professionals must be CPR-trained or -certified; skills assessment and written test required; conducts aide/homemaker training in several offices.

Care Plan: In-home RN assessment in all cases.

Supervision: In-home visit every two weeks.

Payment: No minimum; accepts American Express.

Superior Care, Inc.
287 Northern Blvd
Great Neck, NY 11201
(800) 645–6270

Superior Care, Inc., was established about 1977. It has grown to 31 offices in 16 states; 13 are Medicare-certified.

Superior Care admits to having some past problems, but a full-time nursing director has been hired to help standardize procedures among branch offices.

Services: Standard plus occupational, physical, and speech therapy nationwide. Medical social services, respiratory therapy at some offices; no dietitian services; high-tech services at some offices.

Personnel: Aides and homemakers must comply with state regulations; professionals must show experience in their specialty areas.

Care Plan: In-home RN assessment in all except nonmedical cases.

Supervision: In-home visits not provided in all cases; weekly telephone contact.

Payment: Some branches may have minimums; no credit cards; will bill monthly.

SELECTED COMPETITORS

The profiles that follow broadly describe three "generic" competitors to the national for-profits which may be available in your community. Note that these groups operate *independently,* although they share commonalities. The names and addresses listed are those of their national membership organizations.

Visiting Nurse Association or Service (VNA/VNS)

American Affiliation of Visiting Nurse Associations and Services
21 Maryland Plaza, Suite 300
St. Louis, MO 63108
(314) 367-7744

As a group, the VNAs/VNSs are the oldest large-scale home care organizations, having been set up in the late nineteenth century. Most have been in existence over fifty years, and they have a rich tradition of providing high-quality, consumer-oriented home care. Currently located in most states, they number 500; most are Medicare-certified. Don't let the name "visiting nurse" fool you; these agencies provide a full range of services.

Services: Standard but generally no live-in options. Many still do not provide services on weekends or evenings; social services available at all agencies; most therapies available at most agencies; chore and dietitian services, high-tech, specialized rehabilitation at many agencies; will coordinate DME; strong emphasis on community case management and patient teaching; some offer hospice and special programs for the elderly, teen mothers, or pediatric home care.

Personnel: Standards vary; generally very high for professionals and paraprofessionals.

Care Plan: In-home RN assessment for all cases is the norm.

Supervision: Varies; generally biweekly in medical cases; may be less frequent in other situations.

Payment: Competitive rates with sliding scale (see page 143); accepts insurance assignment; generally no credit cards.

Hospital-Based Home Care Agencies

American Hospital Association
Division of Ambulatory Care
840 N Lake Shore Dr
Chicago, IL 60611
(312) 280–6216

Hospitals are in home care to stay. Between December 1, 1983, and December 1, 1984, there was a 52 percent increase in hospital-based Medicare-certified agencies. Of the estimated 6,000 hospitals, about 2,700 offer (or plan to offer) home care; 861 are Medicare-certified.

When you consider a hospital-based agency, remember you are not obliged to use its services simply because you are hospitalized or because your doctor has patient privileges there.

Hospital home care at present is a mixed bag for consumers. Many top-notch hospital-based agencies have been in business ten years or more, long before hospital home care was fashionable and profitable. In Albuquerque, New Mexico, for example, Hospital Home Health Care has been serving the community since 1973. In the Los Angeles–Orange County area, the Hospital Home Health Care Agency of California has been hard at work since 1970. Similar outstanding hospital-based agencies could be cited. Evaluate newcomers carefully. Look for JCAH accreditation. Some hospital-based agencies handle only skilled care cases. Check.

Services: Standard but often no live-in or bed and bath options; most or all therapies, social services, DME sales or coordination uniformly available; some offer mental health services, long-term care, hospice care, and physician care (see Chapter 19); high-tech services increasing in availability.

Personnel: Standards vary; will follow federal and state regulations at a minimum.

Care Plan: In-home or hospital assessment for medical cases; others vary.

Supervision: Generally biweekly in-home visits for medical cases; others will vary.

Payment: Competitive rates; sliding scale often available at non-profit hospital agencies; accept insurance assignment; some accept credit cards.

Homemaker–Home Health Aide Services

National HomeCaring Council (NHC)
235 Park Ave S
New York, NY 10003
(212) 674–4990

According to NHC estimates, about 5,000 homemaker–home health aide services exist nationwide. These services by definition do not qualify for Medicare certification. Some operate as independent agencies; many, however, exist within multiservice community organizations such as Councils on Aging or Family Service agencies. Their services are geared toward social services and home support for the frail elderly, the disabled, and families in crisis or in need of guidance.

Services: Nonskilled home support services including chore; heavy emphasis on social services is the norm; may coordinate DME; no therapy or skilled nursing; some experimental programs available in high-tech pediatric home care.

Personnel: Standards vary; NHC-accredited have high standards.

Care Plan: In-home RN or social worker assessment standard practice among professional services.

Supervision: In-home visit at least every three months at minimum; many provide much more intensive supervision.

Payment: Sliding scale available at community nonprofits, services generally not insurance reimbursable; generally no credit cards.

——8——

Do-It-Yourself Home Care

If you need home care, you may wonder, "Do I really need a home care agency?" Why not just do it yourself and hire help through an employment agency, a nurses' registry, or a newspaper ad?

Hiring outside help this way may appear to be an easy or less expensive option than using the services of a good home care agency. If this is your line of reasoning, before you decide you should be aware of the possible perils and pitfalls of do-it-yourself arrangements.

First, this option may *not* always be cheaper. To evaluate costs, itemize the extra expenses, including insurance and taxes, that you will incur as an employer (see pages 132–134). Add these figures to your proposed wages and total. Then compare your *actual* cost with the agency's rate. Very often the difference is marginal if you consider the built-in services (assessment, supervision, doctor consultation, insurance, billing, etc.) that a professional agency will provide.

On the more important and personal side, realize that the care is seldom as good as what a professional agency can provide. The majority of home care abuses involve fly-by-night agencies or do-it-yourself situations. In a *New York Times* interview, one woman who had hired help independently to care for her father (elderly, sick, living alone, out of town) summed up the all-too-frequent frustration: "After a while you get to depending on the caretakers so much, that even if they are stealing, you don't want to confront them on it, because you're so tired of training new people." She concluded: "There are times when I feel totally helpless."

Like this woman, many consumers are often willing to

accept very poor employee performance. Employee lateness, poor work habits, indifferent care, or worse may be overlooked because people are grateful for any help at all. Certainly once you hire someone, you want that situation to work. If it doesn't, you must start the hiring process all over again. In the interim, you are left stranded without any help at all.

Before you do it yourself, soul-search and answer this question: Are you sure that you want to, and can, act as an employer for several weeks or indefinitely? Remember that an employer must screen personnel, evaluate care, provide day-to-day supervision, and more. This is a tall order to fill, more so if you are sick or failing. Even if the care you seek is for someone else, these tasks are not simple when you have your own life—a home, family, and/or a job—to contend with, plus the added stress that a loved one's decline and its related problems bring.

IF YOU HIRE

If you answer "yes" and are motivated, organized, self-directed, and understand the basics of proper care, you can make do-it-yourself work. In California's In-Home Support Services (IHSS) program, several thousand disabled individuals prefer to, and successfully, hire, train, supervise, and fire, if necessary, home attendants who provide mainly personal care that makes independent living possible.

Mrs. Julie Beckett, whose little daughter Katie is on a life support ventilator, has trained neighbors as well as nurses to provide this high-tech care for Katie. "I had a twenty-year-old neighbor who was the best person I ever had," recalls Mrs. Beckett. "She took care of Katie all the time I taught school that first year after Katie's coming home from the hospital. I taught her how to suction; taught her how to bag; taught her what to do in case of an emergency. I trusted her." However, Mrs. Beckett agrees this has worked for her "because I am a strong person. People must be ready to assume responsibilities and risks," states Mrs. Beckett.

In order to make this arrangement work well for you, be

prepared to become deeply involved in your own care. Here are guidelines to assist you. Also review Part V, "How to Get the Best Care," for additional advice.

Select Employees Carefully

You may need home care in a hurry, but don't shortchange yourself on the time needed to tackle this critical area properly.

Registries are a step up from classified ads, but don't count on them to do real screening for you. Most registries stay in business by dealing in personnel volume. Therefore, practically any health worker can join a registry just by filing a form and paying a fee. Registries only check for current licensing, if needed, and ask for references. These references may be given to you, but they are seldom checked by the registry. Nor do registries evaluate or test would-be workers for proper skills. In the end, it is *you* who must make the evaluation.

One simple rule: Employ personnel whose skills match your home care needs. Improper matching, a common mistake, invites problems. If you hire an aide to handle skilled tasks such as changing a sterile dressing on a wound, you court infection. Likewise, don't employ a nurse simply to help bathe and dress, or to monitor temperature or blood pressure—tasks less skilled employees can do.

You don't ensure better care by hiring a nurse to do an aide's job. When people don't use the skills they've been trained for, they often become bored and careless. Nor do you save money by employing a homemaker and nurse rolled into one. Most good nurses will not perform non-nursing tasks except those incidental to skilled nursing care. Nurses who regularly serve as glorified aides may lack the professional skills needed to provide competent nursing care. Keep in mind that solid experience becomes very important, since you won't have professional nursing supervision as a backup.

After back surgery, Debbie K., a young mother, thought she had the ideal home care solution. A friend, a part-time hospital LPN, agreed to change her surgical dressing and assist with personal care for a small daily fee.

Once home, Mrs. K. started running a fever and felt worse instead of better. Though her friend assured Mrs. K. the stitches were healing nicely, the wound felt inflamed; small drops of pus oozed, and she felt very uncomfortable.

After a week, her nurse-friend had to return to her regular job. The same night, Mrs. K.'s incision burst, releasing enough fluid to soak more than one bath towel, and creating a large open back wound.

Mrs. K. was promptly rehospitalized so the infection which had been festering since her discharge could be properly treated. Afterward, Mrs. K. learned that her friend was a hospital "floater," someone who fills in where needed, and had no real experience in surgical care.

To avoid problems, before you select personnel use the self-assessment checklist on page 386 to itemize your needs. Use the caregiver descriptions in Chapter 4 as an initial guide to personnel. Get advice from your doctor or from nursing professionals about needed skills and experience. If nursing care is advised, get your doctor's recommendations about the specifics of care in writing, if possible. Take whatever extra time you need for screening potential employees.

If you use a registry, look for one that is hospital-affiliated or nurse-run, which may be better than your run-of-the-mill employment agency. If employment agencies or registries must be licensed in your community, deal only with those licensed agencies. Contact your local Better Business Bureau or Consumer Affairs Office to learn if any complaints have been lodged against the registry.

As an alternative to using an unknown registry, contact the personnel office of your local hospital. It may maintain a list of available personnel. Or ask friends who may have used home care agency personnel. Some good agency personnel moonlight. Check with your clergyman or other trustworthy sources, such as the social service staff at senior centers, for their suggestions.

When You Check References

Before you interview anyone, ask for the names and telephone numbers of at least two references from former employers—not co-workers or personal friends. Make sure you get references that you can check.

Talk to these references; take notes. Briefly explain the reason for your call, and ask plenty of questions:

- What was the relationship between the applicant and the reference? (supervisor? co-worker? family member of a home care client?)
- What type of patient(s) did the applicant care for? (bedridden? elderly? children? diabetic? cancer?)
- What specifically did the applicant do on the job? (personal care? meal preparation? basic or skilled nursing? exercise?)
- How much responsibility did the applicant have for patient care? (full? minimal? helped family?)
- How much supervision was provided or needed? (Remember, home care personnel must be able to work well without direct supervision.)
- What was the applicant's overall job performance? (good points? weak points? attitude toward care?)
- Was the applicant frequently late or absent?
- Why did the applicant leave the job?

The Interview

When you interview job applicants, ask the professionals to bring proof of *current* license and any malpractice insurance; paraprofessionals should bring proof of any training completed. Note whether applicants arrive on time and their general appearance (neat, sloppy, heavily perfumed, etc.).

Briefly describe the job, work hours, and the person (if other than yourself) needing care. If care is for someone else, have your loved one review applicants too, if possible.

Have applicants briefly describe their work experience and tell you a little about themselves. If yours is not a full-time position, ask why they want a part-time job. You could find yourself without care if a better job with more hours comes along.

If they have family responsibilities, discuss what arrangements they have made so you can rely on regular services. Ask some of the same questions you asked their references and compare the two answers.

You may want to ask a few open-ended questions that any capable employee should be able to handle. Here is a sample:

- What would you do if you found a patient unconscious? not breathing? bleeding? had fallen and couldn't get up? had a fever? (Consult a first aid or home nursing manual so you know the correct answers first.)
- What would you do if a patient swore at you? called you names? hit you? refused to cooperate or deliberately made your job harder? soiled the bed you had just freshly made?

Also ask questions that could apply specifically to the help needed in your situation:

- For a diabetic or high blood pressure patient who will need help with meal preparation: What foods should be avoided? What would you make for breakfast or dinner?
- For a bedridden patient needing help with personal care: What signs of problems would you watch for? How can you prevent bedsores?
- For children: What would you do if the child stays out late? refuses to eat? wets the bed?

If you are concerned about theft, you might ask:

- Would you agree to be fingerprinted or have a police check run prior to starting this job?

Even if you have no intention of following up on this last question, just posing it can have a chilling effect on the dishonest. If someone declines to work for you, claiming this is an insult, consider yourself lucky.

When hiring a nurse, ask him or her briefly to outline and discuss a plan for care and treatment goals based on your doctor's recommendations. As a layperson, you'll be at a disadvantage in fully evaluating their medical answers. Consult with your doctor afterward if you have questions.

Give applicants a chance to ask as well as answer questions. Pay attention to what questions are asked. Do they concern only pay, working hours, and conditions? Potential employees should also ask about the person who requires care and about his or her condition.

Prepare and write out your interview questions beforehand. Take notes during the interview, or record your impressions immediately afterward.

WHEN YOU HIRE

Decide who you will hire based on the applicant's background, references, answers, attitude, and your intuition. Then hope you are right. Avoid hiring someone on the spot unless you have already interviewed several applicants. As an inexperienced "employer," comparing several would-be workers will help you make a sounder choice.

Once you have decided, put your verbal understanding down in writing before care begins. Details of a discussion can easily be forgotten or misunderstood. A written agreement that explains all key employment issues helps you avoid problems. It also helps assure that both parties understand their mutual obligations. Employees may take their responsibilities more seriously if you have a businesslike arrangement.

Employer Obligations

When you hire help yourself, you often become the employer of record. As such you become *legally* responsible for extra expenses:

- Employer social security tax (FICA) must be paid on wages of $50 or more in each calendar quarter. Wages include the amount you pay for employee transit fares, meals, or lodging. In 1985, this tax rate added 7.05 percent to the cost of hiring.
- Federal unemployment tax (FUTA) must be paid on

wages of $1,000 or more in a calendar quarter. As of
1985, this tax rate added 6.2 percent to the cost of hiring.
- Any other employer taxes that apply in your state, such
as workers' compensation, unemployment, and disability,
must also be paid.

In addition to these actual expenses, you are responsible
for a *lot* of paperwork *and* other financial duties. The Internal
Revenue Service (IRS) states you must:

- Handle employee W-4 forms, and compute and regularly
withhold employee federal taxes on earnings as well as
social security taxes
- File quarterly and year-end employee wage statements
and forward withheld taxes to the proper federal authorities

Add to this the paperwork on state taxes, workers' compensation, and so on. If all this sounds complicated, it is. Get
a complete rundown on these tasks, the necessary forms, and
the labor laws from your accountant or the IRS, Social
Security Administration (SSA), and the federal and state
departments of labor (or employment). Many people ignore,
or don't know about, the governing labor and tax laws, and
later run into problems.

Mrs. R. paid a registry nurse her wages in full, thinking
that was the end of the matter. Months later, at tax time,
long after the job was done, Mrs. R. got a call from the nurse
requesting a "W-2" federal wage statement. In the end,
because of IRS rules, Mrs. R. had to pay the full employer's
and employee's share of social security taxes. She never was
able to collect from the nurse her share of the social security
tax. This experience cost Mrs. R. an extra $150, but she was
lucky. The SSA did not fine her as well. Failure to comply
with any applicable tax laws can subject you to financial
penalties on top of overdue taxes.

Whenever you hire outside help, double-check who pays
these employer expenses. Also, watch out for surprise "placement" fees, which some employment agencies or registries
charge once you actually hire someone through their referral.

Insurance Issues

Find out whether the person you wish to hire is self-insured for malpractice or general liability. Professionals may be self-insured; aides almost never are. Insurance won't protect you against all problems, but it will give you some financial recourse if needed.

Carefully check your homeowner's insurance policy for coverage in the case of property damage or loss or personal injury—not just to yourself, but the worker. Without adequate coverage you may have big problems if, for example, your employee slips and is hurt in your household. If your policy is poor, you would be wise to improve your coverage, despite the extra cost involved.

When you consider self-employed personnel, don't overlook the issue of your own health insurance. Check it carefully or contact your insurer *beforehand* to learn if personnel you hire yourself are covered under your insurance policy; and if so, what kind of home care records the insurer will require for reimbursement.

The Employer-Employee Agreement

If you hire through a registry, it may have a standardized form for a work agreement. Don't worry if you must devise one yourself. You don't have to hire a lawyer. All you need is a basic written or typed statement that outlines in plain language the full terms of employment. It should clearly state:

- Your name and address and that of the person you are hiring.
- The weekly employment period. Be specific: State the number of hours per day, per week, and the days of the expected employment schedule: Example: Mon., Wed., Fri., 9:30 A.M.–12:30 P.M.; Tues. and Fri., 1:00 P.M.–3:00 P.M. Total weekly—13 hours.
- Starting date of employment.
- Salary and payment terms. Specify the agreed hourly or weekly rate. Include any special provisions made for evening, weekend, overtime, or holiday pay. Outline how

and when salary will be paid. (cash? check? weekly?)

- Which party—you or the hiree—assumes responsibility for social security payments, deductions for federal, state, and local taxes, and any insurance. If the hiree will assume this responsibility, make sure your agreement clearly spells this out. Remember, if this is challenged later, the burden of proof will be on you to show why you should not be held liable as the employer.
- Description of services to be rendered. For example, you might list "personal care, homemaking," or "skilled nursing plus personal care." If you intend this section to serve as your care plan too, then be more specific. It's always wise to outline all individual employment tasks.
- Any malpractice or liability insurance the hiree carries, with the company name and policy number.

You and your employee should both carefully read and discuss the agreement, then each sign and date it. Make, and keep for yourself, a copy. Give one to the employee.

MAKE A CARE PLAN

Set Sound Standards

When you do it yourself, both you and any employees must also come to grips with the issue of proper care. Do employees provide proper care when they do as you wish and say, or when they render care that is in your best interest? Having your own way may give you satisfaction, but not satisfactory care.

"Patients often do not like to follow the doctor's orders," observes Marie Fiorentino, nursing director for Visiting Nurse Service of New York. "Whether this means taking medicine, following a special diet or an exercise routine, they don't want to change their life style. It's important that the patient have someone who will say, 'This is what the doctor has prescribed'; not 'It's all right, I understand why you don't want to take your medicine today.' Patients need someone who will be accountable to the physician."

Yet it can be hard for an employee to tell you "no" or push you to take prescribed exercise when you'd rather just sit. After all, you're the employer, and you pay that salary. So before you undermine your own care, settle this issue. Set goals and standards for care. Involve your doctor in this process if need be.

Have a Backup Plan

It's almost inevitable in any ongoing home care situation that there will be days when an employee cannot or does not come to work. When you're dealing with a good home care agency, it can remedy this problem promptly. However, when you've hired home care personnel directly, be ready with your own backup plan.

Why plan ahead? If you are fairly able-bodied, need only marginal help, and/or have someone else at home, a no-show day may not worry you. But consider the effect this could have on:

- A partially bedridden person living alone who relies on an aide for personal care and to prepare meals
- A working parent, spouse, or adult son or daughter who depends on hired help to care for a loved one during working hours
- An elderly couple, one of whom needs daily nursing after hospitalization because the other is unable to provide care

The fact is that there are few situations where a no-show makes no difference. Line up your backup assistance in advance. Don't take it for granted that family members, friends, or neighbors will help; ask beforehand.

Remember that you can call on home care agencies in a pinch. Depending on your needs, personnel availability, and timing, agencies can often supply help within a few hours. So even though you don't use an agency regularly, it's wise to screen home care agencies anyway for good professional backup. When you do, ask how quickly they can respond on short notice.

III

THE FINANCIAL SIDE
TO HOME CARE

—— 9 ——

Dollars and Sense

COSTS AND CONSUMERISM

Before you choose an agency, remember consumer rule one: Compare quality before cost. Cost alone says nothing about quality. A big price tag does not guarantee you deluxe services, nor does a lower cost mean you get cut-rate care.

When you contact an agency, first ask the quality-related questions outlined in Chapter 6, *then* ask about the cost. Narrow your choices based on quality first; then you can let a price tag be your guide. Doing otherwise can be one of the most costly mistakes you can make, as one consumer I spoke to discovered.

Several weeks after Mrs. B. returned home following surgery, her health started to fail. Since she lived alone, she panicked, understandably. After talking to her concerned next-door neighbor, Mrs. B. decided she needed nursing care. The two friends looked through the Yellow Pages, made a few quick phone calls, and chose an agency whose price seemed right. Unfortunately, they selected a "mom and pop" agency without professional standards. No one conducted a proper assessment, nor did anyone consult with her doctor. The agency did, however, rush over the nurse Mrs. B. had self-prescribed for a full eight hours a day of nursing care.

As it turned out, the skilled nursing care that the agency charged Mrs. B. for was not even provided. The LPN performed only the tasks of a home health aide. No one supervised. During the week, Mrs. B.'s health continued to go downhill. Finally the LPN became frightened enough to call the doctor, who promptly hospitalized Mrs. B. on an emergency basis.

When Mrs. B. returned home some time later, she found an $800 home care bill on top of her hospital bill. Her insurance company wouldn't pay because her doctor had not authorized the care. Nor had the agency nurse kept the kind of careful, professional notes insurance companies require.

Looking back, it is hard to say how much this experience cost her in both health and dollars. With the kind of proper nursing intervention a professional agency would have provided, hospitalization might have been prevented; or perhaps Mrs. B. would have been hospitalized earlier and received proper care before her health was seriously threatened. Mrs. B. herself fully admits, "I learned my lesson the hard way."

Remember, to get the best care your money can buy, compare quality first!

THE COST QUESTION

What does home care cost? This question is on the minds of most consumers seeking home care. The answer, however, is not as clear as the question. Costs vary by:

- Agency
- Geographic region
- Type of services needed; the more highly skilled, the more costly
- Number of services needed
- Frequency and duration of services; longer hours and more days of care equal higher costs

When most people ask about costs, what they really want to know is what will it cost *me?* This also depends on the availability of any insurance coverage such as Medicare or Blue Cross and Blue Shield or eligibility for other programs that may help offset out-of-pocket costs. If you must pay for part or all of home care services yourself, it's critical that you know all about costs beforehand.

As a starting point, realize that home care rates are subject to many of the same economic factors as other consumer services. Home care costs vary somewhat regionally like other labor services. A study conducted by the U.S. Select Committee on Aging in cooperation with the National Association for Home Care found rates lowest in the New England region (Maine, New Hampshire, Vermont, Massachusetts, Rhode Island, and Connecticut), while rural areas had the highest rates overall. But agencies located in major cities (New York, Chicago, Los Angeles), where wage rates are high, often charge premium rates for their service. In addition to higher salaries, they generally have higher costs for rent, utilities, phone, and other business essentials. But even within the same community, you will find that rates vary among agencies, often by as much as 50 percent or more.

Why such wide differences? Reasons vary. For example, some agencies may have higher administrative costs or may employ more highly skilled or experienced personnel, who command higher wages. Or they may try to market themselves as a "blue chip" agency on the basis of a premium price tag. Other agencies may charge lower rates by keeping administrative costs down while dealing in high client volume. Others may skimp on supervision to keep costs down. In rural areas, travel time and expense increase rates. It's hard to generalize about the comparative rates you will find among agencies within your community. However, a study conducted by the U.S. General Accounting Office (GAO) found that, on average, private nonprofit agencies were the most expensive; visiting nurse and government-funded agencies, the least expensive. But competition plays a hand in the cost equation, too. In communities where many agencies must scramble for the same pool of home care customers, prices may be very competitive, regardless of whether they are private nonprofit, proprietary, or community nonprofit.

When you consider cost, remember that some home care services are free or low cost, chiefly because they are funded through public or philanthropic organizations. Many also operate on a modest budget thanks to volunteer assistance.

Free or inexpensive services include: Meals-on-Wheels, friendly visiting, telephone reassurance, medical equipment "loan closets," bereavement or pastoral counseling.

HOW AND WHAT AGENCIES CHARGE

Home care agencies may charge you strictly on an hourly basis for the services of their personnel. Or agencies may charge on a "visit" basis, much the same way a doctor charges for care. At present, the government pays Medicare-certified agencies on a per-visit basis. Some agencies may charge for services either way, depending on your preference or insurance coverage.

As a rule of thumb, the more highly skilled the home care personnel, the higher the price tag. Unskilled home help, such as the services of companions and homemakers, usually command the lowest rates. Rates for home health aides, considered a semi-skilled service, are often but not always higher. Some agencies charge a flat aide rate irrespective of whether personnel provide "hands on" personal care, basic nursing, housekeeping, or just companionship.

In the nursing category, rates for registered nurses are generally higher than for licensed practical nurses. Some agencies may have a skilled nursing rate and supply either an RN or LPN, their option, depending on the nursing expertise your care requires. Rates for registered nurses are not based on their educational level. So a more highly educated BSN nurse should not cost more than the less educated RN. However, some agencies may charge a premium rate if you need an RN with special qualifications such as high-tech training.

At the higher end of the rate range are fees for social workers; physical, occupational, or speech therapists; and similar professionals. Should "assistants" such as a physical therapist assistant provide simple therapy, the fees charged should be lower than top professional rates. Assistant charges should apply *only* to bona fide assistants who have completed

MAXIMUM AGENCY CHARGE TO PRIVATE PAY PATIENTS

	Per Visit		Per Hour	
Registered nurse	$26–$40	(32%)	$10–$25	(16%)
	$41–$55	(42%)	$26–$45	(49%)
	$56 or more	(12%)	$46 or more	(27%)
Physical therapist	$21–$35	(18%)	$25 or less	(16%)
	$36–$50	(38%)	$26–$45	(36%)
	$51 or more	(16%)	$46 or more	(29%)
Occupational therapist	$21–$35	(9%)	$25 or less	(5%)
	$36–$50	(32%)	$26–$50	(29%)
	$51 or more	(12%)	$51 or more	(10%)
Speech therapist	$21–$35	(11%)	$25 or less	(7%)
	$36–$50	(44%)	$26–$50	(43%)
	$51 or more	(15%)	$51 or more	(13%)
Medical social worker	$21–$35	(5%)	$25 or less	(3%)
	$36–$50	(32%)	$26–$50	(29%)
	$51 or more	(23%)	$51 or more	(15%)
Homemaker–home health aide	$20 or less	(22%)	$10 or less	(16%)
	$21–$35	(37%)	$11–$20	(25%)
	$36–$50	(23%)	$21–$35	(26%)
			$35 or more	(19%)

Note: This information is based on a survey conducted by the U.S. Select Committee on Aging in cooperation with the National Association for Home Care. Data reflect the responses of 292 agencies (Medicare-certified only) and do not total 100% because of nonresponse rate to some survey questions. For detailed data see: "Building a Long-Term Policy: Home Care Data and Implications," U.S. Select Committee on Aging, December 1984, Comm. Pub. No. 98-484, U.S. Government Printing Office, Washington, 1985.

recognized college or hospital training. Aides who receive inservice agency training in rehabilitation therapy are not qualified as assistants. In such cases, you should be charged only the aide rate.

The accompanying table will give you a better idea of the range of rates for home care services.

WHEN YOU ASK ABOUT COST

When you question an agency about costs, you should request more information than just basic rates. The agency's individual policies can affect your wallet too. Any reputable agency will fully disclose all costs and work with you to help conserve your financial resources. If the agency cannot provide a sound plan of care that is within your means, it should refer you to another agency that can.

Here is a breakdown of the cost questions you may want to ask. They are repeated in the checklist on page 397 so you can compare agency responses.

Is there a sliding scale?

Community (voluntary) nonprofit agencies often operate on a "sliding scale" or "part-pay" basis if you cannot afford the full home care rate. The fee is scaled according to your ability to pay, with any qualifying insurance taken into account. The lower your income, the lower your charges. Services may even be free—quite a phenomenon today.

To cite just one example, the Visiting Nurse Service of New York provided $2.5 million in free care in 1984. Among those who benefited from this community service were the employed whose incomes disqualified them for Medicaid or other public services and the frail, low-income elderly who needed the kind of home care help that Medicare won't pay for.

Most voluntary nonprofit agencies receive widespread phil- anthropic support from groups such as corporations, United Way, and foundations, as well as through private donations and fundraising. With this support, they can reduce established fees when you cannot afford the full price. Of course, if you have sufficient income, you will be charged top dollar. For full payers, a nonprofit rate does not mean a bargain. Care through a community nonprofit agency may run roughly the same as a for-profit agency, sometimes more.

How much you must pay can be determined only after a basic financial assessment has been made. This assessment takes into account many factors, including family income, size of household, medical expenses, and outstanding bills. All information is *strictly* confidential. For example, if the agency's standard nurse visit fee is $50, you will be charged this rate. The agency then applies any insurance you may have available against this fee. If your insurer pays 80 percent, this would leave you with a $10 balance. Depending on the assessment, you may be asked to pay only $5, and the agency absorbs the difference.

Is there a charge for a minimum number of hours?

An agency's basic rate may seem attractive, but it often only tells half the story. Be aware that many agencies require that you contract for a minimum number of hours per day and/or days per week of care. Because of minimums, an agency that charges less per hour may cost you more. Here's how it works.

Let's assume you want homemaker services for your elderly mother just two hours a day, three times a week, to help with bathing, dressing, and cooking a light meal. Agency A charges $8.50 an hour, no minimums. Agency B charges $6.50 an hour, a full $2 an hour less. But agency B has a four-hour-a-day, twice-a-week minimum, not an uncommon practice.

If you choose agency B on the basis of its hourly rate, it will cost you $78 a week ($6.50 × four hours = $26 per day × 3 days). You will get extra hours of care that you don't really need but must pay for. Or you could cut back to twice-a-week care. The price tag becomes $52 ($26 × 2 days), but you must decide how you will manage with less help than you need.

If you analyze the cost of home care through agency A, it is cheaper. It will cost $51 a week ($8.50 × 2 hours = $17 per day × 3 days). You will save $27 each week and get only the care you need on a schedule suited to you.

Is there any charge for assessment and supervision?

Professional agencies build the cost of these home care essentials into their standard fees, so there should never be additional charges for the in-home assessment required to develop the care plan, or for a supervisor's periodic visits to evaluate your condition and progress. Nor should an agency charge extra if the supervisor must make extra in-home visits to investigate complaints about care or evaluate reports of developing health problems. This is all part of a professional agency's services.

Agencies may sometimes charge additional fees if you request a service outside the scope of "routine" assessment and supervision. For example, if you request a "special" RN in-home visit for the sole purpose of assessing a relative for nursing home placement and to help complete all necessary application forms, this would probably be extra. If you want more in-home supervision than the agency normally provides, it may also charge extra. However, before you agree, check other professional agencies which may offer more supervision for the same price.

Are there special rates for evening, weekend, and holiday care?

Often aides and nurses prefer to work evenings or on weekends, so if you need home care during these hours, don't automatically expect to pay extra. Some agencies do charge more; others don't.

When you ask about special rates, discuss this for each personnel category in question. If you need physical therapy on a weekend, for example, you might be charged a premium even if the agency has no additional charge for weekend RN care. Or you may be charged extra for an RN, but not for an aide's care.

Don't forget to consider overtime charges when you start to estimate costs. Home care agencies are subject to the same labor regulations as other industries. Agency employees who work more than 40 hours a week must be paid overtime (time-and-a-half), by federal law. However, this cost should be passed on to you *only* when a single employee cares for you more than 40 hours in a week. For example, if you require 48 hours of care in a week and want the same worker to provide it, you will normally be charged 8 hours of overtime. On the other hand, if you are willing to divide time among two workers, say 24 hours of work each during the week, you do not incur any overtime charges. However, in a few locales by *state* law overtime rates apply whenever an employee works more than 8 hours in a single day.

Higher charges usually apply when you need help on certain holidays. Most agencies charge extra—often overtime rates—for holiday care if they provide you with any help at all. Expect to pay more on Christmas, New Year's, Thanksgiving, Fourth of July—all standard holidays. However, agencies make their own holiday schedules, ranging from six to twelve holidays per year. Before you contract for care, check this.

Is there a fee for professional consultation?

This essential of quality home care should never carry an extra charge. An agency should consult with your doctor as well as other professionals, such as a nonagency social worker who may be assisting you. With your consent, an agency should keep concerned family members informed about your health and welfare, without any special charge. Likewise there should never be charges for any home care team conferences conducted to provide you with coordinated care.

Is there a fee for social work service?

This is a gray area when it comes to cost. As a rule of thumb, you shouldn't be charged for the standard in-home assessment and supervision an agency social worker sometimes provides. Agencies should not charge for basic information and referral assistance—for example, identifying and providing you with the names and telephone numbers of helpful community services or calling other community agencies on your behalf when necessary. Personnel should discuss, at no cost for their time, Medicare and Medicaid requirements and application procedures.

But if you need more extensive assistance, such as counseling, expect additional charges. Discuss this fully in advance. Some agencies may provide one social work visit at no cost in order to evaluate whether more extensive social services are needed and appropriate. Additional charges may begin once further services are rendered.

Is there any charge for business services?

All professional agencies view the paperwork end of home

care as an essential service. Therefore, an agency should not
charge you to:

- Fill out insurance claim forms
- Provide written reports to your doctor or other profes-
  sionals involved in your care or to your family, if requested
- Provide copies of any bills sent to your insurance com-
  panies
- Provide necessary documentation for tax purposes

Is there a charge for medical equipment and supplies?

If you need medical equipment, these costs are almost
always extra, unless an agency has a free "loan closet."
Medical supplies are not normally included in basic home
care rates and are usually billed separately. Because costs may
vary widely among agencies, it is wise to compare these costs
among agencies (see Chapter 13 for further advice).

What is the policy on transportation, travel time, and meals?

Transportation costs are almost always paid by the workers
themselves, although there may be some exceptions. For
example, if you live in an urban two-fare zone, the second
fare may be extra. You should not be charged travel time. If
an employee will drive you using his or her own car, expect
a mileage charge. As for meals, while a cup of coffee might
be welcome, you are not expected to provide meal service.
Meals add to your costs and can easily strain a budget over
time. Employees should bring lunch if they will be at your
home all day or through the lunch hour. However, if you
want someone on a live-in basis you are expected to provide
meals, so you should discuss this issue in advance.

THE IMPORTANT "WHAT IFS"

Before you decide which agency is right for you, there are
final questions you should ask the agency and yourself. What
if you lose insurance benefits because you've changed jobs,

or are laid off? What if you use up your benefits more quickly than expected because recovery slows or a setback occurs? No one likes to look for problems, but planning ahead will help prevent them. How constructively the agency responds to these questions can make an important difference to you.

—10—

The Insurance Angle

Before you reach into your pocket to pay for home care, reach for your insurance policy. As growing evidence supports the cost savings side to home care, employers, health insurers, and the government are all taking notice. New benefit programs are being developed and existing ones expanded. The consulting firm of Towers, Perrin, Forster & Crosby found 53 percent of the companies they surveyed offered some home care benefits.

"Insurance companies are encouraging employers to make changes that will no longer drive employees into hospitals," explains Daniel Thomas of the Health Insurance Association of America (HIAA). "The trend is for health insurance companies and their clients to liberalize their payment for home health care." However, this doesn't mean a blank check. Many insurers and employers are still reluctant to offer too much in the way of home care benefits, fearing that home care will be an "add-on" rather than an "instead-of" health care cost.

Still, you are more likely than ever before to find some help for part of and sometimes all home care costs. Though many companies voluntarily offer home care benefits, as of 1985, 17 states mandated or required insurers to do so in their group plans. These home care states are: Arizona, California, Colorado, Connecticut, Kentucky, Maine, Maryland, Montana, Nevada, New Jersey, New Mexico, New York, Rhode Island, Vermont, Washington, West Virginia and Wisconsin.

WHAT HOME CARE SERVICES
ARE COVERED?

Insurance companies almost without exception pay only for health-treatment-oriented home care services. If you just need help to bathe, dress, toilet, and so on because of disability or disease, don't expect insurance to pay for this. Personal care services alone are very seldom covered by insurance. Personal care is usually considered custodial care, not health care. However, in maternity cases some insurance companies are throwing the rule book away. They will allow limited personal care and homemaking service as an incentive for early hospital discharge.

Many insurers now provide hospice benefits, usually apart from home care. Custodial services are sometimes reimbursed under the hospice benefit when provided as part of an overall hospice service (see Chapter 18).

In group or individual policies, home care may be provided under major medical benefits or under hospital insurance. A 1981 HIAA survey of employer health plans found that 43 percent of 36 major insurance companies queried covered home care benefits provided by an agency. The agency-covered services usually include:

- Part-time nursing care under supervision of a registered nurse
- Physical, occupational, and speech therapy
- Part-time home health aide services
- Physician-prescribed medical supplies, equipment, drugs, and laboratory services to the limit that would normally be covered in the hospital

Note that many insurers do not cover in-home respiratory therapy, although respiratory equipment such as an oxygen unit is covered. Unless a respiratory therapist's services are provided gratis by the agency or equipment dealer, this often becomes an out-of-pocket expense.

Also frequently missing are such valuable services as medical social services and dietetic services. When medical social services are provided, coverage usually extends only to the patient—not to the family, who may need as much counseling or more. Family counseling becomes an out-of-pocket cost.

In cases of catastrophic illness or injury such as a severe car accident requiring lengthy, extensive (and expensive) rehabilitation, some insurers pay for the costs of necessary architectural home changes such as widening doorways for wheelchair access to permit patients to go home.

THE GENERAL RULES

Insurance rules on coverage vary tremendously, but some general guidelines apply. The most important rule concerns doctors. A physician must prescribe home care, usually *before* any services rendered will be paid for by an insurance company. In addition, most programs require that you remain under a doctor's *continuing* medical supervision while you receive home health benefits. A doctor's supervision, however, does not mean that your physician must make "regular visits" to you at home or that you must go to the office. Normally, the home health agency must periodically inform the physician about your progress, usually at least once every 60 days.

If you need home care following hospitalization, insurers often require that services begin no later than three to seven days after discharge. Some insurers will allow you, with a doctor's okay, to use home care to *prevent* initial hospitalization.

The majority of plans place limits on the number of covered visits. Don't compare "visits" directly with hospital insured days and become alarmed. Hospital coverage often provides for 120 days of care or more; home care benefits may provide for as few as 20 visits, though most policies are more generous. You have to put the concept of limited visits in perspective.

Let's look at the case of one 16-year-old boy who received home care through the Visiting Nurse Service in Toledo, Ohio. The boy was hospitalized with massive injuries after he had been run over by a train. His left arm and leg were lost. He suffered multiple pelvic fractures and tearing of abdominal muscle walls. He required a colostomy as well as skin grafts to his hip sockets, among other major surgical treatments. After five weeks of hospitalization, he was able to go home early with the VNS special rehabilitation service, which saved 30 hospital days. The VNS home care coordinator, a nurse, coordinated all the treatment, including supplies and medical equipment.

For the first two weeks, the boy received daily skilled nursing visits. Then, after his family had learned and could confidently perform the nursing procedures, nursing visits were reduced to three times a week. Aide services helped with simple nonsurgical and personal care. Intensive physical and occupational therapy were provided during initial recovery and later, when the boy received artificial limbs.

Over the course of a nine-month period, until the boy was able to return to school, he received comprehensive home care services. How many visits? A total of 129—not many if you consider the extent of his injuries. So, your home care coverage may be far better than you would suspect by just looking at the number of visits permitted. One government study of visits needed by Medicare patients showed that only 3.2 percent required more than 100 visits; 76.6 percent required fewer than 30 visits.

Don't let what might appear to be limited coverage prevent you from taking advantage of home care. Your doctor and the agency can advise you of how far your benefits will stretch, given your individual situation.

HOW MUCH IS COVERED?

That answer again varies by plan. Some plans require a "deductible" before fees for home care services are covered; co-payment may be required.

A *deductible* is a fixed dollar amount that you must pay out of pocket for any service before insurance pays out. In recent years, insurance deductibles have increased. However, some insurance policies do not require consumer deductibles for home health services, as an incentive to use home care instead of hospitalization.

A co-payment is the amount the insurer considers your fair share of the bill. Often insurance may pay 80 percent of a charge and require the consumer to pick up the remaining 20 percent. Some policies, however, will pay 100 percent of home care costs as a consumer incentive.

With this as a backdrop, let's look at some major payment sources for home care.

MEDICARE HOME CARE

At present, Medicare, a federal health insurance program, is the largest single source of payment for home care. In 1982, some 2 million people received home care services through Medicare at an approximate cost of $1,268,000,000—over a *billion* dollars.

Medicare is also a source of confusion and distress to the majority of its recipients. One government survey found that by and large, seniors don't understand what Medicare is and how it works. We will look briefly at Medicare in general and at its home care benefits in detail, and address major points of confusion. For more information on the overall Medicare program, call your local social security office for a free copy of the *Medicare Handbook* or contact The American Association of Retired Persons, 1909 K Street, NW, Washington, DC 20049, for its free booklet *Information on Medicare & Health Insurance for Older People.*

Basic Eligibility for Medicare

Medicare is primarily for social-security-qualified seniors aged 65 and over. Seniors eligible for survivor's benefits and railroad retirees also qualify. Note that you do *not* have to be a U.S. citizen to receive Medicare.

When you apply for social security benefits just prior to your 65th birthday, you automatically become enrolled in Medicare. If you elect to receive social security benefits early, at age 62, you are ineligible for Medicare until age 65, when you must apply for it. To apply for Medicare, contact your local social security administration office. If you do not qualify for social security benefits at retirement age, you can still get Medicare for a fee. If you are under age 65, you can also qualify for Medicare provided you suffer from serious, permanent kidney disease that requires kidney dialysis or transplantation; *or* are considered disabled and have received social security disability payments for a two-year period.

General Coverage and Cost

Like most insurance programs, Medicare is divided into two categories: hospital insurance, also called Part A, and medical insurance, also known as Part B.

In brief, hospital insurance (Part A) primarily covers the cost of inpatient care in a hospital or skilled nursing facility. This includes meals, drugs, nursing services, tests, X rays, medical supplies, operating room costs, and rehabilitation therapies. It does *not* cover the cost of doctors' services. Hospital insurance is free to social security recipients; other seniors pay a monthly fee.

Medical insurance (Part B) covers doctors' services, either in or out of the hospital. It also covers outpatient hospital services such as X-ray, lab, or emergency room services as well as outpatient therapy and medical equipment and supplies. All seniors, whether on social security or not, must pay a monthly premium for Part B coverage.

Your local social security office can advise you of the current monthly fees for Medicare Parts A and B. These increase annually on January 1.

Both Medicare hospital insurance (Part A) and medical insurance (Part B) provide *identical* home care benefits. Hospital insurance also covers hospice care (see Chapter 18).

Here is what the 1985 *Medicare Handbook* says about home health care:

> If you need part-time, skilled health care in your home for the treatment of an illness or injury, Medicare can pay for

covered home health visits furnished by a participating home health agency.

Medicare can pay for home health visits only if *all* of the following conditions are met: (1) the care you need includes part-time skilled nursing care, physical therapy, or speech therapy; (2) you are confined to your home; (3) a doctor determines you need home health care and sets up a home health plan for you; and (4) the home health agency providing services is participating in Medicare.

Once these conditions are met, either hospital insurance or medical insurance can pay for an unlimited number of home health visits. When you no longer need part-time home nursing care, physical therapy, or speech therapy, Medicare can continue to pay for home health visits *if* you need occupational therapy.

Medicare does *not* cover general household services, meal preparation, shopping, assistance in bathing or dressing, or other home care services furnished mainly to assist people in meeting personal, family, or domestic needs.

Medicare considers these household services noncovered "custodial" care. The handbook also provides a checklist of those home care services Medicare can and cannot pay for:

CAN PAY FOR
- Part-time skilled nursing care
- Physical therapy
- Speech therapy

If you need part-time skilled nursing care, physical or speech therapy, Medicare can also pay for:
- Occupational therapy
- Part-time services of home health aides
- Medical social services
- Medical supplies and equipment provided by the agency

CANNOT PAY FOR
- Full-time nursing care at home
- Drugs and biologicals
- Meals delivered to home
- Homemaker services
- Blood transfusions

Also covered under medical insurance is ambulance service to get you home from the hospital and, under certain conditions, from home to other health facilities for care.

For Medicare purposes, your "home" may be your own home or apartment (condominium, etc.) or that of a relative. For example, if you wish to recover at your daughter's home instead of your own following illness or surgery, Medicare home care benefits apply. Your home may also be a home for the aged or other institution such as a board and care facility like that described in Chapter 27. However, institutions that provide hospital or skilled nursing home–type care do not qualify for Medicare home care.

The Pluses of Medicare Home Care

One real advantage of home care is that, unlike other Part A or B services, you do not have to pay any deductible or co-payment. Medicare pays the full approved cost of all covered home health visits.* Moreover, you are also relieved of the burden of filing confusing Medicare forms. The home health agency will submit your claim for payment. You don't have to send in any bills yourself. Nor do you have to pay the agency in advance for services and then wait for reimbursement. The agency in effect agrees to accept what Medicare pays for services. The home health agency sends its bills for payment to private insurance companies called fiscal intermediaries (FIs), which work under contract with the federal government.

You may be charged only for noncovered services or those that Medicare just partially covers, such as medical equipment or ambulance services.

Another major advantage of home care that many Medicare consumers do not fully appreciate is its cost savings. By using home care to reduce hospital and nursing home stays, you

---

*In 1985, as a proposed budget measure, legislative attempts were made to impose copayments on beneficiaries starting with the twenty-first Medicare-covered home care visit. Although this proposal was defeated, Medicare beneficiaries can expect similar proposals in the future to undercut home care benefits.

can conserve your hospital insurance benefits and thereby cut down on out-of-pocket expenses.

Under Medicare, you can also use home care to *prevent* hospitalization. If your health starts to decline, with your doctor's okay you can get skilled care at home first, which may eliminate the need for hospitalization. Should health problems arise, keep in mind this important, but little used, aspect of home care.

Important Medicare Rules and Limitations

At face value, the information presented in the *Medicare Handbook* seems straightforward enough. However, Medicare home care has certain rules and limitations that are not apparent in the handbook.

Home care benefits are governed by guidelines developed by the Health Care Financing Administration (HCFA), pronounced "hic-fa," the federal agency that oversees the entire Medicare program.

HCFA rules change periodically. They also are interpreted differently by the individual FIs. Therefore, although Medicare is supposed to be a national program with uniform benefits for all, in practice the benefits you may receive can actually vary from state to state.

If you are ever in doubt about services or eligibility, your best guide is to discuss your questions and your situation with a Medicare-certified home health agency. These agencies are thoroughly familiar with the fine points of the Medicare rules. They keep up to date on the latest changes that can affect you.

Let's look at the most important HCFA rules and limitations that confuse consumers.

The Confinement Rule

You must be confined to your home, or "homebound," as one of the four preconditions for receiving Medicare home benefits.

This does not mean that you must be bedridden. However, your condition must be such that your ability to leave home would require considerable and taxing effort on your part. For example, you might need the assistance of crutches, canes, wheelchairs, or walkers; the use of special transportation; or the assistance of another person. It is also expected that if you leave home, such absences would be relatively infrequent or for periods of a short duration. Most absences from the home must be for the purpose of receiving medical treatment. If you are absent *occasionally* from home for nonmedical reasons, such as a trip to the barber or hairdresser, a walk around the block, or a drive, you can still be considered homebound.

Once you are able to leave home frequently for any reason, you are no longer considered confined to your home. You could obtain health care in outpatient facilities rather than in the home, so home care eligibility ceases. Other examples of homebound patients include:

- A person who is blind or senile and requires the assistance of another person in order to leave his/her place of residence
- A person who has lost the use of his/her arms and therefore cannot open doors or use handrails on stairways and therefore requires the assistance of another person in order to leave the home
- A patient who has just returned from a hospital stay and who is in pain and whose activities are severely restricted by doctor's orders
- A person with severe heart disease who must avoid all stress and physical activity
- A person with a psychiatric problem which is evident in part by his/her refusal to leave the home

Would a person who is feeble, frail, and insecure because of advanced age be considered "confined" to home even if he/she seldom if ever goes out? Generally not, unless he/she meets one of the conditions described.

Limits on Home Care Benefits

The extent of home care services available often confuses consumers. You may reason that the handbook's reference to part-time skilled care and "unlimited" home care visits means you can receive daily home care indefinitely. But this is not the case.

HCFA guidelines allow home care agencies to provide you with part-time professional and home health aide services for a few hours a day, several times a week.

Home health aide visits can last one to three hours a day, several times a week. Nurse's visits are shorter. Therapy visits seldom exceed an hour.

If needed, you may receive more intensive daily care, for periods up to eight hours a day, for a short time, generally no longer than two to three weeks. After that initial three-week period, special permission must be obtained from Medicare if you still need daily care.

Periodic care can continue indefinitely as long as you need *skilled* care for an *acute* condition. If you require *only* the help of a home health aide, not a skilled nurse or other professional, Medicare will not cover your home care. Also, once your health stabilizes or you are considered chronically ill, Medicare coverage for home care stops. In effect, Medicare does not cover home care when it is needed simply for health maintenance.

This limitation is perhaps the most difficult for consumers to understand and the most frustrating for certified home health agency staff. To illustrate the point, let's look at one extreme, but real, example which was presented in one of the government's own studies of Medicare home health care. One elderly consumer, no longer eligible for Medicare home care under this limitation, described his situation in the following manner:

> I am totally blind, I have two stumps for legs, I am a diabetic and have high blood pressure. I need to have my blood tested, my urine tested, and have insulin once a day. I have just learned I am no longer covered by the nurse practitioner service and if I want to continue it, it will be on my own payment. This is not right as I need the services and if they are not performed, I will land back in the hospital; then the government will have to pay, and pay through the nose again. This is ridiculous for me to have Medicare render me no longer eligible for the services now

that I am in a "maintaining" stage. If my diabetes gets out of hand (or my high blood pressure), then the government will pay, but they won't help prevent it from getting out of hand. That's crazy.

In this case, his frustrated nurse practitioner stated: "The irony of Medicare stabilization is that it is home health services that cause the stabilization; without the services, the patient deteriorates. The patient is not really stable if he can't maintain his health status without us."

This limitation is truly the Catch-22 Medicare rule. Senior citizens' advocate groups, the National Association for Home Care, and concerned legislators such as Senator John Heinz (R–Pa.), chairman of the Senate Special Committee on Aging, and Congressman Claude Pepper (D–Fla.), have been working to liberalize the rule.

When you receive Medicare-covered home care services, your home health agency can advise when you are approaching the "maintenance" stage and discuss any alternative care arrangements you may wish after Medicare stops.

If you disagree that you are in the maintenance stage, a HCFA official suggests you do two things. First, contact your doctor. Sometimes a certified agency may stop services because of your doctor's orders. Discuss your condition personally with your doctor and request a revision of your care plan. Second, if you need the service and intend to continue at your own expense in any case, insist the agency submit the bills to Medicare. The FI will probably automatically "deny" the bills. But, advises the HCFA official, once your claim is denied, you can then appeal your case. (This is a fairly simple paperwork process). Appealed cases receive a sound medical review. If you win, the agency will be paid those bills and it in turn can provide a rebate to you. There is some risk, but if consumers intend to buy home care services from the agency anyway, said the official, "These consumers have nothing to lose by appealing."

MEDICAID/MEDI-CAL

Sometimes referred to by its authorizing legislation, Title XIX, Medicaid, or Medi-Cal as it is called in California, generally helps low-income families or individuals meet health care expenses. In some states, Medicaid may also assist middle-income people when situations such as job loss, sudden income drop, unusually high medical bills, or catastrophic illness occur.

Both the federal and state governments share the cost of the program. However, Medicaid is administered by individual states, usually through the department of social services or welfare. Therefore, each state makes its own rules on eligibility, which services are covered, and which providers are authorized for payment for covered services.

There are two important points you should understand about Medicaid. (1) Medicaid operates independently of other health insurance. You can be eligible for, and receive, Medicaid even when you are covered by Medicare or other health insurance programs. In this case, Medicaid can pay what Medicare does not. (2) Medicaid is a *medical assistance* program that operates apart from public assistance. You do not have to "go on welfare" in order to receive Medicaid/Medi-Cal.

General Eligibility

Your individual or family income and assets are the principal factors that determine Medicaid eligibility. Each state sets its own permissible income and asset levels.

For the elderly, this usually means approximately $1,500 for a single person; $2,250 for a couple. Assets include cash on hand, bank accounts, stocks, bonds, and real property. Contrary to popular belief, you *do not* have to sell your home to become eligible. Your home, clothing, furniture, and certain personal effects are excluded as assets, as are limited burial funds. But before you can receive Medicaid, most other marketable assets must be liquidated and the money spent until your assets reach the permissible level. This practice is referred to as "spending down."

Allowable state income levels are scaled according to family size. If your income level qualifies for state welfare, income maintenance, public assistance payments, or supplemental social security benefits (SSI), you generally qualify for Medicaid. However, in many states you *do not* have to be welfare-eligible to qualify for Medicaid. Some states also have a "surplus" income program that provides Medicaid coverage even if you have a monthly income above permissible Medicaid levels.

Covered Services

Recipients of Medicaid are covered for the usual home health services. However, depending on state requirements, Medicaid may also provide homemaker and personal care services. In some states, special exemptions to the law, called "waivers," allow Medicaid to provide long-term in-home nursing and therapy for chronic health conditions. Under waivers, agencies can also provide chore, home repair, and even exterminator service.

Why is Medicaid so generous? Basically because the buck stops here. Without these services, those receiving Medicaid would have to be placed in nursing homes or other public institutions. Medicaid would still have to pick up the tab, only it would be much higher. Medicaid also assists families who are in distress; for example, a homemaker may provide round-the-clock help to care for children who otherwise would have to be placed in foster care.

Normally Medicaid will pay only for services provided through agencies that have been Medicaid-certified by the state or that operate under special state contracts. However, arrangements for certain Medicaid home care programs for children or the elderly may have to be authorized or coordinated, in advance, by the local department of social services, public assistance, or health and rehabilitation. But your fastest route to identifying special Medicaid-funded programs for the elderly may be to contact your state Unit on Aging.

HEALTH MAINTENANCE ORGANIZATIONS (HMOs)

In 1964, there were just 13 health maintenance organizations, referred to more simply by their initials, HMO. Today they number over 275 nationwide and service some 12 million people, making HMOs one of the most widely available and widely used alternatives to our traditional pay-as-you-go health care system. Why are HMOs so popular? Because their purpose is to keep costs low, yet still provide quality health care. With this mission in mind, the majority of HMOs provide home care benefits.

How HMOs Work

HMOs combine health insurance *and* health services. HMO members pay a fixed premium in advance, either directly or through their employee health plans. In return for this flat fee, members receive complete, comprehensive health services through the HMO. Most HMOs cover additional services such as drugs, lab tests, X rays, health education, and same-day surgery. Some even provide dental care. Members pay little or nothing out-of-pocket for care, since HMO plans generally do not require any deductibles or co-payments, or when required, such payments are very low. Joining an HMO will not guarantee that you will save money, but studies show that HMO members on an average pay less for health care than do other consumers.

HMOs emphasize preventive care (notice the name—health maintenance organization) in order to keep you healthy and out of costly hospitals. HMOs must provide care within a fixed, predetermined budget based on member fees, so if they practice good, efficient medicine, HMOs operate in the black.

Therefore HMOs want you to seek help early for minor problems when the chances of cure or control are best and when treatment is usually simpler, with less wear and tear on you. Simple preventive measures such as immunizations, blood pressure screenings, or cancer checkups are encouraged. As an HMO member, you are less likely to receive a barrage of questionable tests, X rays or procedures, or undergo nonemergency surgery. Unless absolutely needed, these procedures add cost and expose you to some risk.

With such measures, HMO members are generally hospitalized less often, and when hospitalized go home sooner than non-HMO patients. Of course, if you need hospital or skilled nursing home care, you will get it through your HMO. HMOs usually provide these services at no extra charge to members through special arrangements with local community institutions.

With all this discussion of cost, you may wonder whether HMOs skimp on the quality of patient care. The answer is "no." Numerous studies which have compared HMOs to traditional care find that HMOs generally provide equal and sometimes even better care.

HMO Home Care Benefits

As a less costly quality option to hospitals and skilled nursing homes, home care has a natural place within the HMO concept. Most HMOs provide home care benefits either as part of their basic services, or as an extra service that may carry a small surcharge. For example, a Tampa, Florida, HMO belonging to the CIGNA Corporation, the largest investor-owned HMO chain corporation, charges members a modest $10 per home care visit. All federally subsidized HMOs must offer home care as one of their basic services.

Just as HMOs contract with hospitals for care, they also contract with home health agencies for services for their members. Therefore, if you need home care, you generally will have to use the home care agency preselected by your HMO.

Each HMO plan has its own policy governing home care benefits. Most plans will provide at least the same kind of services as do other major insurance programs.

Before you can receive home care, your HMO primary care doctor must recommend it and prescribe the services you need. Because HMOs are both cost- and quality-conscious, your HMO doctor may be more receptive to home care than other community physicians. However, for the same reason, he or she is more likely to monitor your ongoing need for home care closely.

If your HMO is one of the few unenlightened ones that does not provide any home care benefits or a particular home health service that you may need, ask questions. Your questioning may pay off, as it did for one hospitalized member of a Minnesota HMO whose policy covered only skilled nursing care at home. In order to be cared for at home, this person needed more extensive services. So, backed up by the home health agency, he put in for home care to the HMO director. As a result, the member was sent home with the physical and speech therapy he needed, as well as skilled nursing.

HMO Options

Two HMO options exist. *Group practice HMOs* are organized as mini-medical centers staffed with primary care doctors, medical specialists, nurses, and other personnel. Patient medical records and lab, X-ray, and pharmacy services are usually housed here as well. This type of HMO offers a one-stop shop for most of your health care needs.

One common misconception about HMOs is the notion that you can't choose your doctor and must see "the next available" physician. In a group practice HMO, you select one of the primary care doctors on staff, who then becomes your personal physician and coordinator for other HMO services you may need, including specialist care. When you need to see your HMO doctor, you telephone for an appointment just as you would arrange for any doctor's services.

Individual Practice Associations (IPAs), though HMOs, more closely resemble traditional health care. This type of HMO has only a central administrative office. Its doctors each maintain individual private offices within the community and usually care for HMO and non-HMO patients alike. However, when an HMO member visits the doctor, the

HMO—not the patient—is charged. Members choose their primary care doctor from a list of participating doctors who work under contract with the HMO. The IPA approach is less likely to offer the full range of services normally available through the group practice HMO. However, many community doctors participate in these HMOs, so you may have a greater choice in your physician selection.

Should you consider an HMO? If you join an HMO, you usually "give up" your present doctor (unless he/she is an IPA associate). If you have an established relationship with your doctor, this may present the major disadvantage. Also, if you need specialist, hospital, or other care, you will have to use the HMO-affiliated providers. You won't be able to choose. If you travel a lot, check the HMO policy carefully on *nonemergency* care outside your locale. It may be very limited or unavailable. However, if you join, remember that an HMO is not forever. You can quit at any time with notification. Since most HMOs operate on a monthly fee basis, you seldom lose much, if anything.

If You Are on Medicare

Some HMOs are participating in a federal government demonstration project aimed at reducing Medicare costs, while maintaining quality in health care for seniors.

The project works something like the DRG system. For each Medicare enrollee, the government pays the HMO a lump sum equal to 95 percent of the average community Medicare bill. If an HMO can provide quality care for less, it pockets the difference. Therefore, HMOs have an incentive to participate in the demonstration. The government automatically saves 5 percent, so it is ahead. If you are a Medicare senior, you will probably come out ahead too.

The Advantages

When you join, you must "turn in" your Medicare card. However, the HMO must offer benefits equal to that of traditional Medicare Parts A and B. You lose absolutely nothing in benefits, and usually you gain in several ways:

1. *You may save money.* You will no longer have to search for a doctor or other health provider who accepts Medicare assignment as payment in full. Nor will you have to worry about Medicare's payment policy, which is based on what *it* considers reasonable and necessary charges. Because it is an HMO plan, you pay little or nothing out of pocket, just a monthly premium. Some HMOs do not require any monthly premium at all. However, in any case you must still pay your Part B medical insurance premium each month. Gone are the usual Part A and B deductibles. Co-payments, when required, are small.

2. *You may receive better benefits.* Some HMOs offer a high-option plan that provides better benefits than traditional Medicare for a slightly higher monthly premium. Other HMOs automatically offer higher benefits as part of their basic senior HMO plan, and do so without any extra charge. Typical nontraditional extras include routine foot care, eye-glasses, hearing aids, and even basic dental care. These benefits translate into dollar savings for you.

3. *Your care may be better coordinated.* Your HMO primary doctor coordinates all the care you receive. This can help prevent the problems that often occur when consumers use the services of more than one doctor. For example, without coordination, lab tests may be duplicated. Or drugs prescribed by one doctor may interact harmfully with drugs ordered by another doctor.

4. *You will be freed of troublesome Medicare paperwork.* As an HMO member, you will not have to worry about completing complicated Medicare forms. Any necessary paperwork is handled by the HMO.

As of 1984, more than 95,000 seniors were HMO-enrolled in Florida. Yet fewer than 1 percent of these members lodged any complaints whatsoever with the government about their services. However, for seniors who enroll and then choose to drop out, one word of caution: Before you see a doctor again, make sure Medicare has notified you that you are officially reenrolled in the traditional Medicare program. Otherwise,

Medicare will not pay for care and you will be stuck with the doctor's bill. Until you are sure you are in the fold again, you should use the HMO plan.

SOCIAL/HEALTH MAINTENANCE ORGANIZATIONS (S/HMOs)

When you see the prefix *S* with an HMO, the *S* stands for *social*; in practice, it means senior in capital letters. The social/health maintenance organization or S/HMO (rhymes with "snow") is a bold new experiment that provides *long-term* home care.

Unlike other demonstration HMOs, S/HMOs are 100 percent senior membership. Where HMOs provide seniors with home care according to Medicare guidelines, S/HMOs provide home care when seniors have a chronic health problem where health restoration is not likely and maintaining function and independence become the primary goals. In the S/HMO system, personal care services of a purely custodial nature can be provided according to a preset budget limit. S/HMOs also provide garden-variety HMO services, as well as the extra services offered by experimental HMO plans.

If all this sounds too good to be true, in a sense it is. At present, it's unlikely you will find a S/HMO if you look for one. There are only four nationwide:

- Elderplan, Inc. (Metropolitan Jewish Geriatric Center), Brooklyn, NY
- Kaiser-Permanente Medical Care Program, Portland, OR
- Medicare Partners (Ebenezer Society/Group Health, Inc.), Minneapolis, MN
- SCAN Health Plan (Senior Care Action Network), Long Beach, CA

Despite their scarcity, S/HMOs are making health headlines because, for the first time, they will test several key questions:

- Can a S/HMO effectively provide seniors with complete, coordinated health packages (basic sick care, wellness

programs, Medigap extras, long-term home care)?
- Can it provide this package at a cost that does not exceed the public costs of Medicare and Medicaid?
- Will senior consumers view S/HMO as an attractive alternative to the traditional pay-as-you-go care system and pay the premiums for its unique services?

If, as S/HMO planners believe, the answer to all these questions is "yes," S/HMOs may start another home care revolution. Up to now, Medicaid, which forces consumers to spend down, has acted as the only "health insurance" available for long-term care. Traditional health insurers have been afraid to touch long-term care, since they cannot predict consumer demand for this service, consumer willingness to pay premiums, what such benefits might actually cost, and how to price the premiums.

S/HMOs, as the first free market offering of long-term care insurance, will provide such data. They will show insurers whether consumers are willing to pay for such benefits, and if they will like what they get in return. As S/HMOs go, so may the health insurance industry. A S/HMO success story may mean that such benefits will become universally available. And within five years or so, you (or your employer) may be able to purchase long-term home care and nursing home benefits as you would any other health benefit.

PREFERRED PROVIDER ORGANIZATIONS (PPOs)

If you are covered by a group health insurance plan, you may find that home care benefits are offered through preferred provider organizations. PPOs essentially work this way. Your employer, union, or insurance company (like Blue Cross and Blue Shield) works out ongoing contracts with local providers—hospitals, doctors, or home care agencies—to provide services to group members at preset discounted fees. In return for their discounts, these providers are "preferred" or favored by the group plan.

What does this mean to you? Usually your group plan provides you with some financial incentive to use optional PPO services rather than those of other community providers. It may charge you a lower deductible for PPO care or require a smaller co-payment.

VETERANS ADMINISTRATION

If you are a veteran, your chance of getting home care through the Veterans Administration (VA) is getting better each year. The number of veterans age 65 and older will rise dramatically between now and the year 2000, from roughly 3 million to 8.9 million. The VA, which serves about 10 to 12 percent of the veteran population each year, realizes that this trend requires changes in the system in order to respond to the needs of an older, more chronically ill veteran population.

Change is already underway. The number of hospital-based home care units is growing in the 172-hospital VA network. As of October 1984, 49 units were providing home care to veterans, and by 1990 the VA plans to have 77 units operational.

Mary Shirashi, chief of VA hospital-based home care, explains that VA home care services "provide care to try to minimize reinstitutionalization and cut down on emergency visits at VA hospitals." The VA is also interested in the cost effectiveness of home care. "We are undertaking a well-designed scientific case control study," Chief Shirashi reports, "which will give us vital information on home care for future planning."

If the VA finds home care a cost-saver, this may further boost the availability of VA home care nationwide.

Who Qualifies for VA Medical Care?

Before you can be considered for VA home care, you must first qualify for VA medical care. You may qualify for such care regardless of whether you have a service or non-service-connected medical condition. Ninety percent of all veterans who receive VA care, both home care and hospital care, receive help for non-service-connected medical conditions.

For all veterans with service-connected medical conditions, the VA provides hospital, nursing home, or outpatient care. Even veterans without an honorable discharge can qualify if the disability was incurred or aggravated during active service in the line of duty.

If you are a veteran with a non-service-connected medical condition, to qualify for VA care you must require hospitalization *and* generally meet any *one* of the following conditions:

- 65 years of age or older
- VA pensioned
- Medicaid-eligible
- Former POW
- Military-retired due to disability aggravated in the line of duty

If you don't meet any of the above requirements, you can still qualify if you cannot pay for the cost of comparable care in the community and sign a statement to this effect.

Qualified veterans are admitted to VA hospitals on a space available basis. Your local VA office can provide further details on eligibility and how to apply.

Home Care Eligibility

If you are a VA-qualified veteran, as just described, you may also qualify for home care when needed and without charge, through community home care agencies or through home care units at selected VA hospitals. But certain conditions apply.

By special authorization, the VA will pay for community home care only if you are a former POW, World War I veteran, have a 50 percent or more rated service-connected disability, or are enrolled in a VA vocational rehabilitation program. Otherwise, all home care you receive must be provided through a hospital-based VA home care unit.

If your nearest VA hospital does not have a home care

unit, for the present you are out of luck. The VA will not authorize you to use a community agency. "We've talked about allowing it," says Ms. Shirashi, noting that "all VA hospitals won't be able to support home care units. With the number of patient discharges some have it would be inefficient." Such authorization would require legislative changes.

VA Hospital-Based Home Care

Home care units serve veterans who are in the VA hospitals or nursing home units or who receive VA-authorized community nursing home care.

As a precondition for home care, you usually must live within a 30-minute drive of the VA hospital. Also you must usually have a relative or friend who will agree to help care for you at home. This caregiver does not necessarily have to reside with you, but he or she must live reasonably nearby so that regular, ongoing care is assured. In very short-term home care situations, this requirement may be waived.

Your VA doctor, social worker, or discharge nurse can refer you to the VA home care program. An assessment is conducted, and if recommended, home care is then authorized and a comprehensive care plan developed.

VA Home Care Services and Coverage

If you are eligible for VA home care, you should be pleased to know that the quality of that care is generally high. All programs are JCAH-accredited, and the team concept of care is strongly promoted. Except for a few shortcomings, the VA provides better home care coverage than is available through Medicare and most private health insurance.

Basically, the VA program is designated as a patient-family self-help program. Although the VA program is geared toward rehabilitation and recovery, many of the veterans served are terminally ill. Available services include:

• *Doctor's visits.* These are chiefly provided by the VA

doctor responsible for the patient's admission, medical care, and discharge from the VA hospital or nursing home.

- *Skilled nursing by registered nurses.* The nurses provide care as needed, but their primary role in the VA system is to teach you and your family how to perform home nursing procedures and manage the patient's condition.
- *Rehabilitation therapy by a corrective therapist.* These therapists teach and assist with exercises designed to increase mobility and independence. Therapists also order equipment that can be adapted to home use to assist the patient in self-care activities.
- *Physical, speech, respiratory, or occupational therapy.* Available only at selected units. When unavailable, therapy must be obtained through outpatient clinics.
- *Home health aides.* These services are not available through all VA home care programs.
- *Social services.* The social workers work with you *and* your family to ease problems related to illness.
- *Nutrition service.* This is provided by a dietitian.
- *Supplies and medical equipment.* Whatever is medically necessary for your care at home is provided.
- *Drugs.* Whatever drugs are needed to treat the patient's condition are provided.

All covered services are provided free of charge. However, the family may be responsible for picking up any needed drugs, supplies, or medical equipment at the VA hospital. A unique feature of VA home care is that home improvement and structural alterations, if needed, are paid for within certain dollar limits so care can be provided at home. Respite care for families is also available at the VA hospital for varying periods up to one month.

There is no limit on the number of visits that may be provided. Daily nursing care or therapy sessions are specifically excluded. High-tech services would require special authorization.

Unlike Medicare or other available insurance-related programs, care may be "open-ended," depending on the needs of the patient and family. The laws governing VA home care stipulate care up to one year, but extensions can occur after that on a case-by-case basis. "We have some patients for years," Ms. Shirashi points out. "We are a long-term program."

CHAMPVA/CHAMPUS

These acronyms stand for Civilian Health and Medical Program of the Veterans Administration and the United States, respectively. CHAMPVA provides health insurance coverage to surviving spouses and dependents of deceased veterans who were permanently and totally service-connected disabled. CHAMPUS covers dependents of the active military, the retired military and their dependents, and the surviving dependents of deceased or retired military.

CHAMPUS/CHAMPVA provides limited home care benefits. Its home care services may be provided through a home care agency. Currently, home health aide services, occupational therapy, and social services are not covered. No personal care services are covered even if incidentally furnished by nurses as part of patient care. Physician-prescribed medical equipment is covered, and respiratory therapy can be provided as an outpatient service. Physical therapy is limited to no more than two visits per week.

HOME EQUITY CONVERSION

"Use your own home to stay at home" really sums up the concept behind *home equity conversion* for home care. It is a method to help home-rich but cash-poor consumers pay for goods and services they want, home care included.

Consider Mrs. G.'s case. At age 84, she lived alone, was very frail, suffered from several minor chronic conditions, but was otherwise healthy. However, in order to remain in her home, where she wanted to be, she needed homemaking and personal care services. On her small income, she couldn't afford to pay for these home care services. Fiercely independent, she steadfastly refused community services. Home equity conversion solved her problem. She now receives a $400 check each month—a loan against the value of her home (home equity)—that she can use to pay for home care and whatever else she needs.

Home equity conversion basically unlocks the value (equity) of your house or condominium and converts it into cash or credit. The beauty of the conversion program is that you receive cash or credit while you continue to live in your home. Prior to home equity conversion, the only way homeowners could get income from the equity in their homes was to sell the home itself. If you need home care, this is clearly a self-defeating proposition.

Two types of home equity conversion plans exist: a loan plan and a sales plan. Let's see how each plan works.

The Loan Plan

The loan program allows you to borrow money, using your home as collateral. Let's say you own a home now valued at $100,000. If your remaining mortgage is $50,000, you have a $50,000 net balance or equity in your home to work with. In a loan program, a lender will allow you to borrow 60 to 80 percent of your $50,000, or $30,000 to $40,000. This really amounts to a second mortgage.

The loan plan is often called a "reverse" mortgage, or a reverse annuity mortgage (RAM)—a loan that pays you monthly. In a conventional mortgage, the interest you owe on your loan decreases as the loan balance is paid. In a RAM, the amount of interest owed rises as the amount of your total debt increases each month.

Loan repayment may be deferred until death, sale of the home, or a specified date. One elderly woman who participated in the San Francisco Development Fund RAM Program received a four-year loan of $95,000. The term was based on her life expectancy. Until the time of her death only a year later, she received a RAM check of $1,400 a month, which allowed her to purchase home care and pay for other living expenses. Prior to RAM intercession, she was awaiting nursing home placement following leg amputation. After the woman's death, the house was sold, the bank loan repaid, and the remaining funds distributed to her heirs. The interest rates charged in this loan program are normally much lower than consumer loan rates.

In a loan program, you may receive monthly loan payments, or you may get an open line of credit up to your equity limit. With your credit line may come an equity credit card that you can use to purchase goods and services as you would any other consumer credit card. The idea of an equity credit card may seem strange now, but financial experts predict that such cards will become commonplace in the near future. You can even expect to find automated cash machines where you can push in your card and dip into your home equity with the same ease with which you can now dip into your bank account.

The Sales Plan

In a sales plan, you do not receive a loan or incur a debt. Instead, you actually sell your home but retain your right to live there until death, or in the case of a couple, until both die. Houses sold this way are generally sold at a negotiated discount, perhaps 20 percent below market value, so a $100,000 home would receive an $80,000 price tag. You may receive payments for your home in monthly installments or as a lump sum that can be reinvested to provide monthly income. Often the sales plan includes a leaseback provision under which you are granted lifetime tenancy at a specified rental rate.

A variation of the sales plan is sometimes called a "split" equity or life plan. You do not have to give up title to your home until your death. You remain in your home and receive monthly payments toward the sale. However, the equity is considered a "split" because with each payment, the buyer owns a greater interest in your home. When you die, and the buyer makes payment in full, the buyer receives title to the property. Should the buyer fail to make proper payment at any time, he or she forfeits the rights to the house.

Benefits and Pitfalls

Should you use home equity? Clearly home equity is not for everyone. If you have accrued little equity in your home or have other existing debts, this may not make much sense. However, if you are a senior homeowner, you may want to give home equity serious consideration. Approximately 12.5 million homes are owned by those age 65 or older. Of these, four out of five are owned free and clear. So it is likely that if you are older, you have a hefty amount of equity available. For most seniors, their home is their single most valuable asset. You can leave this asset alone and simply pass it along to your heirs. Or you can put it to work for you so you can remain at home and independent.

Anyone interested in home equity conversion should proceed cautiously and get sound legal advice. Participation could affect anyone receiving SSI or Medicaid benefits. Full disclosure and full understanding of all loan and sales terms are essential. Before plunging ahead, learn more about home equity conversion options.

Currently, there are special equity conversion programs operating in the states. Most operate as nonprofit social service community programs. With an estimated $600 billion in home equity now held by older Americans, and the increasing need for in-home long-term care, home equity programs are expected to grow.

For more information on conversion plans and state programs, contact the National Center for Home Equity Conversion, 110 E Main St, Room 1010, Madison, WI 53703, (608) 256–2111.

WORKERS' COMPENSATION/ LONG-TERM DISABILITY

If you become disabled, no matter for how short or how long a period of time, because of an injury or sickness related to your job, you are probably eligible for workers' compensation. Workers' compensation is insurance paid by your employer that provides "medical" care, including home care, when needed. The benefits available vary somewhat from state to state. The program is administered by the state Workers' Compensation Board.

To apply, you should report any job-related illness or injury promptly to your employer, and obtain and complete the necessary forms. You must receive medical care from a physician authorized by your state board. If appropriate, home care can be prescribed. The agency, in some states, may also have to be board-authorized as well. Depending on the nature of your condition, the home care services provided can be quite extensive. For example, the rehabilitation home care for the trauma patient described on page 257 was paid totally by workers' compensation. Your employer, worker's compensation representative, or state board can give you the necessary details.

Some employers also provide long-term disability insurance that may provide cash payments and rehabilitation services. Rehabilitation often covers home care if it may restore a person to gainful employment.

OLDER AMERICANS ACT/ SOCIAL SECURITY BLOCK GRANTS

The Older Americans Act, Title III, funds many home care services for Americans age 60 and older. These funds are administered through the Area Agencies on Aging (3As) described in Chapter 5. Contact the 3As directly for more information.

The social security block grants, Title XX, are monies that go from the federal government to the states. Many states use these funds for special home care programs, primarily for personal care and homemaker services. You cannot apply directly for these funds. However, if you contact your local office of the state Department of Social Services or Aging for home care services, it can direct you to any Title XX funded programs for which you may qualify.

Two Dozen Dollar-Savers

When you try to plan financially for home care, the maze of insurance requirements, government regulations, and confusing forms may seem overwhelming. As the experts, home care agencies can usually help you cut quickly through the financial red tape. But you can help yourself develop a sound financial plan if you learn as much as you can in advance about the financial side to home care.

For some consumers, the biggest problem in home care is how to meet its cost at all, particularly in situations where long-term care is needed. While no simple solutions exist, some of the strategies outlined here may help if you face this situation.

These tips will help put you on a better financial track for home care. Some suggestions will help you avoid payment pitfalls; others should help you cut costs or otherwise save money.

Know thy insurance policy.

When you plan financially for home care, this truly becomes the first cost commandment. "Most people have no idea of what their insurance policy covers," Carolyn Fitzpatrick, a hospice agency director, emphatically states. "If you can get them to look, you'll do a public service."

To check your coverage, review a current copy of your policy and/or benefits booklet. When you check coverage, don't forget to look under hospital *and* medical insurance benefits.

Even if home health care is not mentioned by name, you may still be covered. Home care benefits can often be provided under provisions such as private duty nursing, outpatient care, "miscellaneous," or "other" clauses. Remember too that home care benefits are mandated in certain states (see page 149). However, frequently insurance material prepared for national distribution for unions or employer groups never mentions these state variations. Complete the insurance worksheet on page 400, which outlines the key coverage points of which you and the home care agency should be aware. If you are not sure of coverage details, contact your employer, union benefits or personnel manager, or health insurance representative. Professional agencies will also perform this service for you prior to care if you wish.

Don't overlook any coverage you may have on your spouse's health insurance or other insurance such as your homeowner's policy, auto, or disability insurance, if appropriate.

Negotiate with your insurer if you are not covered (or covered adequately) for home care.

If your policy does not cover home care, don't give up. It's true that many policies still retain old language that does not specifically cover home care, or a policy may not provide the coverage for services that would allow some hospitalized patients to go home. Despite this, Daniel Thomas of the Health Insurance Association of America counsels: "Health insurance companies can be convinced to pay for services, under appropriate circumstances, on a case-by-case basis."

How do you convince an insurer? First, with sound economic arguments. If the cost comparison, in your case, of inpatient versus home care is presented clearly, this will get the insurer's attention. Also you should provide evidence that: (1) quality of patient care at home can be assured; (2) services and care are medically appropriate and relate to the diagnosis.

To negotiate, you will need medical support and documentation from your doctor. The home care agency and the hospital discharge staff can provide support for the care and cost arguments. Often, the agency becomes your advocate with the insurer. Your employer can also be a supporter if the cost side of the issue is understood.

You can start, but don't stop, at the lowest level in the insurance company. Mr. Thomas advises: "Every company has a medical director. If at some point you don't get satisfaction, go there." The medical director is often fairly inaccessible. It may help, at this level, if your doctor intercedes directly in your behalf.

Make sure the agency you choose qualifies for your health insurance coverage.

Just because an agency's advertising states it "accepts insurance coverage" does not mean *your* insurance company will cover the services of that agency. For example, unless it is Medicare-certified, Medicare will not pay for home care under *any* circumstances. Many health insurance programs reimburse only for home care provided through licensed or certified agencies or through agencies with which they contract. Sometimes insurers may cover the services of other agencies, but with limited benefits—such as higher co-payments or fewer covered visits.

Use health insurance benefits prudently to your best advantage.

Work closely with the agency so your care plan and bills are structured to make sound use of *any* available insurance benefits, so you do not needlessly pay for care out of pocket. For example, many insurance plans define a "visit" as each service period up to four hours. Knowing this, to conserve limited benefits arrange with your agency to schedule only four hours of care on a given day (one visit), instead of six or eight hours, which would count as two, unless absolutely necessary.

Whenever RN assessment and supervisory visits are built into basic rates, you should not be charged for these visits simply because insurance may cover it. This would unethically use limited visits and may, if you must co-pay, cost you more than need be. Also, when your insurance plan reimburses services on a "visit" basis, instead of at an hourly rate, you should get the full value of the care you need, not a quick token visit that is just enough for the agency to bill for insurance purposes.

Some insurance plans cover private duty nursing care under a separate provision apart from home health care. In this case, an agency may be able to charge your aide and therapy visits under home health care visits, and your skilled nursing separately as private duty, if you need to stretch your coverage. However, don't insist on benefit usage merely because coverage may be available. "Some people demand eight-hour-a-day private duty nursing," says James Booth, RN, director of nursing and quality assurance for Superior Care. "We try to advise them it is not needed, but when they are aware that the insurance provides for it, they insist. In the end, we provide private duty because they will just go elsewhere."

Choose an agency that limits its fee to "reasonable and customary" charges.

The "reasonable and customary" charge is the going rate charged by most providers for a particular service within the community. This rate becomes the yardstick insurers use as a base for their payment for services. The reasonable and customary charge is commonly used for doctors' fees, but it applies to home care too. For example, if most home care agencies in your community charge $40 to $50 per skilled nursing visit, your insurer may set $50 as its reasonable and customary rate. A home care agency is under no obligation to charge this amount. But if you choose an agency that does charge more, you should realize up front how much more this can cost you.

Let's assume that your insurance plan pays 80 percent of the agency's fee; you pay 20 percent. Assume also that you choose an agency which charges $60 per skilled nursing visit. What will each visit cost you out of pocket? If you expect to pay a $12 balance per visit based on 80 percent of the $60 agency fee, you are in for an unhappy surprise. You will owe the agency $20, not $12. Here's why: The insurance company bases its fair share payment on the reasonable and customary charge or the agency's actual charge, whichever is *lower*. So in this example, the insurance company would pay 80 percent of $50, which is $40, leaving you an unpaid balance of $20 per visit.

Most professional agencies should agree to limit their fees to reasonable and customary rates. When an agency won't, you may well wonder why. Unless it provides some special service that justifies this extra cost, be prepared to spend more for the care than you have to. If there is any question about the insurer's reasonable rate, check with the claims office beforehand.

Look for an agency that permits assignment of benefits.

Assignment of benefits is an agreement among you, your insurance company, and the home care agency. In this agreement, you transfer or "assign" the agency your right to receive any payment from the insurance company for the insured services you have received.

Such an arrangement is very beneficial to you. With it, you do not have to pay the agency 100 percent and then collect your insurance reimbursement from the company. Instead the agency only bills, and you only pay for, your fair share of insured home care costs. So if your insurance is a 20–80 percent split, the agency bills you 20 percent and your insurance company the remaining 80 percent.

If you have ever had to wait for an insurance reimbursement, you will understand how assignment can take the hassle out of paying for home care. Insurance companies are often very slow to pay. If an agency does not permit assignment, you may wait weeks for reimbursement on home care bills you have already paid.

Before you ask the agency about assignment, check your policy. Some plans, sometimes union-related, do not allow assignment and insist all payments go to you directly. If your insurer allows assignment and the agency agrees, the procedure is simple. You sign a standard agreement (which the agency will provide) which has you list the policyholder's name, the home care client's name if different (for example, a spouse), the insurer's name and address, and the correct policy number.

Once the agency verifies that you are covered for benefits, assignment begins.

Ask the agency to accept your insurance assignment as payment in full if you cannot otherwise afford the full home care rate.

In this era of growing agency competition, you may find some agencies, proprietaries as well as community nonprofit, which may agree to accept your assignment as full payment. This is more likely if your insurance company pays 75 percent or more for home care and/or there is a good chance that the agency will at least break even in providing care.

Why would an agency agree to this arrangement? For public relations and/or community service reasons. In fact, your chance of making such an arrangement is much better if you ask your doctor, a hospital discharge planner, or a social worker to intercede in your behalf. Such professionals can be an important referral source for further agency business.

Home care agencies are looking for ways to "woo" professionals and distinguish themselves from the agency pack. Some for-profits have even established small "free care pools" in which the agency adds a certain number of free service hours each month so it can occasionally help those in financially troubled situations. Such exceptions to normal business practices can make a very positive impression. Word of mouth among doctors, other professionals, and patients can be an important source of goodwill and good business.

Coordinate home care benefits to increase coverage when appropriate.

When you are covered by more than one group health plan—for example, first through your own employer's health plan and second as a dependent on your spouse's employer's plan—you can combine or coordinate benefits. This has advantages for you and for the insurance companies.

From the insurance company's view, coordination of benefits (COB) saves money, since neither company duplicates the payment of the other and together they do not pay more than 100 percent of the covered cost. COB can help you get more coverage than either plan alone provides.

Say you are covered by two group insurance plans. After you submit your claim to your primary plan, and it pays, you can then submit your claim to the secondary insurer. It will pay too, up to the amount it would normally pay without COB or up to your unreimbursed home care expenses, whichever is less. Eventually, with COB you will have your costs *completely* covered, including your out-of-pocket deductibles. Also with COB, you may find that one plan covers a home care service such as respiratory therapy that the other plan might not. Again, it's to your advantage to coordinate benefits.

Appeal any claim denials.

If you are covered for home care and your insurance company denies any claims for care, don't let the matter rest there. Many legitimate claims are initially rejected because, says Daniel Thomas of the Health Insurance Association of America, "too often the information supplied to the insurance company was insufficient."

Your care must be clearly related to a medical diagnosis. The progress notes your agency keeps must show that skilled nursing or therapy was provided, not just health aide services.

Professional agencies will always assist you with insurance appeals. If the agency accepts assignment, it will automatically go to bat for you, contacting your doctor if necessary and resubmitting the additional information to support your claim.

If you are on Medicare, the agency will advise you of Medicare procedures. Also, staff at most senior centers or social service organizations can assist. If you are handling the insurance problem yourself, check first with your insurer, if possible, about the claims denial. Don't talk to a clerk; request a supervisor or claims manager.

Once you understand the nature of the denial, then contact your doctor and the home care agency for the necessary supporting information. If your claim is rejected again, you can go to the next administrative level, where you may get satisfaction.

Of course, as you go through the appeals process, document your efforts in writing. Keep copies.

If you find that you have repeated insurance problems because of the agency's failure to keep professional, detailed notes, then switch agencies. You are dealing with a second-rater.

Maximize the help you get from your insured home health aide visits.

If you live alone, take note of this tip, since it is likely you will need some household as well as health care services during recovery. Insurers have strict guidelines for the services of home health aides. When you qualify for insured home health care, aide visits are not covered when they are provided mainly for general household services, meal preparation, laundry, and so on. However, do not interpret this to mean that home health aides can never perform these tasks. The question of payment hinges on how much time the aide spends on these activities.

If these activities *substantially* increase an aide's time in your home, then the visit is not covered by insurance. But if these tasks are *incidental* to your care, they are okay. For example, an aide could put a load of laundry in the wash while she assists you with bathing. After the bath, the aide can wipe the bathroom floor and tidy the room. While you rest after exercise, an aide could make a meal, or do some quick grocery shopping or light housekeeping.

Experienced and motivated aides might structure work activities like this on their own. More realistically, you should expect to work with the agency supervisor to maximize the services you obtain from the aide's visit.

Keep track of services and check all bills carefully.

If you're not in the habit of keeping records and checking medical bills, start. It may save you money. Insurers and employers who double-check hospital and other medical bills regularly find cost-increasing errors. One accounting firm that audits hospital bills found that 93 percent contained such errors, suggesting the existence of a major problem, at least with hospital bills.

In home care, the chance for mistakes is less. Agencies provide fewer services, so bills are much simpler. Still, errors can occur.

Keep your own records of services, equipment, and supplies as a double check. This record is also helpful for insurance and tax purposes. Use a calendar to keep track of care. For example, jot down RN for nurse, HA for health aide, or devise your own system. If you sign a weekly time sheet that verifies personnel attendance, always review this carefully before signing. Your signature indicates you agree that the statement is correct. Make sure the time slip correctly lists the *total* number of work hours; otherwise extra attendance can be logged after signing. Ask for a copy of the time sheet if it is not automatically offered, as well as copies of all bills on your account, including those sent to your insurance company. Bills should be itemized.

Check all bills for accuracy. Ask for an explanation of anything you don't understand. Should you spot errors, bring it to the agency's attention without delay. The longer you wait, the harder it becomes to correct mistakes.

Discuss the agency's standard billing procedures in advance and request adjustments as needed.

As standard practice, most agencies bill weekly for services. If you are paid or pensioned once a month, this may cause problems. However, if you discuss billing in advance, you will find that many agencies will work out more flexible arrangements to accommodate you. For example, an agency may still bill you weekly, but agree to accept payment on a semi-monthly or monthly basis.

Also discuss the agency's procedures for the processing of insurance claims, particularly if the agency does not permit assignment of benefits. Some agencies complete forms only after you have made payment in full and your check has cleared. This practice could mean a delay of several weeks before you can even file your insurance claims, and weeks more before you receive payment.

Ask for an adjustment on your bill when you are dissatisfied with services.

As a consumer, treat home care agencies just as you would any other community business. When you have a valid reason for dissatisfaction, ask for and expect an adjustment on your bill.

All professional agencies consider this reasonable business practice and will adjust bills when situations warrant. For example, one agency administrator said that, should a scheduled worker fail to report for work, he does not always charge the client for the necessary replacement.

Don't hesitate to use basic consumer action. You should not, however, expect an agency to make adjustments in every case. For example, if you are dissatisfied with an assigned aide because of personality differences, but the care provided to date has been competent and respectful, the agency should change your aide, not your bill. Valid reasons for adjustments include any breach of basic business practices such as frequent or serious employee lateness or failure to perform contractual duties. Certainly any agency would also be at fault if it provided unqualified or otherwise unprofessional personnel. In such cases, you should not be charged at all.

Notify the agency promptly should any payment problem occur.

When you contract for care with a proprietary agency, you sign a binding agreement to pay for services provided. If you cannot make your payment for any reason, don't avoid this situation. Discuss the matter with the agency right away. It can often help. For example, agency personnel may help you apply for financial assistance for which you may qualify, or you may be referred to an alternate community service. In a sliding scale agency, the fee may be reduced further or waived entirely. If slow insurance reimbursement is the problem, the agency can contact the insurance claims supervisor to help correct this situation.

Ask if the agency accepts credit cards for payment or gives discounts for cash.

If you haven't already noticed, many hospitals, doctors,

laboratories, and other health services accept major credit cards. Some home care agencies do too. Whether or not you prefer to pay with plastic is your decision. But a 30-day or more delay between credit card billing and required payment can be helpful indeed, especially if you are waiting for insurance reimbursement. It may have tax advantages too (see page 200). If an agency takes credit cards, also ask about a discount for cash. Many consumer businesses do extend a 3 to 5 percent discount, roughly equivalent to the credit card company's surcharge.

Supplement professional home care with informal care networks.

Because payment for professional home care is often a problem, informal grassroots networks for care are springing up in many communities. They may be church-centered or outgrowths of senior community centers or advocate groups.

Maggie Kuhn, founder of the activist Gray Panthers, cites an innovative concept her group is testing in Philadelphia. "We are organizing 'healthy blocks' and getting neighbors [young and old] to look after neighbors."

Some informal systems have evolved from support groups formed to help individuals and families deal with problems such as Alzheimer's disease. The kind of assistance provided reflects community or group needs and ranges from shopping, transportation, and chore services to regular personal care or respite help for families.

Assess your home care needs carefully and in advance.

When you practice this strategy, you are more likely to contract and pay only for essential and appropriate care. Through this process, you may realize that you need more reassurance than real help. An emergency response system may be an answer that reduces the need for help.

Use the assessment checklist on page 386 as a guide. Discuss to what extent family or friends will help with individual tasks and analyze the time when regular help is available. For example, can you get some help evenings during the week and/or weekends, when family members may be freer? If so, fewer weekday visits may be needed. Advise the agency about this outside help when your care plan is developed and personnel are scheduled.

Pay reliable friends or neighbors for supplemental help.

Often nonfamily members will volunteer to run errands, make a meal, and so on for a while. But when you need assistance indefinitely, even the best-intentioned neighbors may want out. A more businesslike arrangement may prevent this from happening. Don't be concerned that an offer of money may offend your neighbor. You may very well find that some reimbursement, even if only a token, will be accepted and appreciated.

Train interested family members to provide care when practical.

Family help can reduce home care costs, particularly in high-tech, special rehab, and long-term care situations. It may also help conserve limited insurance benefits. Professional home care agencies encourage family care whenever practical and actively teach family members to perform skilled procedures from the simple to the complex. Most local chapters of the American Red Cross offer a basic 16-hour course in home nursing for a very modest fee. Some community hospitals or self-help support groups sponsor self-care programs to help family members learn the basics. Several excellent self-help guides are available, but supervised instruction is usually needed to master skills.

When you use family help, realize that most insurance companies do not reimburse care provided by family members, even those who are health professionals themselves. This rule holds even when agency health professionals would otherwise have been paid to render this care.

In situations where money is tight, look for a sliding scale agency.

When the cost is a major barrier to obtaining care, consider these agencies first. Visiting Nurse and Family Service organizations and home care units of county health departments are among the nonprofit agencies that usually function on a sliding payment scale. Use the suggestions outlined in Chapter 5 to locate such agencies. With some effort, you should be able to find one in your community.

Substitute or supplement paid home care with free or inexpensive community programs.

Look at Chapter 5 again and thoroughly explore the home care options that may be available in your community. Transportation and escort services, friendly visiting, Meals-on-Wheels, Carrier Alert, and senior companions all can help you stretch your home care budget. Don't forget that some organizations like the 3As provide free or low-cost homemaking or personal care services. Consider using home care alternatives like adult day care (see Chapter 25) when appropriate and practical.

Ask the agency for advice on cost-saving measures.

Reputable agencies, whether nonprofit or for-profit, understand the financial problems some consumers face when they need home care, so don't hesitate to discuss your financial needs frankly. Ask the home care experts to suggest cost-saving measures.

For example, people often request costly round-the-clock care. This could mean two employees on 12-hour shifts, or three employees 8 hours a day. A professional agency will evaluate this situation from a cost and care viewpoint. For example, if the person needing care retires early, sleeps late, seldom gets up at night, and has no serious skilled nursing needs, round-the-clock care would probably not be advised at all.

Some agencies have developed special lower-cost services geared toward the elderly. "Bed and bath" and "tuck-in" services are available when just a short visit is needed to provide the small needed boost for someone at home.

In short, ask the agency what it can offer that will help you economize without sacrificing the quality of care.

Ask agencies to waive the minimum policy.

Don't assume that an agency's general rules never bend. Many agency administrators told me they do make exceptions to help a particular individual. One proprietary agency administrator whose agency had a four consecutive hour minimum once a week cited such a case.

For years, an elderly man had paid a next-door neighbor to stop by daily for an hour to help him shave and bathe. This arrangement worked fine until the neighbor became sick and eventually died. The old man was devastated by the loss of his friend and his much-needed help.

"When I heard about him from my coordinator," the administrator said, "I decided that we had to find a way to help him." She did. She searched through the agency's large roster of aides and located one who lived near the man. Now, the aide leaves for work a bit earlier and assists the gentleman before her other assignments begin.

This arrangement benefits everyone. The senior receives the services he needs. The aide gains a regular hour of work each day without any additional carfare costs. The agency has the satisfaction of helping someone in need and receives a small but steady revenue from the transaction.

To locate a willing agency, you may have to make several calls. Professional agencies that operate mainly within your immediate area may be more flexible, since they are more likely to have a larger roster of available workers who live near you.

If your service need is likely to be long term, you have more buying power. Make agencies aware of this fact when you call and ask for a concession. Who you ask is as important as what you ask. Talk to the administrator of operations or a supervisor. The coordinator who handles incoming calls can seldom make such discretionary arrangements.

Consider the tax savings of home care.

Under certain conditions, home care expenses may qualify for the medical deduction or a tax credit on your federal income tax return. The next chapter outlines complete details.

—12—

Tax Tips

You cannot complete your financial plan for home care unless you consider the potential tax effects as well. A few states* now provide tax incentives for the care of elderly or disabled family members. However, most tax planning will involve your federal income tax return. Here home care expenses may translate into tax savings in two situations:

- When home care expenses for yourself, your spouse, or your dependent qualify as a medical expense and exceed 5 percent of your adjusted gross income, you can take a tax deduction on an itemized return.
- When you pay for home care for a disabled spouse or a dependent who lives in your home, so that you can work or look for work, you can claim part of your home care expenses as a tax credit. The disability may be *temporary* or permanent, mental or physical.

Furthermore, in certain circumstances you can take a medical deduction or receive a credit even when the home care expenses incurred are for someone whom you cannot claim as your dependent.

This might apply, for example, if you provide more than half of the support of an elderly parent, including medical expenses. If the parent has an income of $1,000 or more, you cannot claim him or her as a dependent. Nevertheless, you can use the expenses incurred for care of the parent when calculating your tax credits or deductions.

*In 1984 Arizona, Idaho, Iowa, and Oregon provided tax incentives.

THE MEDICAL DEDUCTION FOR HOME CARE

Medical expenses, home care or otherwise, are deductible within certain limits. You can deduct allowable expenses not reimbursed by insurance when they total more than 5 percent of your adjusted gross income. The Internal Revenue Service (IRS) calls this rule in its tax booklet the "5 percent limit." You can determine your 5 percent limit if you take the adjusted gross income figure listed on Form 1040 and multiply by .05.

The result is your limit. For example, if your adjusted gross income is $20,000, your 5 percent limit is $1,000. Anything below the $1,000 limit is *not* deductible; anything above the $1,000 limit *is*. So if your medical expenses for yourself, your spouse, or your dependents total $500, you do not qualify for the deduction. But if your expenses total $1,500, for example, you can take a $500 medical deduction provided you itemize expenses on your tax return.

When you compute this tax deduction, be sure to include *all* deductible medical expenses. Most people overlook several legitimate expenses and thereby reduce the deduction and sometimes miss out on it altogether.

According to the IRS, medical expenses are "payments you make for the diagnosis, cure, relief, treatment, or prevention of disease." They also include payments for "treatment affecting any part or function of the body." Also included under medical expenses is the cost of transportation to and from medical care and also payments made for medical insurance, including Medicare, that provide coverage for yourself, your spouse, and your dependents.

Note that the IRS does not state you must receive the treatment in a hospital or nursing home. Under the IRS definition, many home-care-related costs qualify as medical expenses. Don't overlook the following home care costs when you tally medical expenses. Also remember that all legitimate expenses qualify; you do not have to select the cheapest products or services.

Personnel Expenses

In the IRS information booklet, you will see repeated references to *medical* care or *medical* services and *medical* expenses. Do not let the term "medical" mislead you here.

The care provided in your home by medical or osteopathic doctors, including psychiatrists, of course is an allowable medical expense. But also allowed are the professional services of other health care personnel who do not provide "medical" services or care. Foremost in this category are registered and licensed practical nurses. Covered also under this catchall category are the services of physical, occupational, respiratory, and speech therapists, as well as therapy assistants, medical social workers, and dietitians.

You are on solid IRS ground when the cost of these professional services is claimed as a deduction. But you must be more careful when you consider allowable deductions for paraprofessional personnel.

In repeated IRS rulings, the services of nonskilled personnel have been allowed, but only for basic nursing and/or personal care related to a health condition. Housekeeping services are not deductible. When home health aides, homemakers, or companions perform household chores as well as basic nursing and personal care, you can deduct only the cost of the time they spend performing nursing and/or personal care.

Note that the IRS looks more carefully at what kind of services are provided than at who provides them. If a nurse also performs housekeeping chores as part of his/her duties, the same rule applies. You cannot deduct the full cost of the nurse—you must divide the cost of service between nursing and household duties.

On the basis of *what* not *who,* you may also deduct expenses when you pay a family member or other person to render these nursing and personal care services.

In one tax case, a taxpayer was advised by his doctor to seek care for his arthritic wife. The taxpayer hired and paid his daughter to provide basic nursing services. The daughter provided care according to the doctor's direction. The taxpayer claimed his daughter's salary as a medical deduction, which the IRS disallowed because the daughter was not a "trained nurse." The tax court, however, ruled otherwise, stating a person's job title and qualifications did not determine the deduction, the nature of the services provided did.

The nursing and personal care services must be provided to treat or care for someone with a health problem. Healthy infant or childcare, for example, is not allowed as a medical expense even if needed because the parent caregiver is ill or disabled.

If you hire someone on your own, not through an agency, you may also deduct the cost for social security and other employer expenses. You may also deduct the cost of meals provided for medically necessary personnel whether you go through a home care agency or not.

Drugs, Medicines, Medical Supplies, and Equipment

Prescription drugs are deductible. Over-the-counter medicine such as vitamins or minerals (such as iron supplement to treat anemia) may qualify *provided* they are physician-*prescribed* (in writing) and then *registered* and filled at a pharmacy. The pharmacist may charge you extra for this service. Special sterile IV solutions, though not technically "prescription drugs," also qualify, as do necessary irrigating solutions for wounds, catheter care, and so on. Any other physician-prescribed products for home use, such as blood or oxygen, are also legitimate medical expenses.

Whereas general household first aid supplies such as gauze, tape, and antiseptics do not normally qualify as medical expenses, such items are when they are specifically needed for physician-prescribed care and treatment.

Under certain circumstances, incontinent supplies such as disposable diapers may be allowed. In one case, the IRS allowed disposable diapers for a brain-damaged 4-year-old child. Absorbent paper diapers were advised by doctors to help prevent skin breakdown. Following this line of reasoning, adult disposables may be allowed if the situation dictates.

You can deduct all costs for medical equipment such as

hospital beds, lifts, wheelchairs, walkers, crutches, and similar devices used for the relief of sickness or disability. IV poles and other supportive equipment needed to provide treatment can be claimed. Of course, more sophisticated equipment such as infusion pumps, oxygen units, respirators, or monitors are all deductible too.

Even nonmedical equipment may qualify if a medical case can be made. For example, a separate refrigerator may be necessary for drug and solution storage of hyperalimentation products. If rented or bought and used solely for this purpose, this may become a medical rather than a household expense. Likewise, a special mattress needed to prevent skin breakdown can qualify.

Once equipment is considered medically necessary, any repairs and maintenance costs become allowable expenses too.

Home Improvements and Adaptations

Sometimes disease or disability necessitates changes in the home environment. The expense of special equipment installed in the home, such as grab bars, special plumbing devices, air conditioning, home elevators, or even an extra room, may be allowed, provided they are medically justified and not just for convenience. For example, an elderly person who has already suffered a serious fall or has a condition causing dizzy spells could deduct the cost of grab bars if they are prescribed by a physician.

If a permanent improvement increases the value of your home, you cannot deduct the entire amount. You must subtract the increase in the value of your home from the improvement cost, and then claim the difference. For example, your doctor recommends an elevator for a heart condition, which costs you $2,000. An appraiser states this improvement increases the value of your home by $1,500. You can deduct only $500 as medical expense ($2,000 − $1,500 = $500). Again the maintenance and repairs of such medically necessary items are deductible expenses.

Utilities

Some medically necessary equipment, such as respirators or elevators, may increase your utility rates significantly. You can claim the cost differences between normal household usage and the increased rates. One good way to calculate this figure for IRS purposes is to ask your utility company for a written standard *kilowatt* (not dollar) estimate of normal household usage for a home and family of your size.

You can compare this estimate against your present kilowatt usage and compute your increased cost. If your utility rates rise because of necessary live-in medical help, you can also deduct this increase as a *medical* expense.

Special Diets

Illness may require special foods. However, you cannot claim special food or drinks that replace your normal diet. For example, if your doctor prescribes a low-sugar diet, low-sugar canned goods that substitute for typical store-bought products do not count. However, you may deduct special food or drinks that you need in addition to your normal diet. For example, if your doctor prescribes two ounces of whiskey or a glass of wine each day to relieve heart pain, this qualifies.

Hyperalimentation products that are physician-prescribed are considered special diets or "medicines" for tax purposes.

Wigs

If you undergo chemotherapy or other treatment that causes serious hair loss, the cost of a wig or other hairpiece may qualify as a deductible item. One taxpayer received a favorable ruling when the wig was advised by a physician to help the patient cope with the psychological aspects of illness.

Emergency Response Systems

Like home improvements, ERS costs (see Chapter 14) may qualify as a medical deduction if the taxpayer establishes medical necessity. This means the physician must recommend

ERS use in the *individual* taxpayer's case. Andrew Dibner of Lifeline has received an IRS ruling to this effect.

What applies to one ERS system should generally apply to all, *provided* proper documentation of need is obtained. Should an audit occur, taxpayers using hospital or other health-facility-sponsored programs should have less trouble supporting medical necessity than taxpayers using stand-alone or digital systems marketed to the general public as security as well as medical emergency devices.

THE TAX CREDIT

This is the tax credit that most people think of only as a childcare credit. However, if you pay for someone to care for your disabled dependent or spouse who lives with you so you can work or look for work, the IRS also allows you to take a credit. The rules are complex, and you should check with IRS and/or your accountant on all the details.

You must have job income to claim the credit. The credit you receive is scaled according to your income and number of dependents. The maximum credit permitted was $1,440 in 1984.

The dependent or spouse does *not* have to be permanently disabled for you to claim credit. When the physical or mental disability lasts less than a month, expenses can be calculated on a daily basis. To qualify for the credit, the dependent or spouse must be incapable of self-care. For example, persons who are not able to dress or feed themselves, as might happen if someone suffers a stroke or a debilitating illness, would qualify. Likewise persons who need constant attention to prevent injury to themselves, as in the case of an Alzheimer's patient, are considered disabled.

The care provided must be for the dependent's well-being and protection so that home care such as services provided by a home health aide would qualify. However, expenses *do not* have to be medical in nature. Housekeeping and domestic services provided by homemakers and companions qualify too.

Note that this tax credit can also apply to the cost of care outside the home provided in adult day care centers. However, to qualify the day care center must meet any applicable state and local regulations.

Since tax credits are more advantageous than tax deductions (your accountant will tell you why), you should apply home care expenses as credits first if you can. Any home care expenses that exceed the tax credit limits can be applied as tax deductions for medical expenses.

TAX TIPS

When you think about the tax credit or deduction, think doctor. A doctor's written recommendation is essential to avoid IRS problems. If your doctor provides you with a clear statement indicating your condition, the type of care you need, and the reason why, it is unlikely that you will have IRS problems. You must, however, comply with the rest of the IRS regulations. For example, no matter what your doctor writes, don't expect to get a medical deduction for household help. If you want to know in advance if certain unusual expenses will qualify for the medical deduction, you can request an IRS "letter ruling." Write the IRS with the details, including any supporting medical statements. After a review, the IRS will give its opinion in writing. The ruling is administratively binding on both parties. Write to: Commissioner, IRS, Attn: T-PS-T, Washington, DC 20224.

Keep careful records. IRS decisions depend on these. Here is another area where a professional home care agency can make life better for you. The careful patient and personnel records the agency can provide will relieve you of tremendous record and paperwork burdens. In the event of an audit, for example, a well-documented plan of care would clearly show an IRS auditor that your home health aide was not domestic help or that your homemaker provided many more services than housekeeping alone. You are also less likely to run into IRS problems on allowable medical supplies when these are billed through the home care agency as part of its service.

If you charge home care services on a credit card at year's end, you can claim the charges for the current tax year even if you actually pay the credit card company after January 1.

For more information on medical deductions, see IRS Publication 502, *Medical and Dental Expenses.* Publication 503, *Child and Disabled Dependent Care,* provides detailed information on the tax credit. Some consumers may also find Publication 907, *Tax Information for Handicapped and Disabled Individuals,* useful. You may obtain all these publications free by contacting the IRS.

On page 406, you will find a tax checklist that can help you identify possible medical deductions for home care. Use it as a supplement when you itemize your other medical deductions.

IV

SPECIAL
SERVICES

—13—

Equipping Your Home for Care

If you need home care, you may also need medical equipment or supplies. The list of products now available for home use is indeed staggering. In general, *durable medical equipment* (or *DME,* as it is called in the trade) is a product that can last and withstand repeated use. Wheelchairs, walkers, and hospital beds are examples. Braces, artificial limbs and eyes, pacemakers, and similar items, though durable, are considered *prosthetic devices,* since they replace a normal body function.

Medical supplies are nonreusable products. Typical items include incontinence pads, syringes, dressings, and disposable catheters. However, some items, such as elastic stockings, are also considered medical supplies even though they are reusable. The reason? Because they have little or no value to someone else and are generally discarded after a period of normal use. Also included as supplies are items such as oxygen or irrigating solutions.

A HIGH-GROWTH FIELD

The business of selling these home care products has become a rapidly growing multimillion-dollar industry. According to the New York City market research firm Frost and Sullivan, sales for medical equipment alone are expected to exceed $384 million by 1987. This figure represents a healthy 53 percent jump over 1983 sales figures. The opportunity for high profits is one key reason for the anticipated growth.

The high profit potential has lured many newcomers to the business. Hospitals which traditionally were medical equipment and supply customers are now becoming equipment dealers themselves and selling or renting their products to patients, as are many home care agencies. Even major retailers such as Sears Roebuck and Montgomery Ward have joined this home care market with special in-store departments and a large mail-order catalog business.

The competition among dealers is becoming fierce. From a consumer viewpoint, this should translate into better service and better quality products at the best price *provided* that you shop around.

YOUR SHOPPER'S GUIDE TO EQUIPMENT AND SUPPLIES

Despite the billions consumers spend on medical equipment and supplies, there's little printed information to guide your shopping other than what the manufacturer or dealer provides. That information may be sound advice, too. But most savvy consumers would not rely on such potentially biased advice when out to purchase a high-ticket item like a car or a personal item as important as a bed mattress.

To remedy this situation, this shopper's guide provides basic guidelines on the key aspects of selection, as well as some pointers on specific items most often used by consumers in their own homes.

General Guidelines

Your most important rule of thumb? Apply the same normal consumer standards you would use on *any* purchase to medical equipment. First ask yourself: Why am I purchasing this equipment? What *basic* functions do I want it to perform? Where will it be used (at home only; or in a car or office)? Also, think about basic comfort and equipment care. Consider cost based on the essentials. Look at optional features and frills second. Don't forget any special needs you may have. Most equipment is constructed for the "average" person. If you are very tall or small or very heavy, the standard model may not suit you.

Check all equipment warranties carefully. Make sure you know the coverage and limitations for installation, inspection, maintenance, and repairs initially and in the future. Manufacturer guarantees vary.

Get professional advice—other than the dealer's—before you shop. If you do, you will have a much better idea of what to look for and what you really need.

Resources for Product Information

Are there devices that can help a partially paralyzed stroke patient groom, cook, or dress? What kind of reading or hearing aids are available for the impaired? Is there specially designed clothing for those with disabilities? What kind of bathtub benches or stools are available? What emergency response systems exist? These questions and hundreds of others on products for better living for the ill and disabled can be answered for you through two available computer services.

The Accent on Information system, PO Box 700, Bloomington, IL, (309) 378–2961, is an outgrowth of *Accent on Living* magazine, written for disabled Americans. For a nominal fee, it searches through a databank located at Illinois State University.

Abledata, a service of the National Rehabilitation Information Center (NARIC), 4407 Eighth St NE, The Catholic University of America, Washington, DC 20017, (202) 635–5884, TDD (202) 635–5884, is the most comprehensive database on product information available nationwide. It lists well over 10,000 products with continuous updates. Products are identified by the following categories:

- Personal care
- Vocational/educational
- Seating
- Communication
- Ambulation
- Orthotics/prosthetics
- Home management
- Mobility
- Transportation
- Recreation
- Therapeutic aids
- Sensory aids

Each listing provides the product's common name, brand

name, manufacturer, cost, a brief description, and any formal or informal product evaluation available. If you don't need equipment immediately, this service is a wonderful start to comparative shopping that can save you time and money.

You can access the Abledata information directly through NARIC or through a network of NARIC information brokers who often maintain lists of local equipment distributors and repair services. NARIC services are low cost, about $10 per search, unless an extensive computer search is required. NARIC also has a research service that provides publication lists on rehabilitation and independent living. Though geared more toward professionals, the service contains many consumer-oriented publications.

Commonly Used Products

The Hospital Bed

If you need a hospital bed, you must consider more than just the mattress. First, where will the bed be placed? Make sure that the room is large enough to handle the bed comfortably along with other essential furniture. If a wheelchair will be needed too, check to see that the room allows enough space so you can turn the wheelchair full circle once the bed is in place. Don't forget to check doorway widths so you know for sure that the bed will fit. Is the floor solidly constructed? Hospital beds are often much heavier than regular beds because of their motor weights.

Most hospital beds are standard twin size, the size most insurers will pay for. However, larger beds, which a larger than average person may need for comfort and easy positioning, are available.

Adjustable siderails in half or full lengths are a standard feature. Half lengths are usually easier for the patient to raise and lower unassisted. Some half lengths tuck away when down, giving the bed a more normal appearance. Test tuckaways to make sure that they hold securely even when not in a locked position. Should you forget to lock, a sudden recess could mean a potential accident.

Manual or electric controls that elevate the top and bottom of the bed are also standard. The frames and mattresses of many beds can also be elevated, a convenient feature to look for. Bed controls placed on side rails are impractical unless you have good hand control. Nor are they recommended for patients who become easily confused. For those with poor finger strength, hand controls are much easier to use. More sophisticated breath-controlled units are available for the totally disabled. They are costly and you must be cautious about selection, since a breakdown may mean difficult repairs.

A proper mattress is very important when you are ill or disabled. For someone who can hardly move, the proper mattress can mean the difference between normal skin and painful bedsores. (These sores develop when the pressure of the body weight on the skin greatly slows normal circulation to the tissues. Skin breakdown begins and sores quickly develop, particularly around the joints.)

Repositioning a bedridden person at least every two hours prevents bedsores. A proper mattress helps too, since it distributes body weight evenly, lessening skin pressure.

The standard foam mattress offers comfort, but does not prevent bedsores. For those at high risk of developing these sores, a water, air, or gel mattress is advised. Also available are special electrically controlled air pads that can be placed on a standard mattress and serve the same purpose. When considering a water or air mattress, test the mattress "feel" on the whole body, since these mattresses may impair movement. Look for a mattress with vinyl or stain-resistant covers for easy care.

Wheelchairs

If you need a wheelchair only occasionally, you can probably buy one "off the rack" to meet your needs. But if you must live in it many hours a day, get a custom fit by a physical therapist. Good dealers have physical therapists on staff or on call to provide this service—usually at no extra charge. Also, check with other regular wheelchair users who can supply a lot of practical advice.

When you select a wheelchair, consider:

- *Width* for doorway access and turning. Standard wheelchairs measure 24½ inches across, with an 18-inch seat width. Narrow versions are available.
- *Portability.* Weight, foldup ease, and removable arms are important to many customers. Standards weigh about 35 pounds; narrows about 29.
- *Transferability.* Some models make transfers from bed or commode much easier than the standard chair.
- *Back, head, seat, and foot support.* Models vary considerably in these features, which are important to conserve energy and prevent unnecessary body stress.
- *Ease of propulsion and stability.* Some models are easier for one-armed persons to use. Removable foot rests allow you to propel yourself with just your feet. Make sure that the wheelchair turns safely.
- *Ease of maintenance.* Many-spoked wheel versions are hard to clean. Electric versions may require special care.

Walkers, Crutches, and Canes

If you need any of these mobility devices, simple as they seem, you may also find a therapist's advice useful. Many versions of these items are available beyond the standard, each with special features and functions that can make one a better choice than another for you.

Walkers help if you need some assistance walking because of easy fatigue or poor balance. They may be made of lightweight aluminum or heavier steel, a factor to consider. If not properly sized, you may bend too far forward or stand too straight so you cannot easily lift and move the walker forward. To compensate, some walkers have adjustable heights. Models with backend wheels are available if you cannot lift a conventional walker.

Crutches, which are available mostly in lightweight aluminum or wood, require more strength than walkers to use. Underarm models provide better support, while forearm models are advised if you have reasonably good coordination and arm strength. Crutches may have adjustable height and arm lengths. If improperly sized and used over a long period of time, they can place needless stress on muscles and nerves and create problems. The type of handgrip provided is important for both safety and function.

Canes are useful if you need assistance walking, but have good balance. If balance is poor, stick to a walker to avoid falls. Proper height and handle are important considerations for good support. Canes are available with special four-pronged bases to provide greater stability.

Oxygen at Home

If you have a heart or lung condition, you may require special oxygen support.

Dr. Thomas Petty, past president of the American College of Chest Physicians, has seen home oxygen therapy produce dramatic results. "Some of my chronic respiratory disease patients who had been resigned to lives in nursing homes have gone hunting, fishing, and camping at altitudes of 10,000 feet with the help of oxygen systems that they took along in mobile vans," states Dr. Petty in the *American Lung Association Bulletin.* "A 62-year-old homemaker with emphysema who had suffered a heart attack and had been hospitalized was able to go back to taking complete care of her home." Dr. Petty believes that with proper home oxygen therapy, "many emphysema patients are able to live at home, instead of a nursing home. And most of these patients can even manage without the help of a homemaker." Strong testimony indeed to the wonders of respiratory care at home.

Home oxygen therapy, which must be physician-prescribed, has three equipment systems:

- *Oxygen tanks* store oxygen under high pressure in cylinders.
- *Liquid oxygen systems* store oxygen in reservoirs in a liquid state. As room heat vaporizes the liquid gas, it passes through a thin nasal tube and delivers high-concentration oxygen. This system can be used to fill small, portable units for greater mobility.
- *Oxygen concentrators* separate oxygen from other gases present in normal air and then deliver high oxygen concentrations to the user.

No one system is right for all patients, so sound professional advice and a reputable dealer are critical. Often a doctor will just prescribe "oxygen," leaving the choice of equipment system to the dealer. If you have chosen a reputable dealer, you should get the best system for you.

Let's take the case of a severe headache sufferer who requires oxygen a few times a week for a couple of hours a day. In such cases, unethical dealers have recommended and installed costly liquid oxygen systems. Left untouched between occasional uses, the liquid oxygen soon evaporates and needs constant replacement. This method is designed specifically for patients requiring heavy daily or continuous oxygen use. Therefore, a tank which can be used only when needed and keeps oxygen indefinitely would be much less costly and far more appropriate.

Avoid such problems by discussing the cost and quality pros and cons of oxygen or other respiratory devices with your doctor and respiratory therapist. Don't hesitate to mention cost, so your doctor won't recommend a more costly unit when perhaps a less expensive device might do.

If you require an oxygen concentrator, some dealers will supply a portable backup oxygen unit at no cost. Also, make sure you register with your local utility company as a priority electrical user in the event of power failure.

Incontinence Products

According to market analysts Frost and Sullivan, incontinence product sales in 1987 are expected to exceed $1.5 billion, outselling all other kinds of medical equipment and products. Advertising may suggest diapers and special undergarments are the answer to wetting problems. But medicine says many causes of incontinence are correctable.

Dr. Neil Resnick, a urologist and specialist in geriatrics, Harvard Medical School, offers this message of hope to consumers. "Incontinence is transient in many patients; and with those it isn't, at least a third may be cured, another third can be dramatically improved, and another third can be improved significantly."

So if you or someone you care about is incontinent,

practice health care consumerism. Don't accept this as a natural part of illness or growing old, and just go out and buy disposables. See a doctor first, preferably a urology specialist.

If you need incontinence products, which can be expensive, try generics. If you don't see them about, ask. Most dealers carry generic brands.

The Dealer Difference

Who you buy from is almost as important as what you buy. The sheer number of dealers who provide medical equipment and supplies may overwhelm you. On top of the many traditional equipment dealers listed in the Yellow Pages, you can also choose among the many hospitals, home care agencies, local pharmacies, and household retailers that have joined this business. For simplicity's sake here, we'll use the term "dealers" to refer to this group as a whole.

What should you look for first when you need equipment? In a *Coordinator* magazine survey, hospital discharge planners, home care agency personnel, and other professionals who regularly order DME for patients cited service—not cost—as their number one priority.

Why is service stressed? "When your oxygen equipment alarm goes off in the middle of the night," said one agency nurse, "it's the service that counts most, not a marginal difference in cost." Always keep service and quality in mind first. Your local pharmacy may offer convenience, but as with all dealers, weigh service against the price.

Patient service staffs of organizations such as the American Cancer Society, United Cerebral Palsy, or the Muscular Dystrophy Association may help you to identify dealers with a top-notch reputation for service. Get several recommendations from professionals—therapists, discharge planners, home care agency personnel, senior center staff. Remember to ask professionals *why* they recommend the dealer. You don't want simply a name. Also ask other consumers who may have purchased medical equipment for advice.

As a safeguard, double-check any dealers under consideration with local consumer organizations such as the Better Business Bureau or city or county consumer affairs offices. This industry operates almost without any consumer safeguards, save those that might apply to *any* household retailer. Put another way, this means that without careful consumer checking, you can easily select a "lemon."

If you are on Medicare, you can contact your local social security office or state or local agency on aging to find dealers that accept Medicare assignment.

Should you rely on the "dealer" hospital or home care agency for equipment? This option can offer convenience that may be important to you. Nevertheless, you would be wise to contact at least one other reputable dealer for comparison, especially on costly items. Also, review this dealer option as carefully as you would any other, using the consumer guidelines that follow.

What to Ask

As with choosing a home care agency, you must be prepared to ask questions. Look elsewhere when any dealer tunes out to your questions, acts put off, or tries to intimidate you with a fast sales pitch or technical "equipment" jargon. The following questions are repeated as a checklist in the resource section, so you can compare dealers.

Medicare Certification

If you are a Medicare consumer, inquire about this first. No matter how good a dealer is, you won't be reimbursed by Medicare unless the dealer is Medicare-certified and has a Medicare provider number.

Customer Service

- Is the dealer a full-service provider? You may prefer to work with one professional dealer who can handle all your needs.
- How soon can deliveries be made?
- Is delivery, repair, and maintenance service available 24 hours a day, seven days a week if needed?

In the case of a hospital bed, round-the-clock services may not be critical to you. However, these services can be very important when oxygen or home nutritional equipment supplies, for example, are necessary.

- Will the dealer assist with inventory control? Professional dealers help monitor regularly needed supplies such as oxygen so you are not caught short.
- Can the dealer supply your needs if you must travel? If so, how?
- What happens if repairs are needed that cannot be done on the spot?
- Will the dealer supply equipment replacement or loan at little or no cost?
- After the equipment warranty expires, what service will the dealer provide?
- Does the dealership do its own repairs and maintenance?

The dealer has less control over solving repair or maintenance problems if these services are farmed out to maintenance companies via contract. The more complex the equipment, the more important this answer becomes. For example, a hand-held inhalator, like a hair dryer, seldom breaks down. A ventilator often requires special servicing.

- Will dealer personnel make free in-home visits when necessary to aid in proper equipment selection? To train you and/or family in proper equipment use and care?

Often it's necessary for a dealer professional (a physical or respiratory therapist) to evaluate your needs, given your unique home environment, so the most appropriate equipment can be recommended. A tiny sickroom, for example, may not comfortably accommodate certain equipment, or electrical outlets may be poorly placed. A wheelchair or bed may not fit through a doorway. There may be many special considerations which you, as a layperson, may not think of beforehand. Therefore, an in-home visit can better assess your needs. Top-notch dealers do this, and without charge.

If you are hospitalized or in a skilled nursing facility,

professional staff may help guide your selection. The home care agency should consider any needs you may have for medical equipment and supplies when it conducts its first in-home assessment. But how specific the agency's recommendations may be depends on the experience of its assessor. To make the best choice, your physician and the agency often rely on sound dealer advice provided by a professional staff familiar with your situation.

Once that equipment arrives, its use and care are at least as important as the choice of equipment. Again, the services of dealer professionals may be needed so you learn to use the equipment properly and to your best advantage. In the high-tech or special rehab equipment area, ongoing assistance may be needed. Proper use and care of such equipment cannot be learned through a one-visit follow-up.

Personnel

- What kind of training and experience does the dealer require of personnel who service equipment? The professional staff?
- Are personnel regularly employed, or part-time only?

Look for dealers who employ well-trained equipment technicians and service personnel. Proper technician training is provided by schools run by equipment manufacturers or the military, and by biomedical equipment technician programs offered by community colleges. Professionals such as respiratory therapists or nutritionists should hold professional credentials in their field. Nurses who advise on equipment *must* have special training.

As a rule of thumb, you are more likely to get better service from a dealer who employs at least some service and professional staff (when needed) on a full-time basis. Full-time professional staff, for example, can help trouble-shoot the day-to-day questions or problems that patients may sometimes have even after their initial orientation period is over. Dealers who employ only part-time professionals can honestly state to prospective customers that they do provide professional follow-up consultation. However, often this initial consultation service is a one-time only visit, with little provision for ongoing help.

Costs and Payment Terms

- Are delivery, repair, and maintenance included in the equipment cost or rental fee? If so, subject to what conditions or limits? Is there an "after hours" charge when service is needed evenings or on weekends?
- Is there any charge for an in-home visit by dealer staff to recommend equipment? For setup or installation, training in equipment use, or consultation?
- Is payment due upon delivery, or can you be billed later?
- Can you pay by check or credit card? In installments? Are there interest charges? Are all bills itemized and detailed?
- Can equipment be returned for full credit or exchanged? What conditions apply?
- Does the dealer offer a free trial period? (Some do provide at least 24 hours free trial.) What conditions apply? Can you apply rental fees to purchase price? Some companies will allow you to rent for a month to try equipment, and apply the rental to the purchase price.
- Will the dealer accept assignment of insurance benefits (Medicare, Medicaid, or private insurance) and allow you to pay just the difference?

The answer to this key question may decide your choice of a dealer if you are on a tight budget. Once you meet any applicable deductible, assignment keeps money in your pocket (see page 183).

Watch out for dealers that expect or demand cash at the door. Professional dealers never use such strong-arm tactics.

When you look for a dealer, realize that the best companies will go to great lengths for their customers. Therapist Terri Guild, Home Respiratory Care (Worcester, MA) explains: "We had one patient who was on oxygen, which Medicare disallowed, because of her blood test results. Despite the test, I knew that if we removed that oxygen she would be in the emergency room within a few hours. Instead of taking the oxygen out, we went back to her doctor for more medical documentation. Then back to Medicare. We went back and forth for six months while waiting to get paid. Finally, a Medicare review accepted the patient for needed oxygen therapy."

Other Hints

The dealer's answers to your questions on customer service, personnel, cost, and payment may be all the information you need to make a sound choice. As a prudent shopper, there are some additional measures you can take before you decide.

If you can, drop by the dealer's equipment showroom (or ask someone to do so on your behalf). See firsthand if the dealer offers a good selection of up-to-date equipment in clean, ready-to-use condition.

Contact the customer references the dealer provides. Confirm with them the dealer's statements about customer service, payment terms, and so on, and their overall satisfaction. Phone after hours or on weekends any after-hour service numbers that the dealer maintains. Note whether you reach company personnel or an answering service. If the dealer relies on a service, leave your telephone number and time how quickly company personnel get back to you.

COSTS AND PAYMENTS

The price list in the accompanying table will give you some idea of the cost of some common DME and supplies. It is based on Medicare allowable charges.

Costs can vary a lot among dealers. Deluxe versions of standard items may cost more than twice as much. If you need high-ticket items, it can certainly pay to shop for price; but shop only among professional dealers. If you need low-cost medical supplies, price can also become a factor for frequently used items. To make this point about price, one Chicago doctor examined equipment and supply costs for his high-tech respiratory patients. He found differences in equip-

AVERAGE COST OF COMMONLY USED MEDICAL EQUIPMENT

Equipment	Rental (Month)	Purchase
Bedpan	NA	$ 9.00
Canes:		
Standard	$ 2.00	16.00
Quad or three prong	4.40	37.50
Commode chair (standard or mobile with pail or pan)	18.00	74.50
Crutches:		
Forearm	5.50	40.00
Underarm	2.50	25.00
Enteral pump	100.00	NUP
Heat lamp (standard)	4.00	40.00
Heat pad (standard)	1.70	17.00
Hospital bed (standard)	54.39*	444.85*
(Florida)	65.00	650.00
Oxygen equipment:		
Concentrator	290.00	2,425.00
Liquid	79.62*	NUP
Portable (used with concentrator)	40.00	45.00
Oxygen:		
Gaseous per cubic foot	NA	.12
Liquid per pound	NA	1.44
Patient lift (hydraulic with seat with sling)	60.00	685.00
Seat lift chair (easy lift chair)	85.00	840.00
Side-rails for bed:		
Half length	16.00	109.30
Full length	23.00	109.30
Suction pump	45.00	235.00
TENS (two or four lead to stimulate one or two areas for pain relief)	75.00	499.00
Trapeze bars (patient helpers, free-standing with grab bar)	25.00	155.00
Urinal (male standard)	NA	6.75
Walker	16.87*	57.24*
Wheelchair (standard)	28.76*	294.48*

Note: Most costs are based on 1984 Medicare prevailing allowable charges for the State of Florida. The prevailing charge is the amount which is within the range of charges most frequently and widely charged for an item in a given locale.
* Denotes *national* average Medicare allowable charges for an item as identified by the Health Care Financing Administration. DME dealers may charge more for these items than the allowable charge. Medicare pays 80% of the allowable charge.
NA: Not applicable.
NUP: Not usually purchased.

ment costs of 200 to 300 percent among dealers, and 300 percent for disposable medical supplies. Consider the effect of cost on a small disposable at 30 cents per item versus 98 cents should you use hundreds a month.

Whenever you need expensive equipment, always seek professional, nondealer advice from your doctor and appropriate hospital or home care agency staff.

In the doctor's investigation mentioned above, he found that one dealer's equipment plan totaled $40,000. Working with the hospital staff, the doctor developed a plan priced at $24,000 that was also simpler and safer.

Buy or Rent?

Respiratory equipment, hospital beds and wheelchairs, canes, or any DME you can buy can be rented for a monthly fee. In some cases, renting equipment may be a better option than buying outright. To decide, first have your doctor or therapist estimate how long you will need the equipment. Then compare your total expected rental costs against the purchase price. In many cases, if equipment is short term (10 months or less), renting may be more economical. Rental usually covers basic maintenance and repairs, while the purchase price may not.

Before you invest in any equipment, thoroughly investigate the warranty and your insurance coverage. Medicare, Medicaid, and most insurance plans with home care or outpatient benefits cover medical equipment and supplies, but certain rules apply. Find out in advance whether the products you require will qualify.

Also, some insurers may require that you rent rather than purchase equipment, even if purchase will be more economical. Others may require you to buy if it is cheaper. Some may leave the choice up to you.

Clearly it's important to "know thy insurance" first so you can factor in any special conditions, plus the size of the insurance reimbursement, when you consider equipment costs.

Outlined below are general insurance questions and guidelines, with a special focus on the Medicare rules for equipment and supplies. Other insurers often pattern their DME policies after Medicare, so this information generally applies even if you are non-Medicare.

INSURANCE COVERAGE

How Much Does Insurance Pay?

Most insurance will not pay for 100 percent of the equipment cost. In Medicare, DME and supplies are both covered under Medicare Part B, medical insurance. After you meet the annual Part B deductible, Medicare will pay 80 percent of the *approved* purchase or rental price of these items.

Most insurers use a "reasonable" or "allowable" charge system upon which DME payments are based. However, private insurers are usually more generous than Medicare in what charges they deem reasonable.

With Medicare, the approved price often falls below the actual price tag. The approved price is based on the average reasonable cost charged by DME dealers in your area for the standard "no frills" version of the item. For example, the upgraded wheelchair you may wish to purchase may carry a $500 price tag. The 1984 approved Medicare charges for a standard wheelchair average only $294.48. If you have met the deductible, Medicare will pay $235.58 (80% × $294.48) toward the wheelchair's purchase, bringing your out-of-pocket payment to $264.42. On a rental basis, the chair may go for $50 per month. Medicare averages only $28.76 a month rental and would pay 80 percent, or $23, toward the monthly fee. Again, you pay the difference.

If you want to know in advance how much Medicare allows, you can ask the dealer, who should have the information on hand. Or if you prefer, you can check with Medicare directly in most locales. Get the dealer's Medicare-certified number and the equipment code, then call Medicare

Part B's 800 telephone number (ask your operator or your local social security office). The Medicare clerk can usually quote the allowable charge.

What Products Are Covered?

Don't assume that *any* home care product on the market will be covered under Medicare or your insurance policy. Some items will not qualify even on your doctor's orders.

For insurance purposes, durable medical equipment must be for use in your home and: (1) primarily and customarily used for medical purposes and generally not useful in the absence of illness or injury; (2) medically necessary and reasonable. Let's look at what insurers mean.

Medically Useful

Wheelchairs, hospital beds, breathing machines, commodes, and so on are considered medical by their very nature. Other items used generally for nonmedical purposes are not covered even when they serve a direct medical purpose.

Take the case of a heart patient whose doctor has prescribed a sickroom air conditioner. The unit keeps room temperature low, which reduces body fluid loss and helps maintain proper fluid balance. Though the unit serves an important medical function, most insurers, including Medicare, would not consider it "medical" equipment and won't cover it. Similar items—room heaters, humidifiers, electric air cleaners—which help control the home environment do not qualify as medical equipment.

Physical fitness equipment such as an exercycle is not usually covered, nor are useful safety home devices such as preset oxygen units, safety grab bars, and first-aid kits. Medicare even considers equipment such as speech teaching machines or Braille training texts "nonmedical."

Items used primarily for the patient's comfort or convenience are definite Medicare no-nos. These include elevators, posture chairs, and cushion lift chairs.

It's true these items may have general medical value. A lift, for example, can get stroke patients on their feet more

quickly. But Medicare still rules this as comfort and convenience, although some other insurers might not.

Exceptions to this rule exist and are worth noting. An item
such as a seat lift that does not normally qualify as DME
may be covered if the doctor clearly states why the item
serves a definite *treatment* purpose in your case and then
supervises its use during treatment. Thus, a seat lift might be
covered if you have severe arthritis of the hip or knee or a
nerve-muscle disease, provided the doctor states why it will
improve your health or prevent decline.

Likewise, a pressure or water mattress, which Medicare
generally disallows as an anti-bedsore precaution device, can
be covered when prescribed for someone who already has
bedsores or is at very high risk of developing them—for
example, a bedridden diabetic. In either case, the device
would have a recognized treatment purpose. Heat lamps,
normally considered a soothing comfort device, can be covered
when the doctor explains why heat therapy is needed.

Medically Necessary and Reasonable

Though an item unquestionably is medical equipment, it
won't be covered unless it is necessary for treating or improving
your condition. Therefore, not every home care patient
qualifies for the insured use of a hospital bed. In most cases
your doctor's prescription is all that is needed to prove that
equipment is medically necessary.

"Reasonable" is not so clearly defined. Sophisticated medical equipment such as certain respiratory therapy devices
may not be covered by insurance on the basis that they are
meant for hospital use, not home use, and therefore are not
"reasonable."

Medical Supplies

Covered medical supplies include those products which are
essential to the operation of DME—for example, oxygen for
an oxygen pump. But medications that may be administered
by a machine such as a respiratory device are still classed as
drugs. You must check your policy on drug coverage. Drugs
are not usually covered by Medicare.

Also check your policy carefully for a definition of "supplies" as well as "equipment." Sometimes a product you may think of as a supply, such as an indwelling catheter, may be considered a prosthetic device.

Supplies like needles, syringes, and surgical dressings that may be ordered by your doctor in connection with your treatment are usually covered by Medicare or other insurance. However, when *you* purchase adhesive tape, antiseptics, or other common household medical supplies, Medicare or other insurance will not pay. But if these items serve a recognized purpose in your treatment and are provided by a home care agency, they may be covered. Even general hygienic aids such as soaps and shampoos or comfort or beauty aids like baby lotion or skin softeners or powders may be Medicare-covered. For example, such items may be needed for treatment if you are suffering from a skin condition. The key to coverage lies in: (1) your condition, (2) your physician's prescribed treatment, and (3) the *agency's* provision of supplies.

Do Other Restrictions Apply?

For any insurance, this question is important to answer. Medicare, for example, has one *essential* restriction. *You must buy or rent only from Medicare-certified dealers.* Here are some other restrictions to check.

Equipment repairs, maintenance, replacement, and delivery
   Insurers like Medicare normally pay for necessary repairs and replacement of parts such as hoses and mouthpieces when equipment is purchased. When items are rented, Medicare, for example, expects these costs plus maintenance to be built into the rental fee. If you buy, normal maintenance such as routine cleaning, regulating, and testing are *not* covered. Medicare reasons that you as the owner or a family member should be able to handle the maintenance with the help of the standard owner's manual that comes with equipment. However, unless you are a mechanic or engineer, you may find such "routine" maintenance impossible. This restriction is a prime reason why many consumers opt to rent.

Delivery charges are covered under Medicare for rentals or purchases, provided this is the dealer's standard policy for *all* customers and the general practice of other dealers in your area.

Date when DME coverage begins

Don't get caught on a technicality. Have equipment delivered to your home only when you are sure your coverage has begun. Some insurers, including Medicaid, require prior approval *before* delivery.

Dollar limits

Medicare sets no ceiling on the number of items that may be purchased or their total cost in a calendar year, provided all other conditions are met. Some insurance policies may limit overall DME expenses.

MONEY-SAVING TIPS

You can save money if you remember that the rules that govern insurance reimbursement do not govern your income tax. Check Chapter 12 on medical deductions for equipment and supplies.

Once you have no use for the equipment you've purchased, it's still yours to keep even if it was paid for fully or in part by insurance. This means you can sell it and pocket the money or donate it and receive yet another tax deduction.

If you need medical equipment but cannot afford the sticker price, don't be discouraged. The following suggestions may provide a solution to your problem.

Ask the dealer to accept assignment of insurance as payment in full.

Most dealers do not routinely accept assignment as payment in full, but many will help on a case-by-case basis when such help is needed. Medicare may waive the 20 percent beneficiary charge if dealers show that a good-faith effort to collect this portion from the patient has been made.

Consider usable secondhand equipment.

Under a little-known Medicare benefit, Medicare will pay 100 percent for used and reconditioned equipment. However, to qualify the purchase price must be at least 25 percent less than the allowed charge for the same equipment when new. It also must carry the same warranty.

The American Cancer Society, the Salvation Army, the Red Cross, and other community organizations often have equipment available for free loan or at nominal charges. Some home care agencies, such as visiting nurse organizations, may also run loan programs, sometimes called loan "closets."

Dealers themselves sometimes maintain a small supply of used, reconditioned equipment. You may not see it on display. Don't be afraid to ask. Check this equipment carefully to see that it works properly. Don't be put off by cosmetic problems such as dirt or scratches. Do ask about any warranty that may be available. Discuss what happens should repairs be needed. Manufacturers often redesign equipment every few years. When they do, they may stop producing internal working parts in older models, making repairs difficult.

Ask about discounts when you pay in full.

The paperwork for billing and insurance collection adds to equipment costs. Many dealers stated they will give consumers varying discounts up to 20 percent if they can avoid billing, which reduces the dealer's cost.

Ask for assistance from home care or social service agencies.

Agency personnel are the experts in helping others. They know the sources of local assistance that may be available and can often approach a dealer in your behalf. Dealers are often willing to help when approached this way because of goodwill and the possibility of future business.

Manufacturers sometimes help too, and agency professionals are more likely to know about those that do. Grant Airmass Corporation, for example, offers low-cost air mattresses to patients who have, or are at risk of developing, bedsores through its Needy Patient Record Program. Grant provides an 83 percent discount on its PCA bedsore-preventing pad to financially needy patients without insurance.

To apply, a doctor must certify the patient's medical and financial need; but there are no hard and fast income rules that define financial need. Patients not wishing to claim financial need but who have no insurance can receive a 51 percent discount for participating. Once enrolled, the patient's obligation is minimal. Patients need only keep simple records on their skin condition while using the device and report this information to the company periodically. About 600 patients are now enrolled nationwide. For information, contact: Grant Airmass Corporation, 1010 Washington Blvd, Stamford, CT 06901, (800) 243–5237.

Ask health professionals about lower-cost alternatives.

An occupational, physical, or respiratory therapist or other professional can often suggest low-cost equipment substitutes or ways to adapt existing home items that may serve your purpose. For example, adjustable handrails are available that can be attached to a regular home bed. Depending on your condition, this could eliminate the need to purchase or rent a hospital bed.

Keep receipts for all transactions and fill out all warranties properly.

In order to qualify for insurance or warranty-covered repairs or maintenance, you may have to submit proof of purchase or the warranty. Always keep these items as long as the equipment is in your possession.

Submit detailed insurance forms.

Many consumers have to wait needlessly for prior approval for equipment or for insurance reimbursement because forms are incomplete. Make sure your claim clearly states:

- Your diagnosis and prognosis (expected health outlook)
- The reason why equipment is needed *medically*
- How long it is needed (number of months)
- Your doctor's name, address, *and* signature (or that of the physician prescribing the equipment if different)

—14—

Emergency Response Systems: Electronic Live-ins and No-Cost Alternatives

When Mary Calkins of Bethesda, Maryland, accidentally tumbled from her wheelchair one morning, she fell helpless to the floor. Unable to move and living alone, you might have expected her to panic. Instead, she simply pressed on a tiny wireless transmitter that hung around her neck like a pendant, and within a minute help was on the way.

Mrs. Calkins' pushbutton device is the first link in a personal emergency response system aptly named Lifeline. The device, when pushed, triggers a home communicator, which is a small unit attached to the telephone. The communicator automatically dials a hospital (or other health facility) that is staffed by trained coordinators day and night. When the signal is received at the hospital emergency response center, a simple emergency procedure goes into effect.

- The coordinator retrieves key patient information presented on a card or computer screen which lists the patient's name, address, phone number, medical condition, and "responders." These are nearby family, friends, or neighbors, or anyone the patient selects in advance who will respond promptly when called.
- The hospital emergency receiver equipment sends a return signal to the home that sets off flashing lights and a beeping sound. This alerts the Lifeline user that help is coming.
- The coordinator immediately calls the user to assess what

is wrong. If the phone is not answered, the coordinator calls the first responder listed.

- The responder immediately goes to the user's home to give help or call an ambulance if necessary. (In Mrs. Calkins' case, a neighbor came and quickly helped her back into her wheelchair.) The responder pushes the reset button on the Lifeline unit. This alerts the coordinator that help has arrived.

Lifeline has a backup timer set at 12- or 24-hour periods that will automatically dial the hospital in case the user becomes unconscious or is otherwise unable to trigger the system manually. Each time the phone is used, the backup system automatically resets. If the phone is not used during the time period, the user simply resets it manually, signaling that everything at home is okay.

Psychologist Andrew Dibner, Lifeline creator, started the ERS revolution. Lifeline, as the oldest and most widely used system, is currently available through some 1,000 participating hospitals. But many competitors are on the market, and the emergency response system (ERS) field is expanding and changing rapidly.

WHO USES ERS?

If you think that an ERS is effective only for the elderly, you may be surprised to hear that even infants are among Lifeline subscribers. Many families with children such as those at risk for sudden infant death syndrome (SIDS), who are on special monitoring devices, use an ERS to bring immediate emergency help.

Studies of Lifeline users find the highest group reporting medical emergencies are not the elderly, but those in the 30- to 39-year-old group, whom Dr. Dibner reports are usually "very ill or disabled," with conditions such as severe multiple sclerosis or diabetes. The majority of subscribers, however, are 75 years or older, and are mostly women.

THE VALUE OF ERS

The benefits of an ERS are undeniable. A government-funded study of Lifeline users, most of whom live alone, found that with Lifeline, they felt less anxious and more satisfied about their living arrangements and even slept better than nonusers of similar age and health.

Benefits also extend to concerned family. In a *New York Times* interview, one Lifeline customer, Mrs. Helen Emons, age 86, explains: "It gives them [family] peace of mind. Before, they never wanted to go away for the weekend." Dr. Dibner reports that most people become Lifeline users at the insistence of their families. "Before Lifeline," Dr. Dibner told me, "family members would have to call their loved ones several times a day or sometimes take off suddenly from work if there was no answer at home. An ERS eliminates such problems." Lifeline also proved a money-saver, with users averaging only 1 day of nursing home care compared to 13 days of nursing home care for nonusers. A recent Lifeline survey found it shortened hospital stays as well as reducing nursing home use. With today's hospital and nursing home rates, this would mean an annual savings of over $2,500 per user. The results are so encouraging that legislation has been sponsored to provide these services to select patients through Medicare.

For most consumers, the psychological comfort that an ERS brings is the overriding factor in the decision to use one of these devices. While designed primarily as a medical emergency response system, ERS has wide application. "One subscriber," Dr. Dibner recalls, "pushed her button when her pipes broke and water started flooding her apartment. In New York it's been effective against crime. A user is lying in bed and hears someone trying to break in, so she pushes the button. Of course someone will call back, but in the meanwhile the beeper sounds which can frighten intruders away."

Mrs. Emons used Lifeline when she accidentally became trapped inside her stalled car halfway out of the garage. "It was five below zero and there was no point in honking because everyone was indoors." She pushed her button, which summoned her nextdoor neighbor.

TWO-WAY SYSTEMS

Lifeline is a one-way ERS, but two-way communications systems like Communi-Care, which bring an added dimension to the ERS concept, are available. When triggered, these systems link parties directly. The respond center does not have to return the call.

For Ms. S, a young, West Coast client of Staff Builders, a national home care firm that owns Communi-Care, this ERS meant a steady reduced need for home care. Following an accident, Ms. S., a paraplegic victim, required 24-hour in-home attendant care. With Communi-Care backup, she reduced her care first to eight hours, then to four. During her adjustment to greater independence, Ms. S. triggered her transmitter whenever she was unsure about an activity such as transferring from her bed to her wheelchair. Once activated, her "intercom" communicator telephone unit put her in voice-to-voice contact with home care assistants at the response center. The assistants stayed on the ERS, offering support, encouragement, and advice, until the move was successfully made. Ms. S. felt reassured knowing help would come immediately should a problem occur.

Communi-Care customers are encouraged to call daily and get to know the response center staff. For Mrs. L. of Ohio, another Staff Builders client, this person-to-person feature proved critical.

"What happened," said Staff Builders' Diane Hovan, "was that the Home Care Assistants noticed Mrs. L. had begun to sound very depressed. Fortunately, this client called in every day, so they were able to observe that instead of improving, the sadness was deepening day after day. At that point, they suggested to Mrs. L. that she needed professional help. With her consent, the Home Care Assistants notified us to alert the local consultants for her."

Mrs. L., in discussing the incident later, told the response center staff: "Whether you know it or not, you saved my life." Mrs. L. was indeed contemplating suicide.

Of course, in the event of any emergency in a two-way system, staff can offer comfort until help arrives.

Communi-Care stresses the personal aspects of its system. "About 98% of the calls we receive," says Communi-Care's Thomas Quinn, "are for psychosocial reasons. Customers will often call late at night when they feel anxious or alone. We want people to call daily so they become familiar with the equipment and will feel comfortable with it in an emergency." Lengthy conversations aren't encouraged, but people can check in many times for a brief chat. Communi-Care customers and their family receive, via Staff Builders, a small, folksy newsletter each month that has human interest stories about Communi-Care staff and users. "We try to link people together. It's sort of a family of users," notes Mr. Quinn. Another plus to the system is its portability. You can virtually pack it along with your clothes if you go on a trip. It can be installed easily at your new location, whether it is a hotel room or a relative's house or a vacation site. All you need do is notify the response center that you are leaving, and then check in upon arrival, giving them your new list of responders.

Not all two-way communication systems are this people-minded. Many, like VoicEmitter, do a good job providing emergency response, but do not want customer call-in except on a once-a-week or emergency basis.

STAND-ALONE SYSTEMS

Lifeline and the two-way communications systems are digital systems. They send an electronic signal over the telephone line which is picked up by a computer at the response center and translated (decoded) into a message identifying the user.

Also available are stand-alone systems, which operate without a response center. When activated, they either sound an alarm (like a burglar alarm system), or more commonly automatically dial preprogrammed emergency telephone numbers and send a prerecorded voice distress message.

AT&T's Medical Alert, for example, will dial a first number, and if no one answers, dial a second. The system continues dialing, alternating between the two numbers, until it gets a response. Stand-alone systems may dial up to five numbers; some have a preset timer feature.

These systems have obvious drawbacks. For the alarm-type devices to be effective, you need someone close enough to hear the alarm and know what to do. With all stand-alone systems, you can't be sure your distress call has been received and that help is on the way. If your responders are not at home or their phone lines are busy, help may be greatly delayed.

If you are interested in these systems, check if you can program the numbers yourself. Some require special equipment; sometimes the dealer must program the unit, usually for an extra fee.

FALSE ALARMS

On any ERS, false alarms can occur. You may accidentally touch off the system, or sometimes a power surge or thunderstorm may trigger it. With a preset timer you may simply forget to push the reset button, thereby creating a false alarm.

While embarrassing, false alarms can become a real problem if your ERS automatically alerts the fire department, police, or ambulance-rescue squad. A one-time false alarm may be tolerated, but frequent false alarms may cost you a fine or false-alarm fee. Some states now prohibit consumers from contacting municipal emergency services directly via an ERS stand-alone system. However, two-way systems or a carefully controlled one-way system like Lifeline do not pose such problems.

AVAILABILITY AND COST

Not all the ERSs that have been developed are available nationwide. Some systems like Lifeline are available only through participating local hospitals, home care agencies, or other health providers. With hospitals seeking to discharge Medicare patients earlier than ever before, it is expected that more hospitals will offer patients an ERS on a temporary basis. These hospitals purchase the response center equipment and individual home units, which are then leased to patients. Leasing fees vary.

For Lifeline users, most hospital monthly fees hover in the nominal $10 to $15 range, with some charging as little as $5 or nothing to certain patients, or higher fees up to $25. There may be an installation fee; but if so, it is also usually nominal.

Some systems like Communi-Care or the AT&T Medical Alert may be secured through participating hospitals or agencies or obtained by direct consumer purchase or lease through the company involved or its dealers.

Unless you will need equipment indefinitely, the least expensive option is to lease an ERS through a participating health care provider. Insurance generally does not cover these systems. Purchase or leasing costs vary widely with maintenance, and installation fees are often extra. (On two-way systems, you must still pay a monthly fee; with stand-alones, there is no monthly fee.)

Stand-alones that offer you less security and service were once a less expensive option. However, today stand-alones range from AT&T's 1984 suggested retail price of $250 to Basic Telecommunications Corporation's AbilityPhone, which has lots of special features and costs $2,700. Communi-Care's two-way system costs $525 to own and $350 to lease annually. Consumers who want to use VoicEmitter's effective two-way system pay a modest one-time $99 fee plus $30 monthly for its service.

Standard digital systems like Communi-Care should not

add to your electric bill. Most, for example, use energy equivalent to a 30-watt lightbulb. Phone bills are unaffected, since calls are forwarded through an 800 number.

WHAT TO LOOK FOR

Every ERS claims total security and service. Be wary. Many companies are new and may fall short on their promises. Many traditional security alarm dealers are entering this market. They may not provide the kind of health emergency backup system you desire. If you buy or rent an ERS, get solid answers to the following questions:

- What transmitter styles are available? What is their size? Can the transmitter become wet? Transmitters come in around-the-neck devices, wristwatch styles, belt clip-ons, pocket slip-ins, a signaling pen, or the kind you must carry from place to place. Breath control units are available. Sizes vary, but state-of-the-art devices are small (2 × 2 inches or less) and lightweight.

    Some transmitters are *hazards* when wet; others are perfectly water-safe. Since many falls occur in the bathroom, water safety is a good factor to consider in your choice.
- What is the transmitter range? These vary from about 60 feet to 750 feet. Consider the size of your home and your mobility.
- Will you require only one communication unit, or separate extensions for multiple phones?
- Can the system be triggered even if the phone is off the hook? (Good systems can be.)
- Can the ERS be triggered in the event you cannot activate it manually? If so, how?
- How does the ERS guard against and handle false alarms?
- What are the standard emergency procedures? How will you know if help is on the way? What happens if none of your responders can be reached?
- Who staffs the emergency response center? How have they been trained? Is medical backup available for advice

or screening? Superior ERSs use regular, trained, supervised staff, paid or volunteer, who know how to screen calls and respond to emergencies. A nurse or other appropriate health professional should be available 24 hours to assist as needed.

- What provisions have been made to ensure 24-hour center coverage despite weather or power failures? Adequate phone lines and staff to handle all incoming calls?
- Who "controls" the response center? The hospital or agency? The ERS company? Is the response center service contracted out? When the hospital, agency, or company that provides the services controls the response center system, you have less chance of errors. Be cautious when an ERS company subcontracts this service.
- How much patient information can be stored? How is confidentiality protected? Are calls recorded? In addition to basic identifying data and the available responders, some systems can store important patient information such as diagnoses, medications, and special problems. All information should be strictly confidential, with incoming calls recorded, as is done in any 911 emergency system.
- On two-way systems, are nonemergency calls allowed?
- What kind of volume control is available for the hearing impaired?
- What happens in the event of in-home power problems? How can you know your equipment is in working condition (i.e., batteries still working)?
- Is the system portable, or can you link into the system if you are away from home for an extended time?
- Are special features available? Many systems have a wide range of special features, usually for additional fees. Some use sensors to detect gas leaks or unusually high or low temperatures; some also detect the unusual absence of motion in a room or failure to use common household appliances like a refrigerator, which could signal a problem. In the near future, key body functions such as heart rate or pacemaker activity will be linked to ERSs.
- What does it cost to buy? To rent or lease? Is there a separate charge for the transmitter?
- Is there a charge for repairs? For maintenance? For

installation? What is the monthly fee? How long is the warranty? Does it cover labor and replacement parts? How often is equipment checked and serviced?

- Who repairs the system? Where? How fast? Reports of ERS repair problems are surfacing. Most problems involve independent ERS dealers who do not take responsibility for repairs—nor does the parent company, despite the warranty. The better companies will supply a replacement that same day or overnight so service will not be seriously interrupted.

NO-COST COMMUNITY ALERT SYSTEMS

As an alternative to a regular ERS, you can use community telephone reassurance programs if they are available. These provide for a regular, prescheduled call to check in on the frail, elderly, or homebound. If no one can be reached, a backup system goes into effect to make sure that everything is all right.

Similar in purpose is the U.S. Postal Service Carrier Alert program, which works in cooperation with local community agencies such as the Red Cross. An information card for each participant is filed with the agency. Once registered, the carrier keeps special watch over the participant's mail pickup. If someone fails to pick up mail as usual, the carrier alerts the agency, which then takes action. The program is not yet available nationwide, but most carriers will informally watch out for their customers, if so requested. Contact your local post office about Carrier Alert.

CONSUMER ERS FOLLOW-UP

For information on ERS mentioned in this chapter, contact:

AbilityPhone
Basic Telecommunications Corporation
4414 E Harmony Rd
Ft. Collins, CO 80525
(303) 226–4688

Communi-Care
Americare Health Services
112 E 42 St
New York, NY 10168
(212) 986-9866

Medical Alert
AT&T Special Needs Center
2001 Route 46
Parsippany, NJ 07054
(800) 233-1222, TDD (800) 833-3232

Lifeline
Lifeline Systems
One Arsenal Market Place
Watertown, MA 02172
(617) 923-4141

VoicEmitter
American Medical Alert
3265 Lawson Blvd
Oceanside, NY 11572
(800) 645-3244; (800) 632-6729 (NY)

For other systems, contact Abledata (see page 206).

──15──

High-Tech Home Care

When Margaret M. contracted a hard-to-treat bone infection after hospital hammer-toe surgery, her doctor explained that meant six weeks of round-the-clock intravenous (IV) antibiotic therapy. Two days later, she checked out and went home, where she received successful therapy.

Mike S., a strapping six-foot-tall policeman, lost part of his guts from a gunshot wound during duty, leaving him unable to eat anything by mouth. While his intestines healed, over a period of months, Mr. S. fed himself at home through a special TPN tube that provided nutrition through a vein just above his heart.

Harry R. was stunned when he learned his cancer had spread and he now required more aggressive treatment. He lived over 75 miles from the cancer center, and he didn't know how he could manage the frequent treatments. Just a month later, his cancer seems to be under control. He now gets his treatment daily through a special pump attached to his chest, which he loads with the proper dosage of cancer-fighting drugs.

These are a few examples of high-tech home care in action. Such care, which was once reserved exclusively for hospitals, or skilled nursing or rehabilitation centers, is now being administered at home to growing numbers of patients. For consumers like these patients, this means a chance for early hospital discharge and a reasonably normal life despite a continuing need for sophisticated treatment.

As a movement, high-tech is still in its infancy, but it is growing rapidly. More hospitals, home care agencies, and large health supply and pharmaceutical firms are making high-tech services available to patients. The *Wall Street Journal* heralds high-tech as the fastest-growing segment of the home care industry. One reason high-tech is coming of age is the often dramatic difference in cost between inpatient versus home care.

IV therapy costs 50 to 80 percent less at home than in a hospital. A typical six-week course of IV therapy at home might run about $4,000, compared to $11,000 in the hospital. Home nutrition savings are equally impressive. TPN hospital care may cost as much as $600 a day—almost $220,000 a year. Home costs may be only $125 a day, or about $46,000 a year. The American Association for Respiratory Therapy (AART) reports that the annual average mean cost for chronic home patients on respiratory life support is $21,000, versus a staggering $270,000 for hospital care, almost a quarter of a million dollars difference.

Not surprisingly, these cost discrepancies are catching the attention of insurers and employers who must pay. Some are bending existing rules that exclude high-tech services at home when it can be clearly shown that doing so will save them money.

Hospitals that are being reimbursed under the flat-rate DRG system also have a financial incentive to move patients from hospital to home for high-tech care.

From a patient perspective, the idea of high-tech home care may sound revolutionary and dangerous. But past experience shows that it is neither.

THE ROOTS OF HIGH-TECH

If you believe that "history repeats itself," you need only look at the roots of high-tech home care for evidence that this adage rings true. More than thirty years ago, following the polio epidemic crisis of the early fifties, a pioneering home care program was developed for iron-lung polio victims at Ranchos Los Amigos in Los Angeles.

Here some 150 patients, who could not breathe without the aid of a machine, were undergoing treatment and reha-

bilitation. Of these "ventilator-dependent" patients, an amazing 95 percent were able to return home. The Los Ranchos
staff evaluated each home and suggested adaptations for the
necessary equipment. The family and patient were carefully
trained in equipment use and maintenance until all concerned
were confident of their abilities. As patients returned home,
the hospital functioned as an ongoing lifeline, providing
information and support to patients and their doctors. A
roving Los Ranchos trailer equipped as a machine shop
visited patients regularly to ensure proper equipment maintenance and repair. Home health aides were specially trained
and employed to help support patients and family in daily
care.

Here was proof positive that high-tech patients could be
cared for safely at home and with a high degree of personal
satisfaction. Such care also met the cost test. In 1959, the
then National Foundation for Infantile Paralysis (now known
as the National Foundation—March of Dimes) reported
home care costs for such programs were only one-tenth to
one-fourth the cost of hospital care.

As the numbers of polio patients dropped and health
priorities shifted, funding for such programs dried up, leaving
polio survivors largely on their own to arrange for continuing
care. While the experiences of early polio patients occurred
over thirty years ago, today they make the case eloquently
for high-tech home care.

Jack Genskow, PhD, an associate professor at Sangamon
State University in Springfield, Illinois, contracted polio at
age 19, leaving him dependent on artificial breathing aids in
order to live. Despite this, he completed his doctorate, worked,
married, and enjoyed a normal home life as the father of two
children. "We've traveled as a family unit all over the
country," says Dr. Genskow, "usually driving but sometimes
flying." He credits his success to: (1) good medical care and
planning in the early stages of recovery; (2) ongoing professional support and sound respiratory equipment; (3) an
effective social support system; and (4) "an opportunity to
live in the community like anybody else where I can have
control of my own life."

Dr. Genskow's success points out that high-tech at home is not new, revolutionary, or necessarily dangerous. In fact, the key elements that Dr. Genskow credits for his success apply to success in most of today's high-tech home care situations. But more about that later.

A CLOSER LOOK AT HIGH-TECH

Should you find yourself in a hospital, you'll quickly learn that care is provided *for* you and procedures are done *to* you, mostly without much explanation. The thought of high-tech care at home may seem overwhelming, if not downright impossible. However, a general overview of these procedures can help take the mystery out of high-tech, and make it an option you may want to consider should the need ever arise.

Let's look first at the high-tech *infusion therapies,* so named because they involve one overriding principle—pumping or dripping solutions of various kinds into the body.

How Infusion Therapies Work

Some treatments first require the surgical insertion of a tube called a cannula or catheter into the body. This step is done in the hospital. The cannula or catheter serves as a "hookup" site for removable tubing through which the solution flows. When the site is not in use, it is kept clean and covered with a small gauze dressing or cap. These hookup sites are semipermanent and remain in the body until therapy is no longer needed. Sometimes an electrically powered mechanical infusion device is connected to this system in order to pump and/or control the rate at which the solution flows.

If you picture how gasoline is pumped into a car, you get the idea of how most infusion systems work. The cannula or catheter functions like the opening to the car's fuel tank through which you insert the nozzle of the gasoline hose. The infusion control device acts like the gasoline pump's mechanical hand grip, which helps control gasoline flow.

With these basics in mind, here's a rundown of specific high-tech infusion treatments.

Hyperalimentation

If ill health robs you of one of life's great pleasures and you can't eat, won't eat, or can't eat enough to maintain reasonable weight, your doctor may prescribe hyperalimentation, "being nourished above the normal" way. Two types of high-tech nutrition are used in the home: enteral therapy or total parenteral nutrition therapy, called TPN for short.

If your digestive system can function normally, enteral therapy is the therapy of choice. Patients who are in a coma, are recovering from major surgery, or are suffering from certain cancers, intestinal disorders, or a disabling stroke might be candidates. The thin enteral feeding tube may be painlessly threaded through nose into the stomach, or may be placed directly into the small intestine through a surgical opening in the abdominal wall. In either case, a liquid food preparation containing proteins, fats, vitamins, or other nutrients is pumped or dripped through the feed tube into the digestive system. Digestion then takes place normally, just as if you had chewed and swallowed the food.

When large sections of the intestines no longer function and a patient's digestive system cannot break down and absorb nutrients, parenteral therapy or TPN must be prescribed. In TPN, a thin tube or catheter is first inserted into a large vein just above the heart through a small opening in the chest wall. Veins in the arms and hands cannot be used for TPN, since the custom-mixed solution of predigested nutrients is very concentrated. Repeated solution use would quickly damage these smaller, more delicate veins. The larger vein, however, has a high blood flow that quickly dilutes the solution as it drips through, thereby preventing any vein damage. Once in the bloodstream, the nutrients are transported, absorbed, and nourish the body.

Unlike the typical habit of eating three meals a day, when you are on either therapy at home nutrition is usually given once a day over a period of several hours. For home TPN patients, this is a big plus over hospital treatment, where TPN is often given on a continuous and confining 24-hour schedule.

Chemotherapy

If you have cancer and must undergo lengthy or intensive drug treatments called chemotherapy, home treatment may be an option. In home chemotherapy, you wear a special pump that contains a reservoir for the cancer drug(s). The pump is hooked to a catheter which, as in TPN, has been inserted through the chest wall into a large vein by the heart. The cancer treatment may be given slowly and continuously for as long as 24 hours or more while you conduct a more normal life at home. For certain patients, this continuous technique may increase drug benefits and decrease drug side effects. Therefore, some cancer specialists may prefer home chemotherapy to the more conventional in-hospital or out-patient treatment at the doctor's office. In some cases, chemotherapy may be administered by vein, as is commonly done in home antibiotic therapy.

Antibiotic Therapy

Before the advent of home antibiotic therapy, patients on daily IV antibiotics for persistent, lingering infections, but who were otherwise in good condition, had to remain hospitalized for weeks. Not even frequent daily injections, self-administered or given in a doctor's office, could provide a high enough drug concentration in the bloodstream to combat these tough infections. Not so any longer. Antibiotic treatment may be administered at home via a pump and heart catheter. More commonly, however, the drugs are given via an IV cannula placed in the forearm, or in a manner similar to IV hospital treatment, with a nurse changing the IV site every two to three days.

Diabetes Therapy

When a 14-year-old Wichita girl went home from the hospital complete with a high-tech insulin pump, doctors and state officials held their breaths. The teenager, who suffered with severe, hard-to-manage diabetes, had been hospitalized for a total of 8 months out of the previous 12. Her hospital bill had totaled some $59,000, prompting state Medicaid officials to allow the purchase of the expensive high-tech equipment, as an experiment, so the youngster could go home.

Much to everyone's delight, the experiment worked. Over the next year and a half, the youngster remained at home without a single hospitalization.

The insulin pump, which is removable and specially fitted to the patient, delivers a precisely measured trickle of insulin continuously 24 hours a day. The diabetic loads the pump with an insulin syringe connected by very thin tubing to a small needle. The needle is then self-inserted just under the skin in the abdomen.

Over 4,200 diabetics now use the pump, most very successfully. The pump's continuous flow helps keep blood sugar levels constant in patients with previously difficult to control diabetes. The pumps also help some pregnant diabetic patients, since good control means fewer risks for mothers and babies.

With the pump, insulin, if low, can also be self-adjusted, mimicking the body's natural adjustment, whenever strenuous activity, meals, or other life style factors prompt changing demands. With blood sugar at last under good control, users are generally enthusiastic. "I feel better than I've felt in 20 years," wrote pump user Yvonne Fisher to *Diabetes Forecast* magazine. "My daily routine is more flexible than it has ever been. There are hassles in wearing a pump, but the advantages outweigh the nuisance."

Home Dialysis

You may know television star Gary Coleman from his comedy show "Diff'rent Strokes." But what you probably did not realize was that for years this youngster was also a home dialysis patient. After Gary's first kidney transplant was rejected some years after surgery, he needed regular dialysis until his next transplant took place. While awaiting the new kidney, he enjoyed an active life on stage and off because of a new dialysis program known as CAPD (continuous ambulatory peritoneal dialysis).

CAPD is one form of home dialysis, but for those able to use it, this method has definite advantages. Other conventional home or outpatient dialysis programs require that you remain hooked to stationary machines for 4 to 8 hours about three times a week. On CAPD, you undergo continuous dialysis 24 hours a day, seven days a week, but you are machine-free. CAPD provides much greater freedom, and because it closely mimics the kidney's continuous filtering system, it offers another major bonus. The average CAPD patient does not have to follow the standard dialysis diet, which severely restricts fluid intake and food choice. Research suggests that CAPD may place less stress on the heart and blood vessels than conventional treatment, another plus.

The CAPD system is fairly simple. It uses the body as a dialysis machine. A special chemical cleansing solution drains from a plastic bag through a catheter into the abdominal cavity. Once empty, the bag is rolled up and tucked under clothing. As you go about your normal routine, water and blood wastes filter through the abdominal membrane, the peritoneum (hence "peritoneal" dialysis), into the cleansing solution. When the entire blood supply has been cleansed, the bag is unrolled so it can refill with the waste-laden solution. Afterward it is exchanged for a fresh bag, and the cycle begins again.

Most CAPD patients complete four 4-hour cycles in the daytime, and one 8-hour cycle at night. The bag exchange itself takes only 30 to 45 minutes and could easily be done while sitting at a desk, for example, or while watching TV, or doing homework.

With CAPD, you can truly "do it yourself." Other home dialysis programs usually require a home partner. These other home treatments include:

- *Hemodialysis.* Blood passes from the body through a tube into a dialysis machine, where it is filtered and returned to the body through another tube.

- *Intermittent peritoneal dialysis (IPD).* A catheter is attached to a stationary pump that cycles the cleansing solution in and out of the abdomen.

Respiratory High-Tech

When 8-year-old Donnie Wartenberg crossed the finish line in his soap box racer, he proved himself a winner. Donnie, with his respirator-caboose trailing behind, came in last, but that didn't matter. His achievement was one victory for life, meaningful life for respiratory patients.

Donnie lives each breath, each day, tethered to his respirator. While few of us can imagine what living like that would be like, says Donnie brightly, "Mostly I can do more things than I can't."

Until high-tech home care came of age, all ventilator children like Donnie were forced to grow up inside hospital pediatric intensive care units, without any real home life. For many adults, a respirator meant a life sentence in a nursing home.

Ventilators or respirators do the normal work of lungs and literally provide the breath of life. Without the help of these devices, ventilator-dependent patients simply cannot live long—in some cases only for minutes, and in others only for several hours or brief days.

Though polio survivors proved in the fifties that ventilator care could be done at home, in more recent times there have been major obstacles to making such respiratory home care a reality.

The lack of health insurance or other means to pay for such costly and often long-term care has been one prime barrier. Another hurdle has been that in many cases health professionals have been reluctant to send ventilator patients home, believing this was not in their best interests. An AART survey identified over 2,000 patients who could go home if financial and professional roadblocks were removed.

These patients are the most difficult to care for at hospital or home, but for all involved, the challenge is most rewarding. Of home care, Donnie explains: "I think you need family to get better."

Other High-Tech Care

As our technology continues to expand, so does its use at home. Babies at high risk for sudden death now go home routinely with apnea monitors that sound alarms should breathing or heartbeat cease. Hemophilia patients in whom a minor cut can cause uncontrolled bleeding can receive the special blood-clotting factor they need at home instead of at the hospital. Though in-home blood transfusions are not yet widely performed, they can and will be done more routinely as the techniques become refined.

Keep one rule of thumb in mind as a patient-consumer. If you are in fairly stable condition and need high-tech therapy, consider receiving it at home.

WHO'S RIGHT FOR HIGH-TECH?

Not every patient can or should take advantage of high-tech home care. Patients and family that do must be ready for the changes in life style that high-tech demands. They must also be prepared to assume greater responsibility for care than in many traditional home care situations. Though skilled professionals will help to varying degrees, most patients and families eventually perform most of the high-tech procedures themselves. The constant flow of supplies must be managed, inventoried, and reordered. Blood and urine testing and other self-monitoring must be performed regularly. These home care therapies, while safe, are not risk-free. The risks vary with the treatment.

Insulin pump users, for example, may experience blackouts until the pump is custom-primed to meet their fluctuating insulin demands. Where CAPD is used, carelessness can lead to an abdominal infection called peritonitis which, if unchecked, can be fatal. Serious infections can also occur more easily in therapies that require an indwelling catheter near the heart, since contaminating bacteria there can enter the bloodstream directly. Some ventilator patients risk sudden death should serious mishaps, such as machine failure, occur.

Although the risks of high-tech home care are real, so are the benefits. For starters, these same risks exist in hospital treatment, but at home, under your control, care is often better. Terri Guild, a respiratory therapist with Home Respiratory Care, described how one mother was able to painstakingly wean her child from a respirator, though medical doctors had told her he would be dependent for life. Mrs. Doolan, who maintains all care for her TPN husband, notes: "Hospitals are cold. With the staff cutbacks, the nurses try hard, but they just can't give him the kind of care and attention that I do." For Mrs. M, another TPN wife, the financial benefits of home versus hospital care became extremely important. Her husband's hospital and nursing home Medicare coverage was nearly exhausted, and the bills were piling up.

"What it boils down to," says RN Susan Blumquist, a high-tech supervisor with American Nursing in New Orleans, "patients have to want to do it for whatever reason." Motivation is an important factor, but natural fear should never be a stumbling block. Almost all consumers going into a high-tech situation experience understandable hesitancy and anxiety. Mrs. M. says: "I was scared; it seemed like such a big responsibility." But she was able to master it without problems.

Mrs. Doolan agrees. "It was hard at first, but looking back, I could never believe our life could be so normal." She and her husband Scott had just returned from a three-week trip to Scotland. Her husband, a native of Scotland, had not visited his family in over twenty-seven years. Their personal victory in making the trip was even sweeter when she recalls: "Two years ago, they told me to make funeral arrangements."

The success of high-tech depends not only upon patients and families, but as Dr. Genskow pointed out, on early ongoing medical support and equipment.

Most high-tech patients are hospitalized at the time the decision for home care is made. Getting from hospital to home, and remaining home, usually involves several professional links in the helping chain:

- The doctor who prescribes high-tech home care and provides ongoing medical support and supervision.
- A discharge planning team that helps plan and coordinate the activities necessary for a successful release to the home.
- A drug supply and/or medical equipment company (this could be hospital-owned) that provide the necessary infusion solutions, devices, and related supplies or equipment. The company usually also provides patient education and training and ongoing monitoring of equipment and patient.
- A home care agency called in at the doctor's or patient's request, or working under contract with the drug supply or medical equipment company, to provide initial and ongoing professional support or respite help to the family as needed.

When you face high-tech home care, you will need to rely on good professional support even more than in traditional home care. Whether high-tech or traditional care, applying the same basic consumerism will help you overcome the common hurdles that high-tech patients and their families sometimes experience.

THE DOCTOR'S SIGN-OFF
AND SUPPORT

"My medical doctor didn't know anything about TPN," says Mrs. M. "The stomach specialist who was called in suggested it, and only because he had just returned from a conference where he learned about it." "The doctors advised me against taking my husband home," says Mrs. Doolan. "Two years later, some of them are still saying that."

Despite growing awareness among medical circles that high-tech care can be performed safely at home and has many patient benefits, you cannot always rely on your doctor to recommend these services. Often the idea for this specialized home care will come from a nurse or other hospital professional staff, or from the patients themselves. "In antibiotic therapy," says HNS nurse Allyson Faist, "patients will get 'cabin fever' and start demanding, 'I've got to get out of here.' That's when someone thinks about home care."

For ventilator patients, particularly children, the doctor and other professionals may be very resistant to the thought of home care. Dr. Mark Merken remembers: "We had a 9-year-old ventilator-dependent child in the intensive care unit. Her condition was stable, and a meeting was held to figure out a long-term plan for her. I suggested sending the child home and was met with dead silence." "Sometimes we have to remind professionals that these are *our* children," says Mrs. Julie Beckett, a respirator mother, "not *theirs*. My little girl Katie was happy, stimulated, and loved at the hospital where she got care, but she wasn't home."

If you want high-tech care, and your doctor is resistant or unaware, enlist support from the discharge planner or other interested staff professionals. Top-notch drug and medical equipment companies also have physician consultants who can talk to your doctor on a one-to-one basis if needed. Professional home care agencies, equipped to handle high-tech care, can also answer your physician's questions. Often professional assurances that good care can be provided at home, and an explanation of how, makes the critical difference.

DISCHARGE PLANNING

Patients often assume that if you leave everything to the professionals, they will do it well and do it best. This often happens in high-tech home care, but there are no guarantees. One young, single mother and her chronically ill newborn were sent home complete with an apnea monitor and a raft of sophisticated drug prescriptions. When a specially trained homemaker assigned to help the mother arrived some days later, she discovered the mother was not using the drugs or the monitor. Why not? The local pharmacy did not stock the drugs her doctor had ordered. Nor did her bedroom, where she and her baby slept, contain the necessary three-way electrical outlet for the monitor. None of the pros involved in this situation had ever checked these important details or discussed them with the mother.

To make a good transition from hospital to home takes planning; and this planning should always involve you. After all, you know your home situation best, and will have a good idea of a care plan that will or will not work there. It's not enough just to put all the technology into your home. It has to work, and work well, for you.

In high-tech care, many practical details must be worked out. If not thought out in advance, space for equipment, storage, and supplies can be a major problem. There must be adequate electrical wiring for the equipment, as well as a backup generator in case of power failure. In some cases, an extra refrigerator may be needed so you do not have to store IV solutions in with your vegetables.

Proper advance planning is essential for a good, sound assessment to be made, for a thorough care plan to be developed, and for all the necessary supplies and equipment to be coordinated. How much time is needed will depend on the situation. For an adult ventilator patient, this may mean a few weeks; for a child, this may mean months. In a simple case of antibiotic therapy, the planning time may be much briefer—as little as two days or less.

Planning also includes another critical step in successful high-tech home care—patient education and training.

PATIENT EDUCATION AND TRAINING

Don't let the hospital push you out, or don't insist on getting out, until you have had proper high-tech training *before discharge.* "We get calls from a doctor," says high-tech nurse Susan Blumquist, "saying 'We've got a 21-year-old who wants out now. I'm discharging him in six hours on four antibiotics. You can do it; right?' We do," says Ms. Blumquist, "but this is not ideal." Unless you intend to have round-the-clock RN care, even in antibiotic therapy, you and any family caregivers should know all the basics before you go home. This includes how the equipment operates, what happens during treatment, warning signs, and what to do if something goes wrong.

Patient education and training, and that of the family caregivers, takes time. Mrs. M. received only two or three hours before her husband was discharged for TPN treatment at home. Bill Donovan, a TPN nurse specialist at Mt. Sinai Hospital, says: "Good TPN training requires about twenty hours." You will need time to *practice* what you have learned. "Learning how to trouble-shoot is extremely important," cautions Allyson Faist, RN. "Once you get home, not only will everything seem different, but it is. You won't have a nurse standing over you."

When you learn high-tech care, make sure you learn the ropes by using the *same* equipment and supplies you will use at home—none other. Even a different dial can confuse you during your initial home adjustment. In complex care situations, if possible have staff arrange a supervised "dry run" where you provide the care on a 24- or 48-hour basis in the hospital before you commit to a regular home discharge.

TOP-NOTCH PROFESSIONAL SERVICES

Patients and families almost universally agree that you cannot have too much professional support and backup once you get home, particularly during the initial adjustment period. This does not mean you need 24 hours of nursing care, for instance, but it is critical to have 24-hour professional services on call to answer questions, give professional advice, talk you through any problems that can arise, or do more if needed. You will also frequently need the ongoing services of an RN to monitor the care being provided, the equipment, and the patient's condition.

Though it's your right to choose who will provide these professional services, in 99 high-tech cases out of 100, your doctor or involved hospital staff will probably decide. But since this is a decision you will have to live with, it's important that whoever is selected delivers more than just equipment and supplies. You must be assured that top-rate services will be delivered as well:

- *24-hour coverage.* Should a problem occur, how soon will you get a response when you call? Who will respond? Top-notch providers will respond to your call within 30 minutes or less. You should be able, on short notice, to reach a professional—a registered nurse, pharmacist, therapist, or other appropriate *professional.* A superior practice is to have one particular professional assigned to you, a personal professional with whom you can develop a good working relationship. Mrs. Doolan, for example, an HNS customer, cannot say enough about her special nurse Sherry. "I've called her at 3:00 or 4:00 in the morning," Mrs. Doolan says. "I can always reach her. She has even come out when necessary." Learn if there is a professional in-home backup available when needed on a 24-hour basis. Or will you be told to go to the emergency room?
- *Nursing or therapist support and follow-up.* How much support will you actually get once you get home? High-tech education and training should not end at the hospital. When you get home the first day, the professional should be there too. The professional should follow up until you and the professional are confident that you can perform these procedures. Ongoing monitoring must be provided not only of your techniques and skills and care, but of the equipment.
- *Social or other professional services.* Are supportive professional services available? Patients and families, for example, often need social services, since there are many personal problems involved in coping with long-term high-tech situations. Depression and anger are common emotional reactions. Marital problems and difficulties with children may require social service assistance. Other professionals may also be needed. For example, in a nutrition therapy situation, a dietitian should always be available for consultation.
- *Equipment and supply deliveries and inventory help.* Will the same personnel assist you? How often will supplies be delivered? What about emergencies? What about inventory control? In top-notch services, having the same

delivery worker can be important; the person gets to know you and can help out with your supply needs. Delivery schedules are also important. A monthly versus weekly delivery will affect storage space. Managing the endless number of pieces of equipment and medical supplies can be a problem too for most people adjusting to high-tech care. A good professional system that helps you keep track and reminds you of inventory on hand is essential.

- *Special services.* Despite high-tech care, you should be free to live your life. There are special extras that you can look for. Mrs. Doolan, for example, was able to make her trip to Scotland because her company coordinated everything she needed and was able to deliver the nutrition supplies across the seas. Some companies will provide special refrigerators gratis, as a special service.

Whenever a home care agency, not a company-employed nurse, provides high-tech services, you will want to ask most of the above questions—and more. Most home care agencies who provide skilled nursing services say they can provide high-tech care, but many are not properly experienced to do the job. Ask:

- What experience has the agency had with the high-tech care you need? For how long? Just because an agency has done antibiotic therapy does not mean it can handle ventilator patients, TPN, or CAPD. An agency that handles high-tech only occasionally does not have the same experience as a regular high-tech agency.
- Does it have written procedures for *your* therapy? For emergencies? Ask to see these written procedures. They should be specifically for your therapy, not for home care in general. Avoid an agency that doesn't have these written instructions to guide its personnel.
- Are the RNs trained well in the therapy and experienced in *home care?* Good agencies will use highly experienced RNs, often with special credentials in critical care nursing. All should be CPR-trained.

Once services begin, the normal rules of home care still

apply. The agency high-tech nurse should also be agency-supervised. Margaret O'Brien, a nursing consultant on high-tech care, advises patients to watch for inexperienced personnel. "If agency personnel seem unsure or ask *you* for help," says Ms. O'Brien, "this is a tip-off that the agency is not ready for high-tech."

FINANCIAL BARRIERS

High-tech home care, as mentioned earlier, is expensive. Insulin pumps, for example, may cost between $1,200 and $3,000. But these costs finally are being weighed against the savings resulting from home care. In 1981, Katie Beckett made the headlines when President Reagan, calling the Medicaid rules covering her case "hidebound regulations," signed a special order allowing the Becketts' little daughter to go home. Until then, Medicaid covered the cost of Katie's $12,000 a month respirator care in the hospital, but would not pay for the cheaper care at home. The bill now allows state Medicaid programs across the country to take advantage of the so-called Katie Beckett waivers and, on a case-by-case basis, pay for high-tech treatment at home, not just in the hospital.

In the private sector, insurers will often provide care at home on a case-by-case basis, regardless of what the policy states. Often it is the high-tech companies and the home care agencies, together with the hospitals, that advocate and work out financial arrangements with the insurer.

As a consumer, you should be aware that most high-tech companies will take assignment of any insurance benefits. However, you should thoroughly investigate what happens to any balance that may be due. Will you be billed? If so, how much, and when is payment due? Insurance policies will vary, however, on the coverage for drugs, equipment, or other necessary supplies. In some cases, high-tech care comes under special regulations. Medicare, for example, which does not routinely cover outpatient drugs, will pay for chemotherapy drugs administered via the special high-tech pump at home.

RESPITE AND SOCIAL SUPPORT

Ongoing high-tech care for family caregivers is physically and emotionally demanding. In the case of respiratory care, Karen Shannon says: "It is neither fair nor realistic to expect parents to care for their ventilator-dependent/respiratory failure child indefinitely on a 24-hour, 7-day-a-week basis." Without respite and social support, few families can cope even in less demanding high-tech care situations.

Home care agencies provide respite help. But so do friends, neighbors, and the community at large. Self-help groups have been a wonderful source of additional social support, often providing the practical how-to strategies that can help make the caregiving responsibilities and maneuvering of the health care system much easier. Mrs. Shannon, for example, is founder and executive director of SKIP [Sick Kids (Need) Involved People], 216 New Port Dr, Severna Park, MD 21146, (301) 647–0164, which helps families make workable arrangements for children with severe respiratory problems, and helps educate public policymakers, physicians, and others about the special care and services these children require.

Similar groups exist in other high-tech areas. For example, kidney sufferers can turn to the National Association of Patients on Hemodialysis and Transplantation, 150 Nassau St, New York, NY 10038, (212) 619–2727. To locate other groups, contact The National Health Information Clearinghouse, PO Box 1133, Washington, DC 20013–1133, (800) 336–4797, (703) 522–2590 (VA), or the appropriate regional self-help clearinghouse listed on page 417.

—16—

Specialized Rehabilitation Services

They are mainly the accident victims who make the headlines and the evening news, and are then forgotten. But for those who survive, and their families, the long, hard struggle has just begun. Their medical problems may include severe head or spinal cord injuries, coma, or extensive burns. These patients require special handling, both in and out of hospitals. The numbers of these cases once were small. But with higher accident rates and better emergency medicine, the number of rehabilitation candidates has soared. The National Head Injury Foundation reports that over 600,000 persons alone suffer serious head trauma each year. With good medical care, at least half of these patients will survive. But for these patients and their families, life alone is not enough; the quality of that life becomes essential.

Here again, home care—special home care—can make a dramatic difference.

Robert P., age 25, became a special rehabilitation patient of Staff Builders following a crash of the airplane he was piloting. Hospitalized and in a coma for months after losing part of his brain in the accident, he initially did well with hospital rehabilitation once he regained consciousness. But then unexpectedly he regressed. He couldn't form words or ideas. He refused to leave his wheelchair. "The doctor at the hospital rehabilitation unit told me to put him in a nursing home and divorce him," recalls Mrs. P. But this young woman and the entire family stubbornly refused to give up. They brought him home and the family started working with him round-the-clock. At night, a local home care agency helped, but during the day they were on their own. They provided therapy and hands-on care and brought in a private speech therapist. After six months there was some progress, but the family was exhausted and unable to carry on. The young wife needed to return to work, but understandably felt torn.

When her husband reentered the hospital six months after discharge for cranial surgery, a family member stumbled upon Staff Builders' special rehabilitation program. When Robert went home a second time, he went with a comprehensive rehabilitation program in place.

A special coordinator assessed every aspect of Robert's case. A physical therapist trained a team of nurse specialists to provide rehabilitation 16 hours a day. The therapist evaluated Robert weekly, revising his rehabilitation activities as needed. Even Robert's break time was used to improve his coordination. Instead of vegetating in front of TV to relax, the therapist engaged him in constructing a model plane to improve hand-eye coordination.

Meticulous progress notes were kept, and regular team conferences held to which the family was invited. The speech therapist already on the case remained and, though not a Staff Builders employee, was integrated into the home care team.

In just four months' time with this intensive regimen, rapid progress was seen. This young man, who was formerly a champion swimmer and skydiver, regained each day more of his physical and mental abilities. Today he is still making progress and can read and do math at a twelfth-grade level. He can swim, ride a stationary bike, and walk with crutches—all accomplishments both family and the professionals involved are convinced would have never occurred without this specialized home care service.

As he progresses, his level of rehabilitation care is slowly being reduced. Already Robert is making his plans for the future. This young man, who might have remained in a nursing home all his life, now wants to help others with similar problems.

Robert's case is not an isolated success story for Staff Builders, but it is an unusual one, nevertheless. Too many of these patients never experience intensive rehabilitation efforts and never realize their full human potential. Unfortunately, this is due to lack of availability in some areas of such specialized rehabilitation services, and lack of consumer and professional awareness in others.

IF YOU NEED SPECIAL REHABILITATION

Like high-tech home care, this is a highly specialized area. These cases require top-notch case management, solid continuity of care, and highly individualized programs. Margie Polidoro, RN, director of national rehabilitation for Staff Builders, reports: "We may try unconventional programs impossible to deliver in a traditional setting. For example, we may devise a day program of ten one-half-hour therapy sessions that alternate between audio, visual, and tactile [touch] stimulation." Not every agency, though it may have therapists on staff, is equipped to provide the kind of rehabilitation service that Robert received. Like Staff Builders, other agencies, including some visiting nurse organizations, have designed special programs to assist in such cases. Special rehabilitation centers may also provide home aftercare. When you consider this option, interview any agency on the following points, and involve your doctor in your selection process.

- *The agency's rehabilitation experience.* The agency should have written procedures geared to rehabilitation, not general home care, and demonstrated experience in rehabilitation care. Discuss how the agency will ensure the comprehensive case management and coordination that are essential to rehabilitation care.
- *Personnel.* All personnel must be experienced. Rehabilitation is no place for newcomers to home care. Discuss the professional background of all team members, particularly the coordinator of care. Ask if the agency requires

that employees make a long-term commitment before assignment to care. A nurse or a therapist who works a week or two and then requests reassignment can cause a serious setback in rehabilitation care. More than other patients, these patients require consistency of personnel in order to make progress.

- *Psychosocial support.* For patients and families, these situations are extremely difficult. Social and psychological support must be available when needed. In head trauma, for example, brain damage may cause a variety of behavior problems with which family and patient must learn to cope.

As with high-tech care, the agency must coordinate all elements of home care before discharge from hospital, nursing home, or rehabilitation unit. Extensive medical equipment and home structural alterations are often necessary. The agency should also be an expert in insurance matters, since you may have to negotiate with your insurer to get the maximum coverage.

When you consider this option, review the list of barriers that high-tech families encounter. The same problems hold for rehabilitation cases. Your best chance for success with in-home rehabilitation lies in being prepared to handle these problems in advance.

—17—

Case Management

It took eighteen separate phone calls for Margaret B. to find help for her mother in the city Margaret once called home. After her mother had fallen and fractured her hip, Margaret came the thousand miles to help. But now, two weeks later, it was time for her to go home. Her mother was going to need help, mostly custodial long-term help. Mrs. B.'s doctor had suggested nursing home care, which Margaret had staunchly refused. But she privately worried whether she had made the right decision and how long her mother would be able to remain at home.

When Victor King's 16-year-old son Mark had a skiing accident, he suffered an aneurysm and total paralysis. For the next four months, hospital efforts focused solely on life-sustaining treatment. Said Mr. King, "We felt that the care he received was excellent, but that the communication with us about his options was very poor. No one ever mentioned to us the possibility of rehabilitation until four months after the accident. Then a passing remark from a nurse made us realize that there were options to be investigated."

Both these situations are different; but both would have benefitted from the same service—case management. In Margaret's case, her mother's management needs were primarily nonmedical, while Mr. King's son needed a medically oriented management program.

WHAT IS CASE MANAGEMENT?

Case management is a concept as much as it is a service. Conceptually, it involves:

- Assessment of a person's total care needs and all available resources for help
- Care planning that is realistic, provides quality care, and is cost-effective
- Coordination of all services, including making necessary arrangements
- Monitoring the plan and periodically reevaluating it for necessary changes
- Education of all parties involved: client, family and professional caregivers, and other community health and social service providers

To varying degrees, all professional home care agencies provide case management services. However, the special case management services that are increasing in numbers to assist consumers involve a central case management source outside the home care agency. When you use these services, you have a one-stop shop that handles all your health and social needs, no matter who provides them—the home care agency and/ or other community organizations. In a sense, case management operates like a broker and client advocacy system. It helps you negotiate your way through the maze of health and social services to put together a package of the most appropriate, cost-effective care.

WHO PROVIDES CASE MANAGEMENT?

Many of the professional case management services have been organized to assist the ever-growing chronically ill population, mostly elderly, like Mrs. B. Their goal is to prevent unnecessary institutionalization and keep people in the community as long as possible.

Nonprofit Organizations

These nonprofit case management organizations or projects may be sponsored in cooperation with Area Agencies on

Aging, nonprofit community hospitals, or long-term care facilities. Typically, the nonprofit organizations do not charge low-income elderly; for others, there may be a sliding scale fee.

Frequently services are state or federally funded and are sometimes referred to as "channeling projects." For example, in January 1985, the Philadelphia Corporation for Aging started its Long Term Care Assessment and Management Program (LAMP), which will provide case management for every Medicaid client who seeks nursing home placement. Non-Medicaid consumers may also participate. Connecticut Community Care, Inc. (CCCI) is a statewide nonprofit organization that provides a similar service. Case management services like these exist in many communities.

For-Profit Case Management

In addition to these organizations, professional case management services are available through for-profit organizations or through social workers in private practice strictly for a fee. Rates usually run by the hour, with $50 an hour a common fee. You should generally expect a three- to four-hour charge to assess a home situation and make the necessary referrals and arrangements. Ongoing monitoring, if it is desired, would be extra.

For persons who must arrange for care at long distance, these services can offer convenience. However, since the industry is totally unregulated, you should be cautious about choosing with whom to deal. First, decide if these services are necessary. Professional home care agencies will do an in-home assessment free, so unless your situation is unusual, you may be paying for this service needlessly. Professional agencies will also send you written progress notes, or call if so requested, to keep you informed. The best professional agencies will act as a family substitute, making all necessary arrangements for outside services, including chore work, exterminator service, and so on.

Before you use the services of an individual or for-profit organization, check the credentials of those providing the service. As a safeguard, deal only with services staffed by professional licensed or certified social workers. Ask for customer references. Discuss all fees in advance.

Medical Case Management

If you are hospitalized, particularly for a serious problem like Mark King's, your insurer may be your best friend. The leading insurance companies, including Aetna, Equitable, Prudential, Transamerica Occidental, and Connecticut General, have medical case management systems in place.

The individual programs vary. Transamerica's Patient Care Coordination has a specially trained RN who reviews hospital records to spot patients who could be discharged with home care. The coordinator will discuss home care with your doctor, the hospital discharge planner, and the home care agency to help coordinate your care. For patients like Mark, Transamerica has a Comprehensive Medical Rehabilitation Service that assigns a Transamerica nurse specialist to the case. The specialist, at no extra cost, makes sure home care needs are analyzed, keeps communication open among doctor, patient, and family, and monitors all follow-up care. If need be, contacts are made with local public or private agencies in the patient's behalf.

Aetna's Individual Case Management (ICM) Program works similarly. The ICM nurse coordinator reviews your insurance coverage and can authorize, when needed, benefits that aren't even there. For example, costs for special medical equipment, ramps, or access doorways can be okayed.

Programs may target only certain types of problems. Equitable, for example, provides case management for:

- Neonatal high-risk infants
- Cerebral vascular accident (CVA)—severe stroke
- Multiple sclerosis
- Amyotrophic lateral sclerosis (ALS)—Lou Gehrig's Disease
- Major head trauma
- Spinal cord injury
- Amputations
- Multiple fractures
- Severe burns

Steve Putterman of Equitable points out: "These cases of catastrophic injury are very traumatic. One day you're well, the next day you're not. Spinal cord injuries, for example, are not common, so your local hospital may not be fully equipped to handle them."

This is where the case management program steps in and helps patients and families. Aetna has been so enthusiastic about its case management program that it has extended it to all patient illnesses and injuries, not catastrophic ones alone.

If you're not sure your insurance carrier provides these services, check. You may have a home care advocate in your insurer.

—18—

Hospice: Dying with Dignity

Given a choice, most people would prefer to die at home. Yet most people—at least 80 percent—die in hospitals or nursing homes. Hospice care offers an alternative to this American way of death. As the movement grows, it promises to make death with dignity the rule rather than the exception.

WHERE IT BEGAN

The word "hospice" means haven. The concept of hospice care can be traced back to medieval times. In 1443, the Hospice de Beaune was founded for the care of the poor and dying in the Burgundy region of France. Similar hospices, offering wayfarers relief during travel, flourished throughout Europe during the Middle Ages and then died out. In 1968, the hospice concept was reborn when St. Christopher's Hospice in London, England, opened its doors. St. Christopher's quickly proved that the hospice was as welcome in modern times as it was over five hundred years ago.

St. Christopher's was founded by Dr. Cicely Saunders, who decided that dying patients could benefit from a very special kind of care. Despite the objections of her colleagues, Dr. Saunders' patients were removed from the rigid, impersonal, clinical hospital environment and placed in St. Christopher's, which had been specially designed to offer a warm, homelike atmosphere. Supported by staff trained to work with the dying, patients and families could enjoy their remaining days together as fully as possible. Normal hospital visiting restrictions were lifted. People were free to come and go whenever they wished—day or night. Children and pets were welcomed. Pain was relieved by permitting patients as much medication as they needed for comfort. And drugs were given when they were most effective, rather than as prescribed by a rigid hospital schedule. Patients and families were encouraged to express their feelings toward each other and share the dying experience.

The overwhelming satisfaction of patients and families outstripped the skepticism of health professionals. St. Christopher's was an immediate success. Despite overnight acceptance abroad, hospice did not come to the United States until 1974, when Hospice, Inc., of Connecticut accepted its first patient. Today the National Hospice Organization reports the number of hospice care programs has swelled to over 1,800 and continues to grow.

WHAT IS A HOSPICE?

When you think of hospice, do not think of a place. Think of a special concept of care for the dying and their families. This special concept may be applied in several settings: hospitals, the patient's home, or in facilities specifically designed as hospices. In hospices, the focus is on caring, not curing; on life, not death.

Our modern medical system is not equipped to meet the special needs of the dying and their families. The system is aimed at curing at all costs, even if the patients are sometimes forgotten in the process. When medicine cannot offer anything more to fight the disease, the view becomes "the battle is lost." The doctors and nurses, once so involved in curative measures, often withdraw slowly in uncomfortable silence when they feel nothing more can be done. Patients and family are usually left without hope to face countless fears, problems, and uncertainties that increase their anguish—fear of the unknown; pain and the fear of pain; fears of loneliness, abandonment, and isolation; anger, sadness, and confusion.

This is where hospice steps in, proving that so much can still be done, if not for the disease, then for patients and families. Hospice brings true release from pain, help with the trying practicalities related to death, and spiritual and emotional support during the last stage of illness and the grieving period beyond.

"When patients and families finally reach us," says hospice director Carolyn Fitzpatrick, president of the National Hospice Organization, "the overall response is a sigh of relief. Death is unknown territory for everyone. Families and patients don't know what to do or how to proceed. With hospice, you have help to get through it all."

Hospice is a special program of care with three major goals:

- To offer comfort, dignity, and support to those facing incurable illness
- To help the dying remain at home; or if not at home, in a compassionate, technology-free health care environment
- To provide complete physical, emotional, spiritual, and practical care that allows patients and families to live as fully as possible despite terminal illness

As these goals show, hospice is a pro-life movement. It does not hasten or postpone death. Its care helps patients and families live each day and eventually experience death in a way that is meaningful and acceptable to them. The philosophy of hospice is beautifully embodied in Dr. Saunders' words to her patients: "You matter because you are you. You matter to the last moment of your life, and we will do all we can, not only to help you die peacefully, but also to live until you die."

TYPES OF HOSPICES

With over 1,800 hospices providing care now and some 300 in the planning stage, it is not surprising that programs are organized and run differently.

Some hospice programs are grassroots interest groups that provide support to the dying and their families, largely through professional and (mostly) nonprofessional volunteers.

Most programs, however, are highly organized and are now recognized as distinct providers within the health system.

Only a very few hospices operate like St. Christopher's, as self-contained, homelike inpatient facilities separate and apart from hospitals. These free-standing hospices include the Connecticut Hospice, Hospice of Northern Virginia (Arlington, VA), Nathan Adelson Hospice (Las Vegas, NV), and Hospice of the Monterey Peninsula (Carmel, CA).

Most hospice programs operate in the patient's home, with backup care available at local hospitals or nursing homes. These in-home hospice programs may be affiliated with, or a division of, an existing home care agency. They may also operate exclusively as "hospice" agencies.

Some hospices are hospital-based. A patient floor or other area of the hospital is set aside and designated for hospice patients. Care is provided by a specially trained team, not regular hospital staff. In some hospital-based hospices, patients are not cared for in a separate unit, but are scattered throughout the hospital. The hospice team, except for nursing personnel, "floats" to each patient, providing necessary support. Whenever appropriate, hospital-based hospice programs also provide home care. In fact, the trend in all hospice programs today, no matter whether they are hospital-based or not, is to provide as much care as possible in the home, relying on inpatient care only when absolutely necessary.

HOW HOSPICE DIFFERS FROM HOME CARE

Basically hospice *is* a home care program with special extras and a few important differences.

In home care, the family is viewed as an important contributor in patient care, but the patient takes center stage. The goals and services provided in traditional home care are really patient-oriented. In hospice, the concern is for both patient and family, who are treated as "a single unit of care." Hospice understands that what affects the family affects the patient too. Therefore, the plan of care and hospice services focus on meeting family needs as well as the patient's. For example, in home care social work counseling mainly helps the patient cope with illness-related problems. In hospice care, counseling is available to, and encouraged for, family members as a much-needed support during this difficult time. One wife expressed the "unit of care" concept this way. "The consideration given me was really great. Before it seemed that everyone was concerned about John [the husband] and how he was doing; but when the team of hospice people came in, they cared about me also."

For Elliot Locke, who lost his wife to cancer, hospice was an emotional lifesaver. "I will forever be thankful for their help," says Mr. Locke. "My wife and I had no relatives and I was the only one to cope with this problem. Had it not been for these people [hospice staff], I don't know what I would have done."

Hospice Services

Hospice offers the same general health and supportive services as does home care, but the emphasis is on maintaining or improving function, not rehabilitation. For example, in physical therapy the goal may be to help the patient maintain muscle strength and tone as long as possible in order to delay becoming bedridden. Skilled nursing, homemaker, and home health aide services become extremely important in hospice care. The hospice nurses spend far much more time in the home than regular home care nurses. Hospice nurses usually think of themselves as specialists, just as pediatric nurses do in hospitals.

Nonskilled services are considered extremely important, since they provide the vital practical support that makes it possible for families to keep their loved ones at home. Families can rely on the help of volunteers, homemakers, and home health aides for long hours of care and support. Their services also make hospice affordable for patients.

The team approach common to home care is essential in hospice care. The team consists of the nurse, a hospice doctor, the usual home care personnel, volunteers, and clergy. The team confers regularly to make sure that those they serve get all the support they need. Often the hospice team is headed by the nurse, not the doctor, and the nurse coordinates all the individual elements of care. Paraprofessionals and volunteers are valued members of the hospice team. Says Ms. Fitzpatrick: "We, as professionals, often like to think we are important. However, it is the person who really touches the lives of patients and families that is really important. Often it is not the nurse, social worker, or doctor, but the volunteers and aides who make the difference."

Hospice care is often more flexible than home care services. At Good Samaritan Hospice in Battle Creek, Michigan, where Ms. Fitzpatrick is the director, the team doesn't stand on ceremonial titles; members do whatever needs to be done. "We will do the cleaning, for example, and let the family give the bath," she says. It is more comforting to have personal care provided by a loved one than by concerned staff.

Hospice will arrange for necessary medical equipment and supplies and supportive services such as transportation. Volunteers provide "friendly visiting" just to talk, read to patients, play cards, or whatever.

Families provide much of the hands-on care for their loved ones, but always with the help of the hospice staff. When needed, 24-hour hospice care is available seven days a week. Short-term inpatient hospital care is also arranged when needed or requested, to provide families with respite or support patients if hard-to-manage medical problems arise.

One hospice bonus is the practical guidance available to patients and families upon request. Staff will help them grapple with the countless details that life-threatening illness brings—insurance problems, wills, funeral arrangements, legal matters, financial money management.

As important as all these services are, there are two other special hospice services that deeply affect patients and families.

Pain Control

Almost 90 percent of all hospice patients suffer from cancer. While half of cancer patients have no pain at all, the other half experience moderate to severe distress. Often patients and their families feel that pain must accompany terminal illness. However, upon entering hospice, they learn otherwise.

"Patients get better care in hospice," asserts Anne Katterhagen, director, Hospice of Tacoma, "because they have better pain control." Pain is often poorly controlled in those patients dying outside of hospice. Doctors, inexperienced in working with the dying, often needlessly fear that patients will become addicted to drugs. Therefore doctors may reduce needed drug dosages so pain is never fully relieved, or they may withhold drugs until the patient is in deep distress and literally has to beg for relief. Some doctors err on the other side. They order dosages which are so high and so frequent that patients are robbed of real life. As a result, the patients virtually live out their precious remaining days in a drugged stupor.

Not so with hospice patients. They receive drugs in a way that keeps them comfortable throughout the day and yet alert. Hospice nurse Irene Rehberg points out that "Proper pain control lets patients use the time they have left in what gives them pleasure, instead of focusing on pain."

Hospice doctors are pain control experts who understand the many physical and emotional factors that influence pain. For example, through experience they have learned that drug timing often can be more important than drug dosage. It is easier to prevent pain than to relieve pain once it appears. Also the patient's own fear of returning pain is enough to increase the pain itself.

To break this cycle of pain, a drug program is very carefully designed only after each aspect of the patient's pain has been analyzed. Drugs are not seen as the only answer to pain control. For example, if severe headaches are a complaint, higher drug dosages are not automatically prescribed. It may be that, after talking to the patient, what is really needed for relief is simply to elevate the head of the bed. Emotional factors such as depression can also affect a patient's feeling of pain. When the cause of pain is emotional, more psychological support is recommended to help patients obtain comfort and relief.

Hospice patients and families are also encouraged to self-administer drugs rather than always rely on professionals for pain relief. The drugs are frequently provided in a convenient pleasant-tasting liquid form and are taken at intervals that are timed to keep just ahead of the pain. This method controls pain through prevention and also by reducing the patient's anxiety.

The result of proper pain control methods have been impressive. Pain can be controlled in at least 90 percent of all patients. And even patients in very severe pain can get substantial relief.

Emotional Support, Spiritual and Bereavement Counseling

No human experience is more stressful than death. Emotional pain is a very real problem for patients and families during the last weeks and days of life. Patients and families need to express and share their feelings, but often they don't know how. Without proper help and support, a person can still die alone even though surrounded by family.

Patients and families are often haunted by anguishing questions. How long will it be? How much does he/she know? What should I say to the children? What will my family do when I am gone?

Emotions run high during this time. Anger, sadness, guilt, grief, and depression are all natural.

The hospice team has experienced these difficult and complicated situations before and can provide needed guidance and support. The team knows how to listen and encourage open family communication. They can help patients and families come to grips with emotional problems. With the assistance of a sensitive and trained staff, families can resolve their feelings so they are not left with guilt or regrets and unfinished business.

For most patients, impending death raises issues of an afterlife. For many, dying is the time for spiritual growth and renewal; but for others, the reality of death is made even more difficult by inner turmoil. When desired, nondenominational spiritual support and pastoral counseling is provided by hospice clergy or others without intruding on the patient's wishes and beliefs. Patients are encouraged to express their views and concerns about life and death and a supreme being, or personal philosophy, as well as any fears or misgivings they may have. The staff provides emotional support and insight, and helps the person clarify his or her spiritual concepts.

One pastoral counselor helped a troubled middle-aged cancer patient who had never been a churchgoer and who had no church ties. As a result, the woman felt spiritually isolated, and, although she wanted to and needed to, she felt she did not know how to pray. Through discussion, the counselor helped her understand that there were many ways to pray, and that even her daily experiences shared with her God could serve as a prayer without words. The woman was comforted.

For families, death brings an inevitable sense of loss and grief that begins even before the patient dies. Studies have shown that a bereavement without proper assistance can have a devastating effect on families. For example, for men under age 75, death rates from accidents, heart disease, and some infections increase following the death of a parent or spouse. The death of a parent or brother or sister during childhood increases the risk of more serious emotional problems in children. After looking at the statistical evidence, the Institute of Medicine of the National Academy of Sciences concluded: "The well-being of the family and others close to a dying patient is part of a health professional's responsibility to terminal illness."

Through hospice, families are helped to deal with their own grief by taking an active role in their loved one's care. Studies also show this active involvement has a healing effect on the family, reducing feelings of guilt or regret that may occur after death. After death, bereavement counseling and contact with hospice staff continues, providing ongoing support to the family. For the patient, knowing that this help is available to the family is reassuring and comforting.

THE DECISION FOR HOSPICE

For patients and families facing a terminal illness, the decision to seek hospice care is often difficult. Families may feel that by doing so they may "give up." Or that hospice is really the end of the road. Patients may be reluctant to seek hospice help because they want to protect their families from the reality of oncoming death, or they may not want to burden them with care. Some people may feel that the hospital provides safer and better care. Others feel that to participate in hospice would make an already depressing situation even worse.

If any of these concerns raise serious questions in your mind about hospice, there are some answers you should consider in your decision-making process.

"Because you are in hospice," says Irene Rehberg, RN, "does not mean you have to give up hope. We live by the goals we set for ourselves in the future. We help people reach their goals, although the goals may no longer be long-term." NHO president Carolyn Fitzpatrick agrees. "We want people to keep on hoping. We never take that away. No one ever knows about death for sure. Sometimes dying patients stabilize and even go into remission. This happened to one patient of ours who told me, 'I was all psyched up to die,' and we discharged her from hospice. It *can* happen."

Nor does hospice mean an atmosphere of doom and gloom. "People often fear," says Ms. Fitzpatrick, "that you will have to think and talk about death every day. Actually we talk much more about living."

In the hospital-based hospice where Ms. Rehberg works, the atmosphere is far from solemn silence. "We do a lot of laughing here. We look for humor; it is a great way to reduce tension. People can bring their dogs and cats and share their babies with other patients. Sometimes the nurses will even dance around. Our patients," Ms. Rehberg says matter-of-factly, "aren't dead yet, and we don't treat them that way."

Patients who avoid hospice, wanting to spare their families, unknowingly make later family grief and recovery all the more difficult. Most families who choose hospice never regret the experience. Said one woman, "He and I were always close, but with hospice having him in the home added a new dimension to love and caring. I have some good feelings and happy memories because of it."

As for the safety and quality of hospice care, repeated studies have shown that hospice is as good as, and in many ways superior to, hospital care. Patients die with dignity, usually without the intrusive IV line and tubes, or fruitless resuscitation attempts. "Most patients who come to hospice have been through a lot of very aggressive therapy," Ms. Rehberg points out. "They are tired and want a peaceful and natural death."

Families who are concerned about whether they can provide proper care should be reassured. The hospice team is available round-the-clock every day to provide "hands-on" help and emotional support. Inpatient care can always be relied upon for medical backup as a needed break from care. "Many families are understandably fearful about death at home," says Ms. Rehberg. "The media does not give a very accurate view. Most often death is not a physically traumatic experience. The patient may slip into a deep coma; death usually comes peacefully without struggle."

Who Is Right for Hospice?

Hospice care is not right for every terminally ill patient and family. Most programs admit only patients whose life expectancy is six months or less. To get the full benefit of hospice, it's best to seek care as soon as it is appropriate.

Most patients, Ms. Fitzpatrick asserts, "come too late to hospice. We often get patients with only two weeks to live, though the doctor may say three months or more. Even though doctors support the hospice concept, many find it hard to refer patients," she states. "It is difficult for a doctor to say, 'I don't have any more tricks.' " She urges patients and families to consider hospice care earlier in terminal illness. Families and patients need enough time to work through emotional problems and to deal with the practical details of dying.

When families or physicians are in doubt about whether hospice is appropriate, most hospices will do a no-cost family consultation. Families can discuss their individual situation. And the patient's medical records will be reviewed by the hospice doctor, together with the patient's own doctor. "Usually," says Ms. Fitzpatrick, "we can tell within 15 minutes if hospice is appropriate, or whether the patient has any curative opportunities left."

Patients and families admitted to hospice must also understand and accept the "palliative" nature of hospice care. This means hospice provides relief and supportive therapy—not curative treatment. Ms. Fitzpatrick is quick to point out that accepting hospice care "does not mean you have to believe or accept your death." "We all die differently," says Ms. Rehberg. "Some people may not wish to face death and may fight it to the last breath. That's okay. In hospice, it is our job not to make people accept their death, but to open doors and give them opportunities to die at peace."

Anyone—doctor, social worker, family member, clergyman, friend—can refer someone to hospice. However, patient and family must both agree on hospice care. Since most hospice care is given at home, the programs require that an at-home family member function as the primary caregiver. If the patient lives alone, the hospice team will try to involve, teach, and help caring friends, neighbors, and community volunteers to substitute for family.

The hospice physician will work closely with the patient's personal physician. The hospice doctor provides direct care and supervision only if the patient has no doctor or the patient's physician wants to delegate this responsibility. Most often the family doctor and the hospice physician work cooperatively to plan care and achieve pain control.

Once accepted into a hospice program, patients and families are *always* free to change their minds at any time and return to curative care. But this rarely happens.

Hospice and Children

Most hospice programs will accept terminally ill children of any age, from the tiniest newborn through teenagers. But the decision to seek hospice care for a child is truly most difficult for families and physicians, although children accept hospice care more readily than adults. "Children don't have the fears that adults do," Ms. Fitzpatrick explains. "We can do so much to help the families, although children seldom come to hospice until the very end."

In *The Complete Hospice Guide,* author Dr. Robert Buckingham describes one family's experience with their 3-year-old child that underscores how meaningful in-home care for parent and dying child can be.

> Lisa, like the other children we've described, knew she would die when her tumor reappeared after a remission (when her "owie" came back). The child said it had recurred before X-rays confirmed her intuition. After this, Lisa did not want any further treatment. She wanted to be at home, where she was cheerful and unafraid of death. At home, she could continue her normal activities; as her mother says, "Lisa never missed 'Sesame Street,' even on the day she died."
>
> Lisa indeed died at home, in her mother's arms, cuddled in a rocking chair. Her parents were divorced, but her father was present at her death and had a chance to hold her and say goodbye. Lisa's mother recalls her death as a beautiful experience.

Hospice programs for children involve brothers and sisters who often feel angry, isolated, or neglected, as family attention understandably focuses on the dying child. This involvement reduces emotional difficulties that may otherwise follow a sibling's death.

CHOOSING A HOSPICE PROGRAM

Health professionals, such as doctors, hospital social workers, discharge planners, and home care personnel, are usually aware of existing hospice programs in the community. I&Rs can usually refer you to hospice, or you can check the local phone directory. The state hospice organizations listed in the Resource Guide are excellent sources for hospice information.

They can put you in touch with regular hospice programs, as well as any available informal support groups or services should you not want to participate in a regular hospice program. They also provide information on hospice in general and help communities organize local programs.

In many communities, only one hospice program may be available. In other areas, you may have several choices. From a consumer viewpoint, choosing a hospice is far easier than selecting a home care agency. Not only are choices more limited, but quality among hospice programs is uniformly high. Says Ms. Fitzpatrick, "Hospice is not an easy service for agencies to provide. The patients are sickest and require the most demanding care. This makes hospice unattractive to the unscrupulous operator."

As of 1984, eighteen states licensed or regulated hospice programs. Many states are developing or have hospice legislation pending. NHO expects that hospices will be licensed nationwide within the next five years. The hospice licensing laws are essentially "truth-in-advertising" laws. NHO and other hospice groups have lobbied hard to protect consumers at this most vulnerable time of life. In license states, no program may call itself a "hospice" unless it provides three key services:

- Medical services for pain control
- Skilled and basic nursing
- Emotional support, social work counseling, and bereavement services

Whenever you consider hospice, carefully evaluate these three critical areas.

What to Look For

If hospices are not licensed in your state, check the program's experience and background in hospice care. Does it belong to the National Hospice Organization or the state hospice organization? The Joint Commission on Accreditation of Hospitals accredits hospital-based hospices.

When you look at the hospice program itself, you can use

many of the same basic guidelines as for home care agencies. However, check the following points, which apply specifically to hospice care, carefully:

- *Twenty-four-hour coverage.* Confirm the availability of 24-hour help. Nurses should be "on call" day or night not only for advice, but for in-home emergency hands-on help whenever needed. Families should be encouraged to call for assistance.
- *Inpatient care policies.* Learn which hospital(s) (or nursing homes) the hospice uses to provide backup inpatient care. Make sure that the hospice program can arrange for or provide *ongoing hospice-type* care from the time the patient is admitted throughout the patient stay.

  Ask what happens if the patient needs admission suddenly, as can often happen. When hospice policies require that patients go through the hospital emergency room for admission, they will likely undergo IVs, tubes, transfusions, or other common emergency room procedures that are counter to hospice philosophy.

  Ask what happens in nonemergency situations. Many hospices arrange for patients to reenter the hospital without going through the routine admissions process each time. Also discuss what happens after the patient is admitted. How is the concept of hospice care continued? Some hospices may direct and provide patient care even after hospital admissions; but if not, there should be arrangements for care by special *hospice*-trained nurses, not regular staff.

  When the hospice concept is continued inside the hospital, patients can, for example, eat in bed whenever they want to; frequent temperature checks are dispensed with; and hospice nurses talk to coma patients and communicate with touch. Patients aren't simply treated as bodies.

  If there is no special inpatient hospice unit, ask about guarantees for "no resuscitation" orders or other measures that you may not wish which can needlessly prolong life.
- *Pain control.* If a hospice does not have a good pain control program, you do not have a true hospice program. The hospice doctor should be specially trained and

experienced in pain control with the *terminally ill.* Talk
to the doctor about pain control. The doctor's approach
to pain control should be aggressive and should consider
the psychological as well as the physical factors that are
involved.

- *Skilled and basic nursing.* The nursing staff, including
  homemakers and aides, should have special hospice training. Find out if the hospice provides care directly or
  under contract. According to hospice director Ann Katterhagen, "Only 13 percent of all hospices used subcon-
  tractors." But this is a potential problem area. Review
  the home care guidelines on subcontract personnel (see
  page 109).
- *Counseling and bereavement.* When you discuss this
  service, you may find important differences among programs. Look for programs that offer families as much
  counseling as they do patients. Check the length and type
  of bereavement services available. The follow-up bereavement services available will vary from 6 to 18 months.
  Longer is better. Some programs have little one-to-one
  bereavement counseling available and may confine their
  service to less than ideal group work only, usually with
  several families participating at a time. Ask who can
  participate in the bereavement program. Superior programs involve *all* family members, including children and
  grandparents.
- *Physician involvement.* Programs should always work
  cooperatively with your own family doctor. Avoid any
  program that suggests you will have to give up your
  doctor in order to receive hospice care.
- *The volunteer program.* Discuss the services and the role
  of volunteers. A very active volunteer program is important
  to many much-needed supportive services, as well as
  extra hands-on help at home.

THE FINANCIAL SIDE TO HOSPICE

Dying does not come cheap in our country. During the last
six months of terminal illness, bills upwards of $30,000 for

hospitalization are not uncommon. The last few days of life alone in the traditional high-tech hospital system may cost thousands of dollars. As a result, after death, families are left burdened with financial losses as well as the loss of a loved one.

However, studies that have compared traditional care versus hospice care have found hospice is indeed much less costly. Hospice programs generally cost less because room and board and high-tech procedures are eliminated. Hospital-based hospice programs are more expensive than the community hospice home care programs, but still far cheaper than conventional hospital care. Results of the National Hospice Evaluation Study released in 1984 found that the total costs per patient for hospital-based hospices averaged $5,890; for community hospice programs, $4,758 per patient. Blue Cross of Northeast Ohio reported that the average insurance payment during the last two weeks of life with community hospice was $699, compared to $2,140 for traditional hospital care.

Congress was so impressed by the cost-saving potential of hospice that it authorized an experimental Medicare hospice benefit which runs from November 1, 1983, to September 30, 1986. Analysts expect the benefit to continue after that. Many insurers have started, or are planning, hospice benefits that are completely distinct from home care benefits. And a few states now mandate that insurers offer hospice benefits. Many employers now request hospice benefits in their employee insurance programs. Florida, for example, now provides hospice coverage to all state employees through its Blue Cross and Blue Shield plan.

Most hospice programs apply whatever insurance coverage you may have available, such as home care, hospice, or other benefits, to meet hospice costs. Any remaining costs are charged on a sliding scale. Almost all hospices are supported through community sources and fundraising efforts. And for almost every hospice, the financial policy is this: No one is denied service because of inability to pay.

The Medicare Hospice Benefit

Terminally ill seniors can use regular home care benefits to help pay for hospice care, or they may elect to use the special Medicare hospice benefit.

The hospice benefit is provided under hospital insurance, Medicare Part A. To qualify for the benefit, patients must be terminally ill, with a six-month or less life expectancy, as certified by the hospice and patient's doctor. The patient must sign a statement choosing the hospice benefit and giving up standard Medicare benefits insofar as terminal illness is concerned.

Once the benefit is in effect, the patient can receive hospice coverage until death. For reimbursement purposes, Medicare provides coverage as two 90-day benefit periods followed by a 30-day extension. If further care is needed after this 210-day period, a Medicare-certified hospice will continue to provide care, as long as the patient wishes, at no extra cost. Patients may choose to drop the benefit at any time and return to standard Medicare. In doing so, only the remaining days left in a benefit period are forfeited.

For example, if someone elects to use the hospice benefit initially but drops out after 60 days of hospice care, he or she loses the remaining 30 days left in that 90-day benefit period. If the senior elects the hospice benefit again at a later time, 120 days of hospice care remain available.

In addition to the standard Medicare home care benefits, the hospice benefit provides the following *in full,* without deductibles or co-payments required, except as noted:

- Homemaker services
- Services of the hospice physician
- Bereavement family counseling
- Medical equipment and supplies
- Drugs for pain control and symptom management (a small co-payment is required, no more than $5 per prescription)
- Inpatient respite care—no more than five consecutive days each time admitted; patient pays 5 percent of cost up to a maximum $400 (1985 rate) fee per 90-day period.

(If hospice care is continuous, or with less than a 14-day
interruption between benefit periods, only *one* maximum
fee applies.)

The Advantages

For the terminally ill, the hospice benefit offers decided
advantages over standard Medicare coverage for hospital,
medical, and home care. The accompanying table shows the
major advantages. Overall, the hospice benefit provides better
coverage and will reduce out-of-pocket costs.

Note, for example, that the hospice benefit will pay for
drugs. Often the pain-killing drugs a terminal patient requires
are very expensive, so this benefit means a substantial savings.
Another important provision is the availability of much-
needed custodial care and continuous home care, which
standard Medicare home care benefits never cover.

Savings also accrue with needed medical equipment and
supplies. For example, if a terminal colon cancer patient who
has a colostomy elects the hospice benefit, the cost of colostomy bags would become fully covered.

COMPARISON OF STANDARD
MEDICARE AND HOSPICE BENEFITS

Standard Medicare	Hospice Benefit
Patient must be homebound to qualify for home care	Homebound status not required
Prescription drugs not covered	Drugs related to terminal illness fully covered; small co-payment required
No custodial home care allowed	Custodial home care may be provided by homemakers and home health aides
Medical equipment and supplies: pays 80% of allowed charge after deductible	Medical equipment and supplies fully covered if related to terminal illness
No respite care allowed	Inpatient respite care allowed for limited days during each benefit period
No more than eight hours of home care a day allowed	Continuous care available, up to 24 hours if needed
Inpatient hospital care subject to a deductible and co-payment after 60 days per benefit period	Short-term inpatient care, fully covered; no deductible or co-payment ever required

Important Rules

Be aware that the cost of drugs and care provided under the benefit are for *terminal illness only*. Medicare pays for treatment for other conditions not related to terminal illness under its standard Medicare program. Take the case of a diabetic patient who is dying with cancer. The hospice benefit will not pay for insulin because it is a drug not related to the cancer condition. Or suppose a dying patient falls and breaks a leg. Any costs or treatment involved in this case would be applied toward the standard benefit.

Note that the patient's own doctor's fees are still paid for under Medicare Part B. The hospice benefit applies only to the *hospice* physician.

To use the Medicare hospice benefit, the senior must receive care from a *Medicare-certified hospice*. This is *not* the same as a Medicare-certified home health agency. A home health agency or a hospice must be specially certified in order to participate in the Medicare hospice program.

Of the estimated 1,500 hospices eligible for Medicare certification, 165 were certified as of March 1985. Many eligible hospices have declined to participate in Medicare thus far because of disagreements over the government's reimbursement policy. NHO expects the majority of eligible hospices will eventually become certified as these payment problems are worked out. In the meantime, if there is no certified hospice nearby, seniors may use the standard Medicare benefits for home care and hospital care toward hospice care costs. However, the special hospice benefits, such as drug coverage, will not apply.

Other Insurers

Because the hospice concept is still relatively new, many insurers do not provide separate hospice benefits. However, hospice care may be covered under existing home care, hospital, or outpatient benefits. Hospice staff will work closely with you to help determine any available coverage.

Among the insurers providing hospice benefits, some place a dollar ceiling on the amount of reimbursement for hospice care, rather than limit coverage to a certain number of home care visits. Some insurers do not require deductibles or co-payments or pay at higher rates in order to encourage hospice use. Now that Medicare funds hospice care, many more insurers will offer hospice benefits in the future. Many insurers, such as Blue Cross and Blue Shield, are experimenting with hospice benefits for their group policyholders. Here is a rundown of what some major insurance companies currently provide as hospice benefits. Specifics vary according to the employer's choice of benefit packages.

- Aetna Life Insurance Company usually requires a deductible and co-payment; covers all hospice services except a homemaker. Special hospice benefits are available under major medical insurance only.
- Allstate Life Insurance Company provides inpatient hospice benefits up to a $5,000 maximum under its major medical policy. Professional home care visits, medicine, equipment, supplies, and drugs are covered. Homemaker visits are not covered.
- Blue Cross and Blue Shield plans vary. Some provide hospice as an extension of home health care benefits; others have individual hospice benefits. Empire Blue Cross and Blue Shield, for example, provides 200 home care visits, with an extension if more are needed for hospice care. All standard home care services are provided, plus respiratory therapy and chemotherapy/radiation therapy for symptom control.
- Connecticut General Life Insurance may require a small deductible up to $50, with payments for services ranging from 80 to 100 percent. Limits placed on visits range from 40 to 80, depending on employer's choice.
- Continental Assurance Company requires no deductible; co-payment varies according to employer's option. Covers doctor, skilled nursing, all therapies, dietitian, social services; but *no* home health aide or homemaker service. Equipment, lab fees, and high-tech care are allowable, as is respite care for families and bereavement counseling.

- The Equitable Life Insurance Company provides coverage up to $5,000, including inpatient care. Drugs, homemaker service, and bereavement counseling are included as covered services.
- Hartford Insurance Group does not require any deductibles or co-payments for its hospice benefits. Dietitian services are covered; homemaking is not.
- Metropolitan Life's standard approved hospice benefits provides $7,500 maximum for inpatient care with $3,000 maximum for in-home hospice services. Counseling is limited to six months after death. Benefits normally cover 100 percent of reasonable charges.
- Mutual/United of Omaha covers most hospice services except for homemaking; coverage varies by plan, usually paying 100 percent of cost up to $40 per visit, with a 40-visit limit.
- Provident Life and Accident Insurance Company may not require a deductible or co-payment, depending on the employer's choice. Dietitian services are covered; homemaker is not.
- Prudential Insurance Company of America provides maximum outpatient $2,000, inpatient $3,000 for hospice care. Grief counseling for family is covered.
- Transamerica Occidental Life requires no deductible or co-payment; will cover all hospice services, including homemaker. Limits vary by group policy. TPN, enteral nutrition, IV therapy, and ventilation respiration not covered under hospice, as this is considered "treatment" of an illness.

Doctors, Dentists, and Others at Your Door

DOCTORS

If you remember and long for the days of old-fashioned medicine when doctors made house calls, take heart. House calls are making a comeback.

Why the turnabout? One reason is the increased competition among doctors for patients. Since 1970, the pool of physicians has grown about four times faster than our population. By 1990, forecasters declare we will have a "doctor glut." Supply and demand economics says more doctors and fewer patients equal income losses. Increased house calls represent one response to the pressures of increased competition. But the return to home medical care also stems from human concerns.

With the growing number of older Americans, particularly in the 85 and over age group, many of whom are frail, chronically ill, and homebound, a real need exists for in-home doctor care. Talking to a *St. Petersburg Times* reporter about his newly formed proprietary physician service, Dr. Carl Moore declared: "The invalid is really the kind of patient we want to help out. These people have a real struggle getting to the doctor's office."

However, you do not necessarily have to be homebound to receive a house call. Some consumers use house calls if they require medical assistance after hours or on weekends, when their only other choice is either no care or an emergency room.

Types of Services

If you need home medical care, you may have several choices.

1. Your own personal doctor may be willing to make house calls. An AMA survey found 8 percent of the doctors reported making more house calls now than in the past, with younger doctors making them even more often. From a patient care standpoint, your personal doctor is best. To practice the best medicine, the doctor should be familiar with you and your medical history. When you choose a family doctor, ask if he or she will make house calls.

2. You may use a physician home service if one exists in your area. These are usually incorporated businesses that may be doctor-owned or divisions of or affiliated with other health enterprises, such as home health agencies or walk-in clinics. Doctors Home Care, for example, is part of Instant Care Centers of America, which is a subsidiary of National Medical Enterprises (NME). NME also owns hospitals, nursing homes, home care agencies, and a medical equipment business. These services usually advertise to make consumers aware of their availability.

3. Some home care programs, often based at teaching hospitals, integrate medical services into their overall care program. Typically these programs must serve the elderly or the homebound.

For instance, the Home Oncology Medical Extension (HOME) program of North Shore University Hospital, New York, provides care to cancer patients using an interdisciplinary team that includes physician specialists, a psychiatrist, and a neurologist, as well as nurse specialists, a pharmacist, and other health professionals. A five-ton van equipped to store blood for in-home transfusion and perform on-the-spot lab work is a key link in the service.

In New York City, St. Vincent's Hospital, through its Department of Community Medicine, serves the homebound living in the Chelsea–Greenwich Village area of the city. The youngest patient currently enrolled is 31; the oldest, 113. Nine physicians, many resident doctors, serve the professional team, with additional doctors available as consultants in psychiatry, urology, surgery, cancer, neurology, and ophthalmology.

At Boston University Hospital, its Home Medical Service serves about 1,000 homebound patients in the greater Boston area. The program involves medical students as part of the home care team.

Consumer Guidelines

When you consider the house call option through a proprietary physician service, check the following points carefully:

- *Who qualifies for service?* Some programs limit services to the homebound or to persons living within a certain driving distance. Most physician services are quick to point out they are not replacements for your regular doctor. Some will not provide services to patients of other doctors, even if the personal physician does not make house calls.
- *What are the doctor's credentials?* Anyone who holds a medical license can practice medicine. You should seek a doctor who is board-certified in the specialty that matches your need. For example, a board-certified psychiatrist should not be sent to handle medical cases. Also, inquire about the range of available specialists.
- *Is your request for home medical care screened? If so, by whom?* If an answering service operator or a clerk simply dispenses a doctor upon your request for care, you may be in for trouble. A physician, registered nurse, or other qualified professional should screen incoming calls for their appropriateness for home care.

If you delay emergency care to wait for a doctor at home, in some cases your condition may worsen and your safety may be endangered. For example, a middle-aged man with chest pains or severe "indigestion" may be experiencing a heart attack.

Even if your own doctor does not make house calls, you should call and discuss your condition with him or her. Often a doctor can provide sound self-care advice over the phone, or call in a prescription that may solve your problem without a home visit.

- *What diagnostic and treatment services can be provided at home?* If portable laboratory services, X-ray, and EKG (electrocardiogram) equipment are not available for testing at home, the doctor may decide you need hospitalization or walk-in clinic service, thus defeating the purpose of the house call.

- *What backup and follow-up services are available?* Find out if the doctor is familiar with home care in general, and works with one or more agencies. You may require more assistance than a one-shot visit. Also, discuss possible arrangements should you need ongoing medical care; or will you be seen by whomever is on call (a less than ideal setup)?

- *What happens if hospitalization is necessary?* Find out which hospital(s) you will be referred to. Like doctors, some hospitals are better than others. Also, you will probably want a hospital in your own area.

- *Will your personal doctor receive a copy of your medical report?* If not, make sure you get a copy for your own medical records.

- *How long before the doctor arrives?* You will have to determine yourself if the answer is acceptable.

- *What fees are involved?* Some services charge an annual or one-time enrollment fee in addition to the cost per visit. Professional Home Visits in Manhattan, for example, charges a hefty $100 sign-up fee. For this, consumers receive a medical history questionnaire which, once completed, is fed into a computer file and stored for future reference if care is needed. The home visit charge is $80. Doctors Home Care charges $55; no enrollment fee. Expect lab, X ray, drugs supplied, and so on to be extra. However, check if there is a service charge to give you an injection, draw blood, or take a throat culture.

- *What are the payment policies?* Discuss whether you can be billed or pay by credit card. Will insurance assignment be accepted, or insurance forms completed and/or filed for you? Most doctor visits should be covered by insurance, including Medicare, but double-check your coverage. Some policies do have exceptions or special rules.

DENTISTS

The importance of dental care to overall health is often overlooked. If you have trouble eating because of teeth and gum problems, you are less likely to maintain good nutrition, a vital factor in health, even if the most healthful menu is provided.

Left untreated, dental problems can cause needless pain and discomfort. If you are already ill or frail, dental conditions can sometimes lead to serious infections which can complicate existing medical problems.

Many community nonprofit home care programs are recognizing that there is the need for dental care as part of comprehensive home care services. Programs like that of Boston University Hospital include dental specialists in the home care team.

Dentists in private practice are also making home dental care available through a major national program called Access. The program, which operates in 43 states, has about 22,000 dentists participating. Working with local public health departments or other community agencies, dentists provide free or low-cost care to the homebound.

Because home dentistry requires special portable equipment that costs around $1,000, your local dentist is not likely to have a home equipment set. However, the local Dental Society often purchases a few sets of equipment which it then loans to Access or other area dentists when needed.

Also promoting home dentistry is the National Foundation of Dentistry for the Handicapped. Through the foundation, local dental hygienists and dentists are practicing preventive dentistry. They use mobile vans or portable equipment to assist the physically, mentally, or developmentally disabled, who are often homebound or unable to use conventional dentistry because of physical barriers such as office doors being too narrow to accommodate wheelchairs.

To locate any available home dental services in your area, contact your local Dental Society, nearby dental school, or discuss your dental care needs with your home care coordinator.

THERAPISTS

We usually think only of doctors and dentists as private practitioners. However, depending on state laws, other health professionals can literally hang out a shingle and provide therapy or other services directly to consumers.

Physical, occupational, and speech therapists may work independently, often with a doctor's prescription, or they may work cooperatively in special group practices. Like doctors, therapists may make house calls.

Melissa Cohn, occupational therapist and co-founder of Rehab Associates Limited (Clearwater, FL), explains: "We get a lot of referrals from doctors. We will work with any client who has had an injury or disability or who has lost function from birth. Many of our patients are pediatric cases or adults who have suffered head trauma or stroke."

Like similar groups, Rehab Associates Limited has physical, occupational, and speech therapists on staff and uses assistant-level personnel as well. This group practice provides therapy under contracts with home care agencies, or consumers themselves may contact the group directly to arrange for therapy.

When working privately with patients, therapists usually make a home evaluation, develop a therapy plan of care, and discuss all recommendations with the doctor, if involved. Fees average about $25 to $60 per visit. Therapists may not accept insurance assignments. If you are interested in this type of arrangement, check your insurance policy. The services may be covered under outpatient therapy.

Most therapists in private practice are listed in the Yellow Pages under various therapies or generically under Rehabilitation Services.

PHARMACISTS

It's too soon to say whether the concept of home health care pharmacy services will catch on. But the idea has great merit. One study found that 31 percent of all prescription drugs were improperly taken by patients in a potentially harmful way. Each year about 1.5 million people are hospitalized because of bad drug reactions. Many are elderly people who, according to a HCFA study, fill or refill close to 18 prescriptions each year. Another study found that 92 percent of all elderly people used prescription drugs.

At Vaughn Prescriptions (Fort Smith, AR), a staff pharmacist visits homebound consumers on a routine, scheduled basis. The pharmacist explains the drug program, the timing of doses, and possible drug side effects. Over-the-counter drugs used regularly at home are identified, and any possibly harmful interactions are pointed out. Even nutrition is discussed, since when you eat and what you eat can affect which drugs must be taken and how they act in the body. These home visits provide a chance to improve your understanding of proper drug use and the value of drug therapy, and to spot any problems that may prevent you from taking your drugs as prescribed.

Vaughn also uses a blister card drug dispenser, which makes it much easier for consumers on multiple drugs to take their drugs on schedule. The card works like a calendar that has clear plastic bubbles (the blisters), one for each day of the month. Once a month the pharmacist fills each blister with all the pills that you must take at a given time. You don't have to mess with hard-to-open bottles; you won't mix drugs or forget to take a dose. Each card notes the time of the drug dose, and stickers show the day of the week.

Just a glance at the card tells you if you have taken your drugs properly. Drugs dispensed in this manner cost more than bottles per prescription. But most consumers find the system worth the modest extra charge.

After the pharmacist's initial visit, customers are seen once a month until the drug program is established and there are no side effects or other problems. After that, visits are on an as-needed basis, with phone calls in between.

The combination of the dosage system and pharmacist support promotes independent living. It also reduces the chance of drug errors such as accidental overdoses.

V

HOW TO GET
THE BEST CARE

—20—

What to Do Before Care Begins

FROM HOSPITAL TO HOME

If you are a hospital patient, definitely plan early for home care, ideally before or upon admission, or as soon as possible thereafter. During the first phase of hospitalization, this may seem hard to do. You or your family may feel overwhelmed by the problems at hand. But if your goal is to return home again, start the necessary planning as soon as you can.

If you are a Medicare patient, this pays off. Thanks to the DRG system, hospitals are discharging Medicare patients "sicker and quicker" than ever before, as home care agencies around the country can attest. In the hurry to get Medicare patients out, critical details are sometimes overlooked. In one reported New Jersey case, a stroke patient was all set to go home when someone remembered he was a newly diagnosed diabetic. He was taught the art of insulin injecting in the hospital elevator on his way out!

No matter what kind of care you need—routine home care, high-tech, or specialized rehab—your key to a smooth transition from hospital to home requires planning and coordination among: (1) your doctor; (2) the hospital staff and discharge planner; (3) the home care agency (unless you intend to do it yourself or rely on family; (4) the equipment dealer (if needed); and (5) you and your family.

The hospital discharge planning office is the hospital command center for home care. This office helps ensure that patients, upon discharge, will receive any needed follow-up care. Therefore, discharge planners are an important link in your "continuity of care." In fact, planners are sometimes called "continuity of care coordinators."

Every hospital has discharge planning personnel, although in some hospitals the role may be performed by staff nurses or the medical social worker. About 38 percent of hospitals use nurse–social work discharge planning teams. Planners counsel patients and families about home care or other options, assist in the decision-making process, and will help patients and families arrange aftercare.

Contact the Discharge Planner or Home Care Agency Early

Hospitals encourage dependency, so you may hesitate to contact the discharge planner yourself. But if you wait for, or count on, the discharge planner to contact you, you may be missed altogether. Hospitals have too many patients and too few planners (sometimes only one) to make one-to-one contact possible in every case. Planners rely on a review of patient records or referrals from doctors or hospital staff to spot the patient who may need help.

Some hospitals now include a brief patient questionnaire as part of their admissions process to identify the most likely home care patients; for example, anyone who lives alone, particularly if older and with certain diagnoses. If you don't fit a high-risk profile, you may be overlooked. Or you may be skipped at some hospitals if your doctor does not write "discharge planning" on your chart. Many doctors still do not appreciate the importance of discharge planning and home care, so this is a common problem.

If your condition matches any of those in the accompanying table, give serious thought to home care. Even though you may think you are recovering just fine in the hospital, once you are home you may realize that you cannot easily manage. It's often wiser to try home care first and then cut it back or out.

If the hospital does not have a discharge planning office as

COMMON DIAGNOSES FOR DISCHARGE TO HOME CARE

Diabetes (unstable)

Heart/circulatory conditions, including high blood pressure (unstable) and pacemaker implant

Stroke recovery

Arthritis/joint problems

Respiratory ailments

Cancer

Skin problems, including bedsores and wounds

Bowel and bladder conditions

Nerve-muscle disorders

Digestive disorders, including conditions that require artificial feeding

Postoperative recovery

Accident recovery

such, ask your floor nurse or supervisor or hospital social worker who handles this responsibility.

Talk to the discharge planner about any concerns you may have following hospital release. The planner can enlist the advice of other professionals involved in your care, including your doctor, about your possible home care needs. Sometimes a discharge planning meeting is arranged so you, your family, and the professionals can discuss your situation and provide guidance. However, the decision for or against home care or other alternatives should be yours.

Keep in mind that discharge planning is purely optional. If you wish, you can make your home care decision on your own. If you opt for home care, you can arrange for it yourself, or the discharge planner (even if not otherwise consulted) can assist. You are free to use *any* agency, regardless of whether the hospital operates its own or refers to an affiliated agency. Some home care agencies station their own coordinators within the hospital to help patients plan early for home care. But any professional agency you may call will also provide this guidance.

What does the agency do, once called? It will conduct an in-hospital assessment, also consulting with hospital nurses and staff who provide care and therapy. Unless yours is a special case, it's good practice to wait until a few days prior to discharge for an assessment. Done too early, it won't accurately reflect your condition and needs at discharge time.

How Early Agency Action Helps

Early agency involvement has many advantages. If your experience parallels that of many patients, you may be discharged on a Friday. Wait until Saturday morning to decide you need home care, and you will find that many agencies cannot supply any personnel or may just supply "a body."

If you live alone or do not have anyone who can accompany you home, the agency can provide an aide for this service. The aide could, for example, ride with you in the ambulette that takes you home, and then make sure you are comfortable at home, do some light grocery shopping, or fill any drug prescriptions you may need.

Without advance planning, patients often leave the hospital without specific orders for needed services such as therapy. Michele Quirolo, an agency nurse coordinator who is stationed at a hospital to promote proper planning, explains: "By being involved in advance, I can review the patient record and make sure that the agency is alerted to all the special needs for patient care. Or if a patient will be discharged with a wound, such as a bedsore, I will photograph the wound so that the agency nurse assigned can actually compare the photo with the wound, as is, at home and see for herself if it has gotten better or worse. Planning ahead also gives me time to try to link patients with other community services they may need once home. In any case, when patients leave the hospital, their continuity of care is far better."

The agency nurse coordinator can help you with the practical details, such as arranging for medical equipment purchase or rental and delivery. Advance planning also gives the hospital and home care staff a chance to confer about the best care for you. For example, the hospital and agency physical therapists could discuss your treatment progress or problems one-on-one. This would provide the agency therapist with very important treatment information that could never be obtained merely by reading your patient record.

Going It Alone

If you decide against home care for personal reasons, before you leave the hospital for home, do as the agency would do and double-check these important details:

- Medical equipment, if needed, will be delivered on your discharge date.
- Necessary drug prescriptions are provided; if discharge is on a weekend, ask for a small supply to tide you over until prescriptions can be filled.
- A drug schedule is provided, along with special instructions on drug use and potential side effects; ask your hospital floor nurse.
- Any special diet or exercise orders are provided.
- Patient and/or family instruction is provided in basic self-care techniques.
- Transportation arrangements, if needed, are made through discharge planner, nurse, or social worker.

Don't forget to ask the discharge planner for home care agency recommendations should you change your mind and later decide you need home care.

PLAN FOR CARE BEFORE YOU NEED IT

Just as savvy consumers look for a good doctor before they get sick and need one, scout home care agencies before you actually need care. If you (or a loved one) suffer from a chronic health condition, or if you have older parents, or you or your spouse are seniors, advance planning makes very good sense. This will help take the pressure off decision making during stressful times of illness.

When the actual need for home care arises or seems likely, don't delay. Contact your doctor or other key professionals right away. Remember that home care can help prevent hospitalization. So, should a chronic condition worsen, for example, automatic hospitalization or emergency room care need not always be the solution.

CHOOSE YOUR HOME CARE PROVIDERS YOURSELF

Many consumers let the doctor, discharge planner, or social worker choose the agency or equipment dealer.

This is the "line of least resistance" route to a home care provider. You don't have to ask anyone questions about cost or quality. During stressful times, this may seem the easiest, quickest, and best solution. For some consumers, this proves true. But this can also be a chancy proposition.

With increased home care competition, many providers are aggressively pushing their services through a barrage of phone calls, mailings, and face-to-face meetings. Professionals are usually hard-pressed for time too. Like consumers, they can succumb to advertising and marketing tactics and may recommend without solid knowledge. Sometimes professionals do not want to "play favorites," so they keep rosters and rotate recommendations.

Many professionals try to recommend selectively. Unfortunately, if consumer problems occur, professionals often never find out. Hospital discharge planners seldom have contact with patients once they leave the hospital. Doctors do, but consumers are often embarrassed and reluctant to tell their doctors, even when doctors ask, that their "professional" recommendations have proved faulty. Therefore, professionals may unknowingly recommend providers who do not consistently give top-notch service or care.

Finally, because home care is the most personal kind of care you can receive, professionals may suggest a good provider, but that provider may still not be the best choice for you. For example, doctors or hospital staff, if not familiar with outside providers, may lean toward recommending their own hospital service, if one exists. But the professional may not consider certain factors, like payment policies or special services that may be important to you.

There's no question that professionals can provide solid home care guidance. Seek their counsel in your decision making, but choose your providers yourself. Because in the end, you, not the professional, are the person who must be satisfied with the service and care.

ORGANIZE YOUR HOME

Whether you live in a house or an apartment, give your home a quick review with home care in mind. Often even small adjustments can help improve home care, ease home management when you are frail, sick, or disabled, and make the home a safer place to be.

Safety First

Don't minimize the safety issue. Statistics show that whether you are well or sick, at any age your home can be potentially dangerous. About 36 percent of all disabling accidents occur in the home. Each year over 22,000 people die accidentally in the home. The elderly and the very young are particularly vulnerable to injury and death.

Among the elderly, accidents—particularly falls—represent the biggest threat, although *any* person in poor health or fragile physical condition is at risk.

Make a room-by-room safety check. Target first the high-accident areas—the bathroom and kitchen—where wet, slippery floors are common. To prevent bathroom falls, install sturdy grab bars by the bathtub. Don't rely on an in-the-wall soap caddy to steady you as you climb in and out of the tub. Place bars on the outside tub rim and on the inner tub wall. Make sure you have a nonskid mat or strips on the tub floor. As an added safety measure, place a nonskid stool or chair in the tub for safe, easy showering. Install grab bars by the commode if needed. In the bathroom, kitchen, or elsewhere, avoid highly waxed and polished floors. Place a small nonskid rug by the bathtub and kitchen sink to absorb water spills, but make sure that the rug is securely anchored.

Check all scatter rugs throughout your home. Remove unnecessary rugs. Back essential rugs with double-face tape, and tack down or place a small rubber mat underneath to anchor. Look for curled carpet corners or frayed spots that can cause trips and falls. Never run an electrical cord under a rug. Pay close attention to normal traffic patterns. Remove clutter, cords, or other potential accident causes from common pathways and stairs. Also make sure these areas are well lit.

Burns and fires are another household danger. Set water heater temperatures at 120 degrees Fahrenheit to reduce the chance of scalds. Install smoke detectors and, of course, outlaw smoking in bed. Check all household appliances for frayed cords, a source of electrical fires.

Emergency Alert

Everyone should have a readiness plan in case of emergencies. This becomes doubly important if you are living alone. Make up your "safety net" of emergency numbers and keep your list handy by *each* household telephone. Tape the list on the wall or tabletop so you won't have to fumble to find it. Include in your list:

- Police
- Fire
- Poison control center
- Rescue or paramedic ambulance squad
- Closest neighbor
- Closest relative

- Pharmacist
- Utility company (gas and electric), including after-hours or emergency number. This is a must if you have electrically powered DME.

Once home care begins, don't forget to add the home care agency, the supervisor, or other necessary numbers such as your medical equipment repair number. If you live alone, consider an ERS (see Chapter 14).

The Care Room

Consider the sickroom, its location and layout, for noise level, convenience, and psychological needs. If care is for another, include him or her in any decisions about the care room. Your loved one may spend a great deal of time in this room, so personal preferences are very important.

Some people require a quiet location as far away from street or household noise as possible. Other people prefer a room close to the center of household activity so they can enjoy and participate in family life as much as possible. In this case, don't overlook the importance of privacy. When the patient tires, rest and relaxation will be needed. Even a small room divider can help provide privacy.

When you select the care room, also consider its location in relation to the bathroom. Ideally the two rooms should be adjacent, so frequent trips between will be less taxing. In a multilevel home, stairs often present another obstacle. Patients who must use crutches, canes, or walkers can't manage stairs easily and safely. If the patient will have to make daily trips up and down stairs, locate the care room on the main floor if possible.

In order to secure good care at home, your room does not have to be elaborately equipped, just comfortable. Check the room for proper lighting and ventilation. Make sure the bed has enough pillows for adequate support for sitting in bed. Provide several lightweight blankets so you can make adjustments easily for temperature changes.

For those who are not bedridden, place a sturdy nonskid chair close to the bedside to aid transfer from bed. If the room is not carpeted, place a small nonskid rubber mat by the bedside too.

Don't let boredom interfere with recovery. Have on hand recreational items such as books, magazines, playing cards, radio, or TV. Children enjoy age-appropriate puzzles, games, and crafts, and of course visits from friends.

Equip the bedside nightstand with basic comfort items—water pitcher and glass, tissues and small personal items.

Do you need special equipment? If so, you can choose

from among hundreds of medical items for the home. But choose wisely, since many items on the market are for convenience and are not essential for care. Purchase or rent only essential items first; you can add additional items as needed. Guidelines are outlined in Chapter 13. However, many useful items can be improvised at home.

For example, use a small bell to devise a call system, so caregivers can be alerted when needed. If you cut away two sides of a sturdy cardboard box, you create a lightweight stand that can be used over the lap as a small bed table. Cut down low and placed over the feet beneath the sheet, you make a tent that provides more leg room and eases the pressure of the cover weight. Remove the top from an egg carton and you have a medication tray. Fill each egg cup with the correct pill(s) and label by drug name and/or medication time.

Ask other caregivers, patients, and professionals for tips; or consult a good home nursing guide.

Valuables

Any time a stranger comes into your home, there is a chance that property loss—damage or theft—may occur. Don't expect the worst with home care, but don't deny the unpleasant possibility either. Instead, guard against this situation as best you can.

Whenever possible, store expensive jewelry, large sums of cash, stocks or negotiables, and other small valuables in a safe place—not at home, in a bank. Put valuables left at home safely out of sight. Discuss with the bank any extra safety measures to guard against unauthorized withdrawals—for example, prior telephone verification with you.

Take stock of any remaining "valuables" in each room. Include those with sentimental value, not just cash worth. Often the loss of these items may be more important to you than those money can replace.

Next, make a written list of these items, noting their location. When you list an item, don't just identify it generally. Describe it briefly. A "bracelet" might become "ladies' 14K

gold link bracelet." You may even want to photograph certain
valuable items. Include the property owner's name (if someone
else), and date the list. This list will provide documentation
for insurance or other purposes should property loss occur.

If home care is for a parent or relative who lives elsewhere,
particularly far away, a list can be an invaluable aid. It can
help you quickly identify whether household goods are missing
or damaged since service began. It can also give you peace of
mind by confirming that a "missing" item was not there in
the first place.

Often when adult children visit the family home after a
long absence and find a vividly remembered item gone, they
fear it has been stolen. Yet in many cases, the valuable was
long gone prior to care—lost, sold, broken and discarded,
given away—even though the parent may have no recollection
or have never mentioned its disposal.

Once you have made your list, photocopy it and put each
copy in a safe place for future reference. Contact your local
police precinct for advice about safety measures for large
items such as TVs and stereos. Many police departments run
special theft-prevention programs. You may be able to place
the serial identification numbers of such goods on file with
the police. Some departments will loan special equipment to
mark your valuables distinctively and then give you a "crime
prevention" sticker for your doors and windows that will
alert would-be thieves about your program participation.

WORK CLOSELY WITH THE AGENCY BEFOREHAND

Once you select a professional agency, your best assurance
for good care is to work closely with that agency even before
services begin. Review all key issues with the agency.

Confidentiality

Like other medical records, all home care records—the care
plan, any correspondence, progress notes on care, financial
data, and so on—should be strictly confidential. Before an

agency releases any of your records to another party or if it must obtain information about you in order to provide care, your written permission should be secured in advance. Outside of written records, the privacy of your home should be respected too. Personnel should never discuss your situation with neighbors, however well-meaning.

Ask if the agency will advise others on your condition and progress. Often agencies will inform those persons named as relatives or "others interested" on the home care assessment forms. Some agencies, however, will not provide any information routinely to anyone, including family members, unless the client specifically gives his or her consent. If care is for another, be sure to double-check this point. You may have to make special arrangements in advance in order to be kept informed.

Assigned Personnel

Discuss any general personal preferences you may have that differ from the agency's normal personnel policies. Do you want the aide to wear a uniform, or would you prefer that neat street clothes be worn? When practical, most agencies will honor a request to omit uniforms. Do you want to be addressed by your surname, as the agency normally will require, or would you feel more relaxed if employees addressed you on a first-name basis?

Double-check the essential skills of assigned personnel. You can ask for a quick verbal sketch of the specific training and experience of personnel assigned. If you suffered from a heart condition, wouldn't you want to know the aide or nurse assigned has been trained to perform CPR (cardiopulmonary resuscitation)? Don't forget to confirm any special nonhealth needs (bilingual or kosher cooking experienced) you may have requested too.

Security

Discuss security measures in detail in advance with the supervisor. Don't worry that the agency will think you distrustful. A security-minded agency should initiate such a discussion if you don't. If you're in doubt about security for any reason, don't hesitate to put the agency "on notice" that you expect the highest caliber personnel, and won't hesitate to take legal action, should serious problems occur.

Get the names and the scheduled arrival times of any personnel who will be assigned to your care. Ask what identification employees carry that you can look for. Always discuss the issue of house keys, especially if employees will live in or shop for you.

If employees will shop or pay bills for you, review procedures for such transactions. Better yet, get a copy of the procedures in writing. Most agencies have a standardized system that accounts for such transactions. This system should protect both you and the agency against disputes. For example, some agencies employ a simple recording form that notes the amount of shopping money given to, and received from, the employee. Both you and the employee are asked to sign the completed form to verify the accuracy of the transaction. If financial transactions will be made by check or other means, discuss any appropriate safeguards. For example, you could notify the store manager to set a limit on check transactions.

Finally, review the care plan and the service contract. Don't hesitate to question any details that are not clear. Make sure the care plan lists the supervisor's name and telephone number, as well as the specific home care tasks. Check the contract for correct rates, personnel listed, and mutual obligations. Do not sign any contract or permission forms containing spaces that have been left blank. Scratch over the blanks before signing as a protection against having anything added to your contract without your consent later. Get a copy of anything that you sign, as well as the care plan. Store these in a safe place for further reference.

—21—

What to Do
Once Your Door Opens

If you have heard home care horror stories about theft, abuse, or downright dangerous care, you may be anxious on the day home care begins. Before you panic, keep in mind that most reported cases involve do-it-yourself situations or fly-by-night operations where someone is hired "off the street" to provide home care.

If you have chosen an agency wisely, relax. The chances that a serious problem will occur are slim indeed. Professional, quality-minded home care agencies operate with several built-in safeguards. Still, there are some extra steps you can take that will help prevent problems—big or small—and that will assure not just a safe but a more satisfying home care experience.

FOLLOW COMMONSENSE
SAFETY RULES

Criminals who may stalk your neighborhood pose a far greater safety threat to you than most home care employees themselves. But no matter how small the risk, be cautious. As a self-protection measure, *always* check for proper identification on an employee's first home care visit, and whenever unfamiliar agency personnel call. Don't become conditioned to opening your door to anyone simply on the basis of a uniform or a doorbell ring around a scheduled arrival time. Except in unusual circumstances, a professional agency should always tell you in advance when someone must replace regularly assigned personnel. If you're in doubt about someone despite identification, don't hesitate to call the supervisor for verification.

Keep your home properly secured as before. Don't leave doors unlocked or put house keys under the doormat in anticipation of the home care worker's arrival. If you live in an apartment, don't automatically buzz people into the building until you ascertain that they are from the agency. (For example: Can they correctly name the agency, the supervisor, and the telephone number?) Again, don't open the door until you know the person outside *is* the person you are expecting. After employees enter your home, remember to lock up again or ask them to do so.

Be careful not to leave housekeys, credit cards, bank books, and so on lying about. Never give an employee a duplicate key unless the agency supervisor has been notified and gives permission.

Follow the agency's procedures with respect to handling money to the letter. Always get a receipt for financial transactions of any kind. Don't become lax about money matters or make occasional exceptions to agency rules because you like and trust the worker.

If you're in doubt about the worker for any reason, put the worker "on notice" politely that you will call the police should property loss occur. Or you can "drop a hint" that you have filed the names of all personnel assigned with the police as a precaution.

STRIVE FOR A GOOD WORKING RELATIONSHIP

Your home care experience will be more satisfying if you build a good working relationship with those assigned to your care.

Most personnel want to make a good first impression and will make every effort to put you and those in your household at ease. Make a special effort too and welcome first-time personnel to your home. If possible, have other involved family members or caregivers meet personnel when services begin.

You can help get home care off to a good start if you introduce personnel to your home instead of leaving them alone on a search mission. You don't have to conduct a house tour. Briefly explain the layout of key rooms (bathroom, kitchen) and where essential items can be found. Point out where important telephone numbers can be found and review who to call in an emergency.

Help make employees' jobs easier by letting them know that first day any special routines or preferences you may have. What may be second nature to you will be second guessing to them. If you consider certain household areas out of bounds to personnel, say so. If a back rub after a bath refreshes you, speak up. Home care should complement your life style as much as possible. Don't be timid about making your wishes known.

However, when you do so, treat home care workers with respect. Try to make your requests politely, without making absolute demands. If you extend workers common courtesy in the same way you expect to be treated, you will help build a good relationship.

REVIEW THE CARE PLAN WITH PERSONNEL

When personnel arrive at your home, they should have already reviewed your care plan and may actually have a copy in hand. In any case, have your copy ready and be prepared to review it together, so the details of care are clearly understood. Don't hesitate to ask any questions that may be on your mind, no matter how small.

Most professionals will guide you (and your family, if involved) through the initial adjustment to home care, so you won't be left wondering what happens next. Paraprofessionals may not always be this prepared. Set aside a few minutes after you get acquainted to review the plan of care and to discuss how tasks will be scheduled.

PARTICIPATE IN YOUR CARE AS MUCH AS YOU CAN

Why become a passive patient? With home care, you are not bound by the rigid routines of institutional care. Take full advantage of this unique difference and become an active patient. Learn as much as you can about your condition. There is plenty printed today on almost every health problem. You can also learn more about your condition and care if you ask assigned personnel questions. You could even request a list of warning symptoms or treatment side effects.

Your knowledge will help you spot and report any developing problems and also improve your ability to make decisions concerning your care.

Learn to perform yourself (or with a family member's help), as much as you can, any procedures involved in your care. Home care professionals will instruct you step-by-step in the proper methods. They will monitor your ability until both you and they feel confident that you have really mastered the procedure.

Follow your doctor's treatment plan carefully, just as you would in the hospital. Agency personnel will do their best to see that you follow prescribed treatment, but you should assume some responsibility too. If your purpose for home care is a desire to avoid the prescribed in-hospital regimen, you are sabotaging your own recovery.

MONITOR AGENCY SUPERVISION

Quality home care depends on ongoing supervision. Once care begins, regular supervision should start too. If an agency supervisor does not visit you at home within the first two weeks of care, don't wait any longer. Call the agency and find out why. Remember, phone supervision alone is not acceptable. The supervisor should make periodic in-person visits to confirm that proper care is being rendered. Some visits should be made when care personnel are present.

Keep track as best you can of supervisory visits and calls. Note these on your copy of the employee's weekly time sheet, or mark a calendar. Review your records every few weeks to see if supervision is being provided according to your understanding prior to care. Discuss any discrepancies with the agency supervisor right away.

As soon as care begins, confirm the supervisor's availability during service hours, especially in cases where care is provided during evening or weekend hours. Do this by actually calling the supervisor yourself. When you check, don't apologize or make excuses for your call. Express concern about your ability to reach the supervisor. This will not irritate good supervisors. Their job is to reassure you—and it will help keep the agency on its toes where you are concerned.

If you can't reach the supervisor within an hour, you are risking problems. After all, if you can't reach the supervisor, employees will not be able to reach them either should they need advice if and when problems arise.

Put the agency on notice about this situation. Talk to the "supervisor's supervisor," usually a director of nursing or an agency administrator or manager. Then double-check again later. If you still can't reach the supervisor promptly, switch agencies. You're getting second-rate service.

INVOLVE AN ADVOCATE IN YOUR CARE

It's human nature: Most people do their jobs better and more consistently when others review their performance from time to time. This is one reason why the need for supervision in home care has been repeatedly stressed.

When someone who cares about you is also involved in your home care, agency personnel have another incentive for better performance. If you share a household with someone else, you probably have one or more built-in advocates. But if you live alone or with another who is also ailing or is elderly and frail, or if children require care, yours is a high-risk situation. In these cases an outside "advocate"—someone who cares and whom you trust—can help assure that you get proper services.

What must this advocate do? Often very little other than show he or she is concerned about your welfare.

Family members, friends, or neighbors can be effective advocates if they demonstrate to assigned personnel that they are caring presences in your life. For this reason, whoever you ask to assist you as an advocate should be someone unafraid to voice his or her opinions when necessary. Just the knowledge that someone outside the agency periodically checks in on you can subtly help promote better care and deter major problems. One agency administrator whose grandmother had received regular home care services noted, "Whenever I visited my grandmother she always remarked how much more attentive her aide seemed that day. 'Why don't you come to see me more often?' she mused."

Have your advocate show interest by being present, if possible (or at least call), when services, particularly paraprofessional services, *first* begin—if not the first day, then at a service time as soon as possible thereafter. Ask your advocate to stop by periodically as service continues. Prearrange these "impromptu" visits with your advocate, but don't announce them to agency personnel. It's your right to have anyone in your home, even during a caregiving session.

Your advocate doesn't always have to be physically present in your home to exert a caring influence. Occasional phone calls when the worker is present will also convey the message that if something goes wrong, someone else will know.

The purpose of your advocate's phone calls and visits is to help you get better care, not to detract from it. Keep phone calls and visits short so your care is interrupted only briefly and personnel can get their work done.

If you feel the need, and your advocate is willing, he or she can take a more active role with the agency on your behalf. In some hospitals, for example, hospital-employed advocates called "patient representatives" or "ombudsmen" act as trouble-shooters for any concerns that might arise. They help see that any patient questions about treatment or financial matters are fully resolved. Patients can also channel any complaints about hospital services through these representatives and get action without fear or embarrassment.

You may feel more comfortable about home care if you can voice any dissatisfaction or ask questions through your advocate instead of doing so yourself. If that's the case, it's a good idea to put your advocate's name on file with the agency, for the record, as an interested party if he or she is not otherwise listed. Your advocate does not have to call only to report problems. He or she can call with a general observation about your care, or a compliment if deserved— "I wanted you to know that Mrs./Mr. _____ seems satisfied with her/his health aide after the first week of care." A general or complimentary call helps establish positive advocate-supervisor communications.

REPORT YOUR CONDITION HONESTLY

Good care depends on good communication about your health and abilities. Start by candidly answering all questions during the agency's initial phone evaluation and in-home assessment.

"No one likes to be thought of as a complainer," explained one administrator. "Often people tend to minimize their complaints or infirmities or deny their illness." Yet this information is critical to developing a sound plan of care. It also helps alert personnel to other symptoms they should watch for throughout care.

Whenever you are asked about your ability to manage, don't automatically answer without thinking. Does it take 30 minutes now to get out of bed and get dressed, whereas it took only half the time before? Do you quickly become tired and/or short of breath after little exertion? If so, say so.

Keep in mind that the agency personnel are *not* trying to

pry by asking many questions and requesting detailed answers. Each question is geared toward helping you. During assessment, a question about weight, for example, can be important in the care of an unusually hefty bedridden patient. The agency may have to assign different personnel or arrange for special equipment in order to render proper care.

When care is for another, advise the agency of any potential problems you may foresee, any developing problems or changes you notice. For example, if in the past a patient has been careless about taking prescribed drugs or is usually reluctant to follow doctor's orders, notify the agency about this predisposition. Or perhaps the patient is prone to developing bedsores or to dizziness, or is becoming confused. If you are aware that the home care client has often been depressed or suicidal in the past, don't conceal this fact. The agency can assign personnel with the proper mental health background. With warning about any potential or developing problems, personnel will be more alert to these troubles and can work to prevent problems before they occur, or to prevent a more serious decline.

EXERCISE YOUR RIGHTS AS A HOME CARE CONSUMER

The consumer movement in health care has grown far too slowly. Part of the problem lies with consumers who do not realize they have certain rights or fail to exercise them. The other side to this problem lies with health care providers who do not help educate consumers or promote consumer rights out of their own self-interest. For example, though the American Hospital Association adopted a Patient Bill of Rights in 1973, many hospitals today still do little if anything to make patients aware upon admission of these rights and the bill's existence.

When you receive care in your own home, you have basic rights too. In its position on patient rights and responsibilities, the National Association for Home Care states: "The observance of these rights and responsibilities will contribute to more effective patient care and greater satisfaction for the patient as well as the agency." If you want the best care, you should know what these rights are, expect to receive them routinely, and demand them when necessary.

The Home Care Bill of Rights, outlined below, represents an amalgam of those rights advocated by the National Association for Home Care, the National HomeCaring Council, home care agencies that promote patients' rights or a Code of Ethics, plus the author's additions. They have been organized according to consumer issues for greater clarity.

Human Rights

You have the right to:

- Receive services regardless of race, creed, national origin, or sexual preferences
- Privacy and confidentiality, including communications and records about your health, your social and financial circumstances, and what takes place in your home
- Choose or change home care providers
- Be fully informed of your rights and responsibilities as a home care client
- Home care as long as needed and available; if you are denied solely because of inability to pay, you have the right of referral to another agency that can assist.

Care and Treatment

You have the right to:

- Receive considerate, respectful, appropriate, and professional care in your home at all times
- Participate in the development of your care plan, including an explanation of any service proposed, and of alternative services that may be available in the community
- Receive information necessary to give informed consent prior to the start of any procedure or treatment
- Refuse treatment or other services provided by law and be informed of the potential results of your actions

- Receive nursing supervision of paraprofessionals if medically related personal care is needed
- Reasonable continuity of care

Disclosure about Services and Costs

You have the right to:

- Receive a timely response from the agency to your request for service
- Be admitted for service only if the agency has the ability to provide safe professional care at the level of intensity needed
- Be fully informed of agency policies and charges for services, including eligibility for Medicare or other third-party reimbursements
- Receive complete and written information on your plan of care, including the name of the supervisor responsible for your services
- Examine all bills for service, regardless of whether they are paid for out of pocket or through other payment source(s)
- Be informed within a reasonable time of anticipated termination of service or plans for transfer to another agency

Consumer Action

You have the right to:

- Voice complaints and suggest changes in service or staff without fear or restraint or discrimination

ARE YOU GETTING THE BEST CARE?

Ask yourself this question regularly once care begins. You may have no trouble answering if you are receiving care yourself or if you live with the person who does. But when care is for someone who lives far away, the answer may not be so apparent.

Home care should ease your worries about your loved ones, not add to it. If you live at a distance, make sure you get regular progress notes and calls from the agency. Don't forget to call your loved one often yourself. Visit the home or have someone go on your behalf. Observe and talk to your loved ones. Talk to agency personnel. Then evaluate the care. Compare the tasks outlined in the plan of care with the following checklists. After you run through this guide to proper services, you'll have a better idea of whether or not the care is the best.

Homemaking Services

This is a fairly clear-cut area to evaluate. When you're on track for quality care, you should be able to answer "yes" to each of the questions that apply to your care situation.

- Is the home environment as good or better since care began?
- Is the home garbage- and trash-free?
- Are toilets, bedpans, and bathtubs and sinks clean and odor-free?
- Are bed linens and towels unsoiled and changed often enough?
- Is there enough fresh laundry to meet personal needs?
- Is the home safe from obvious hazards such as clutter on stairs?
- Is there enough food in the house?
- Is food properly stored?
- Are meals prepared according to any special doctor's orders and your personal likes and dislikes?
- Is shopping done according to the items needed and the budget?
- Are bills properly paid or other essential errands run?

Personal Care

Now you are in a gray area. You should also be able to answer "yes" to the appropriate questions listed below. "Nos" always point to problems, but you can't always be sure where. Personnel may be providing poor care, or the person receiving care may be on the decline. Sometimes a "no" may signal that other personal factors in the home are amiss. In any case, a "no" also suggests problems with the agency's supervision. Professional agencies should spot these problems before you do and take corrective action, or discuss them with you.

- Is overall personal hygiene as good or better since care began? Consider general cleanliness, body odor, the appearance of hair, teeth, and nails.
- Is the able person encouraged and assisted to get out of bed each day? helped to dress? brush teeth? bathe? comb hair?
- Is the clothing the patient is wearing clean and appropriate for the weather and home conditions? For example, in a cold room, is your loved one dressed in a sweater or other warm apparel?
- Is the skin condition good? You shouldn't see unexpected or unusual marks, swelling, bruises, cuts, or developing sores on the body.
- Is normal body weight maintained? Unexplained weight loss may signal many problems.
- Are assistive devices such as eyeglasses, dentures, walkers, and so on used appropriately? Watch out if they are obviously stored out of sight. This suggests they are not being used as needed.
- Do personnel suggest and perform care extras for comfort when requested, such as a back massage?
- Do personnel try to provide mental stimulation and enlist interest in daily activities, instead of just providing "custodial-type" care?

Nursing and Other Health Services

Even if you are receiving care yourself, this area is tough for consumers to evaluate. Often the results of these services depend as much on your condition and your cooperation as on those providing care. In order to judge the quality of these services, it's helpful to know in advance the immediate home care goals for basic or skilled nursing or therapy. As a general rule of thumb, if your progress is far below these anticipated goals and you've done your part, then question your care. It indeed may be faulty.

Listed below are more specific questions that can help you decide about quality. Except when indicated, your answers to all questions should be "yes."

- Are vital signs (temperature, pulse, respiration, blood pressure) taken regularly, as the care plan dictates?
- Are you reminded, encouraged, and assisted to perform exercises as often as has been prescribed? In the manner prescribed?
- Are special procedures, such as measuring fluid intake and outgo or urine or blood sugar tests, performed according to the care plan?
- Are vital signs, treatment, and progress notes, including any changes observed in your condition, regularly recorded? Are notes on file and available to you, your family, and your doctor upon request? If in doubt about the thoroughness of records, ask to review them.
- Are team conferences taking place? If so, your patient record should confirm this fact.
- Is your doctor kept informed about your care and condition? For fairly stable chronic conditions, the agency should notify your doctor in writing at least every 60 days. For more serious conditions, there should be more frequent contact by letter or phone. If in doubt, ask your doctor about agency contact, or ask the agency for a copy of all physician reports. Doctor contacts should also be noted in your record.
- Do personnel explain all procedures completely? keep you informed about your condition? instruct you in techniques of care as appropriate?
- Are you given (or reminded to take) the proper medication in the proper dose at the proper time?

Also answer these questions, which require a "no" to indicate satisfactory care.

- Do infections recur or linger at sores, wounds, surgical or drainage sites? with catheter use? This usually indicates improper nursing technique.

- Are you running unexplained fevers? The agency should promptly alert your doctor. If agency personnel seem unconcerned, they don't understand good nursing.
- Are bedsores developing, or have they gotten worse since care began? If need be, monitor by counting sores, measuring and recording their size and location. This condition almost always means a lapse in correct nursing care.

General Personnel Performance

If you want the best care, nothing short of "yes" to all the following questions should satisfy you. These are the basics you should expect and get in any home care situation.

- Are personnel normally on time for their assignments? Do they work as long as is required according to your contract or other arrangements made?
- Do personnel complete the tasks outlined in the care plan responsibly and promptly, instead of doing just enough to get by?
- Are personal appearance and habits of workers acceptable? Employees should be neat, clean, and appropriately dressed. No smoking on the job. They should follow basic practices of proper hygiene—for example, washing hands before meal preparation or nursing care.
- Do personnel understand written and verbal directions? Do they take the initiative in performing job duties, or must you give constant directions?
- Are personnel trustworthy? You should not find money missing or property lost that cannot be reasonably accounted for.
- Are personnel courteous in speech and manner? Verbal abuse should never be tolerated. Do they comply with requests whenever possible?
- Is help not just competent, but caring? Home care should never be rough, impersonal, indifferent, or intimidating.
- Are you encouraged to make decisions about and to participate in personal, household, nursing, or other health care as much as you are able?

- Are your loved one's personality, personal habits, and interest in life unchanged or improved since care began? Look for any signs that may indicate unhappiness, fear, or depression. These often include abnormal changes in personal habits—eating compulsively or too little, sleeplessness or sleeping a great deal, sudden withdrawal or unresponsiveness, constant rocking, or agitation.
- Do personnel promptly ask for guidance from their superiors when problems or disputes arise that cannot be otherwise handled?

—22—

How to Handle Problems

If you want the best care, be ready to address any problems that may arise. In the case of a minor, first-time problem, you can point out the trouble to personnel yourself—or, if you prefer, talk to the agency supervisor. But whenever problems repeat themselves or are more serious, deal directly with the supervisor, and do so right away. This is what the supervisor is there for, and this is one wonderful advantage of using a professional home care agency instead of having to do it yourself. Unfortunately, an AARP study found that two-thirds of the home care consumers interviewed never reported to the agency problems they had had with an employee.

Often consumers don't complain out of concern that they will offend or hurt employees' feelings. Or they may worry that a worker will lose his or her job if they question care. Sometimes consumers such as Medicare clients wrongly fear that they will lose much-needed home care benefits if they voice any dissatisfaction. Fear of employee revenge, another possibility, may also prevent action.

Good agencies are sensitive to these complaint blocks, and they try to make it easy for you to make any trouble known. Agencies can discreetly correct the situation, even if this means replacing an employee.

Put concerns about job loss out of your mind. Conscientious workers will not lose their jobs if you complain. But they may need closer supervision, additional training, or perhaps a less demanding work assignment. In any case, you do yourself, the employee, the agency, and other consumers of the service a favor when you alert the supervisor to problems early. Most important, remember you have the right to complain whether you pay for the services directly or not.

COMMON TROUBLE SPOTS
AND WHAT TO DO

In any home care situation, problems can occur even when you deal with a superior agency. What really counts is how the agency responds to your problems. If an agency tries to put you on the defensive instead of dealing constructively with the problems at hand, you have got the wrong agency. Change without delay.

Some problems occur because of simple misunderstandings, nothing more, and better communication is sometimes all that is needed. So never hesitate to discuss whatever is on your mind.

"She won't wash my windows."
It's been said before, but it bears repeating. Aides, home-makers, and companions do not wash windows, scrub floors or walls, clean stoves, or tackle other heavy-duty jobs. That's "chore work." Talk to the supervisor if you need this type of help. Arrangements can be made.

"She just watches TV" or "She doesn't do anything."
These and similar complaints suggest a variety of possible problems. (1) You may have more help than you need. If so, discuss it with the agency and reduce the number of service hours. (2) Your plan of care is not detailed enough, so the worker does not know what to do. Immediate and better agency supervision is needed. (3) The worker is indifferent and is not following the plan of care. Again, better supervision is needed. Notify the agency. Unless immediate improvement is seen, request a replacement.

"It's a different person every day."

This strongly suggests you have the wrong agency. A good agency regularly provides the same personnel—both professional and nonprofessional. It makes changes only when absolutely necessary, and notifies you in advance. Put the agency on notice about this situation. Don't accept the excuse, "This is the way it has to be." It doesn't. If the agency continues to switch personnel, switch agencies.

"I never know when someone is coming."

This can be a frequent frustration if you don't speak up. Even good agencies often fall down here. Remember that home care is *not* hospital care. You should not constantly have to adjust your routine for someone else. When you are getting care at home, you do not have to tolerate: (1) waiting and wondering all day long when personnel will arrive, or (2) unscheduled interruptions at any hour that suits the agency. However, you should view this problem reasonably and realistically.

When nurses, therapists, or others must see several patients in a day on a visit basis, an *exact* time is seldom possible. Sometimes in trying to juggle personnel assignments, agencies forget that home care is supposed to support your life style, not disrupt it needlessly. But you should be given a *general* arrival time, within one or two hours, that you can count on. Remind them more than once if you have to.

Personnel hired on an hourly basis should arrive promptly and depart according to schedule.

"She treats me like a child."

Unless care is for a child, this attitude has no place in home care. Such an attitude can foster dependence and defeat home care goals. Adults should be treated with proper respect, no matter how sick or how old. If you are treated otherwise, politely bring it to the worker's attention. If there is no change, discuss this with the supervisor. The worker needs sensitivity training, and you may need a worker change.

"I don't like her."

This consumer complaint may cover a multitude of problems. (1) The worker chews gum, wears heavy perfume or jewelry, smokes, or has other unacceptable personal habits. (2) She arrives late, uses your phone frequently, eats your food, or disappears constantly. (3) She gives rough or careless service. Let the agency know about any of these telltale trouble signs as soon as they appear. Professional agencies have a strict dress and behavior code that personnel must observe. If service itself is a problem, request a replacement. With supervision, workers can correct their personal habits; but an indifferent attitude or careless, rough care is not easily changed.

(4) A personality problem may exist. Since home care is a people business, personality differences are bound to occur. Sometimes it's a problem of false expectations. "Everyone wants a daughter," says Marilyn Dean, national director of health care services for Medical Personnel Pool. Home care workers will try to please, but you should not expect them to substitute for family. Ask for a replacement if your personalities do not mesh. But discuss the situation frankly with the supervisor so a better match can be made.

Many agencies will go to great lengths to satisfy their clients. But the problem is not always with the worker. Rosina Dapello, RN, of Metropolitan Jewish Geriatric Center, cited this example. "One elderly woman could not seem to get along with her worker. We sent out no less than twenty-five different people, trying to find the right match. On number twenty-six, I finally had to tell her that was it. Suddenly, she and the worker got along."

(5) There can be a racial/ethnic problem. Professional agencies do not discriminate as to whom they hire or serve. Good agencies will work to resolve personality differences, but they do not assign personnel based on racial or ethnic preferences. If care is for someone with deep-seated prejudices, advise the agency so the worker will understand the problem up front. Often the problem is resolved when competent care overcomes prejudice.

"She doesn't know what she's doing."
Whether this statement refers to a nurse or an aide, the

source of the problem is almost always the same—an agency that did not carefully screen its personnel. All personnel assigned should be qualified to do the job. It is the agency's responsibility to screen personnel for proper skills and training, so if unqualified personnel is the problem, report this immediately to the agency. Sometimes incompetent care may occur with alcohol or drug abuse on the part of the employee. In any case, if the agency doesn't promptly provide a suitable replacement, replace the agency.

"No one showed up."

If employees are an hour late or more and haven't called, call the agency right away. A qualified replacement should be provided promptly. Many agencies have aides that stand by at the office in case a no-show occurs. If nursing care is needed and a replacement cannot be immediately found at a good agency, the supervisor will go out when necessary and do the job. If an agency cannot make a replacement within a reasonable period of time *that* day, replace the agency. Note: "Reasonable" depends upon your circumstance. If care is needed for a bedridden person living alone, the agency should respond fast—within the hour.

"She doesn't understand what I say."

This is a sure sign of a poor agency. It's easy to screen employees for basic ability to read, write, and speak English. A professional agency always does so. Even if you need bilingual personnel, English literacy is necessary to follow agency orders and to communicate about proper patient care. Change agencies immediately.

"She won't accept my gift."

That's right. Professional agencies do not allow employees to accept any gifts, money, household goods, and so on, no matter how small. If you want to show appreciation through some small token, discuss this with the agency supervisor first.

"Something's missing."

This does not always mean theft. First look carefully for the missing object or money. Ask personnel about the item(s) in question. Often "missing" items are simply misplaced. If the item can't be found, notify the agency *promptly*. If the item has value, contact the police and file a report right away. Get a copy. Filing such reports are very routine to police, and you should not be afraid or frightened to do so. A properly filed police report is also generally required for insurance purposes.

Never hesitate to file a police report or an agency complaint because you feel employee theft can't be proved. Agency policies vary on replacement of "missing" items. (You should discuss this in advance.) Many agencies will make good on items even if court proof of wrongdoing is absent. Naturally, the agency should replace the worker involved.

"She hints about money."

The agency pays the employee's salary, so it's best not to discuss salary with the worker in any way—what you pay the agency *or* what the agency pays the worker. Remember, though, the employee is paid less than what the agency charges you; the agency is providing additional services, not just a worker. *Never* supplement an employee's salary. Hints about additional pay or hard luck stories suggesting the need for a loan should be brought immediately to the supervisor's attention.

"I want her to work for me all the time."

If you want to hire the worker permanently, as your own live-in or companion, most agencies will make a special arrangement in this case. Discuss this with the agency. Policies vary. Usually it will charge a placement or finder's fee, often roughly the equivalent of 10 to 15 percent of the employee's annual salary.

—23—

Home Care Hot Spots: Fraud, Abuse, and Malpractice

THE INDUSTRY TRACK RECORD

How does the home care industry score on quality of care and fair business practices? Thus far, the "professional" industry scores surprisingly well overall, especially when you compare it to other segments of the health field such as the nursing home industry, where fraud and patient abuse have been rampant.

A search through the files of the Office of the Inspector General (OIG), the watchdog office of the U.S. Department of Health and Human Services (DHHS), revealed only seven convictions since 1965 for Medicare fraud by home care agency providers. Among nursing home operators, pharmacists, physicians, and others who serve the elderly, there have been thousands.

What about individual patient care? It's more difficult to document the extent of individual consumer problems. In September 1983, a *Parade* magazine article, "When the Elderly Are Victims," invited anyone who knew of home care patient abuse or fraud to call the OIG hotline. Hotline director Calvin Anderson revealed that, following the article's publication, his office received approximately 150 extra calls in two days. However, not all the calls received were home care complaints. More than half focused on other consumer problems with physicians, social security, or Medicare.

A DHHS interview study of 245 clients receiving home care through Medicare, Medicaid, or other public money found only five cases of theft or other abuses. In an AARP study, less than 5 percent of the 178 home care consumers interviewed reported definite theft or complained of rough treatment.

Industry spokesman Val Halamandaris contends: "Historically there has been very little evidence of either fraud or abuse perpetrated by licensed, certified agencies, or their personnel." If you consider that there are over 5,000 certified home care agencies which provide over 28 million visits annually to Medicare consumers alone, the home care track record has indeed been a good one.

THE POTENTIAL FOR PROBLEMS

Consumers cannot afford to be complacent about the past. The potential for serious, widespread home care problems is brewing in direct proportion to the growing dollars spent on home care by consumers, employers, insurers, and the government. Just what impact the entry of get-rich-quick entrepreneurs and the outright unscrupulous will have on home care quality nationwide remains to be seen. But concerns are mounting, especially for the disadvantaged. Florence Moore of the National HomeCaring Council says that "quality agencies with long-standing records of community service are being squeezed out in competitive bidding." The government or other funding organizations are awarding contracts for care for the needy based on bottom-line cost, without adequate consideration for quality. "We have a K-Mart mentality prevailing in health care now," notes NAHC president Halamandaris. "The focus is on how you can make it cheaper. That's going to continue only until we see some scandals."

Some states have resorted to coercing welfare mothers into service to provide care to poverty-stricken elderly, disabled, and children, irrespective of their interests and ability. Naturally this use of unwilling and unqualified workers greatly reduces the quality of care.

Another potential threat to quality home care may come from hospitals and nursing homes that are now moving into home care. "Revolving door" treatment, where patients may be flipped from one health setting to another, depending on what may be most profitable to these owners, is a distinct possibility.

Whether the past generally high quality of home care will be maintained depends on responsible action by government, home care agencies, and consumer groups, and of course better consumer education and action.

WHAT IS HOME CARE FRAUD?

Fraud is generally defined as intentional deception or misrepresentation with the intent of receiving an unauthorized benefit.

Take the case of William L. Schwartz, executive director of the not-for-profit Home Health Care, Inc., North Miami Beach, Florida. In 1983, he was suspended from Medicare as a health care provider because of fraudulent activities. Over several years he bilked Medicare, charging the government for the personal use of agency employees for chores such as babysitting, housecleaning, and house repairs. Records were dummied to bill Medicare for autos leased for business but used for personal purposes. In order to increase Medicare revenues, Schwartz okayed agency visits to patients no longer eligible for home care. Medicare was also charged for the expenses of a private non-Medicare agency called Help Is on the Way, owned by Mr. Schwartz and his wife Deborah.

In the Schwartz fraud case, agency employees, past and present, not agency clients, confirmed the wrongdoing after a routine Medicare audit raised suspicions. However, alert consumers can sometimes help detect fraud.

At the Charles Drew Home Health Agency in Dallas, Texas, father-son team Tobbie Jones, Sr., executive director and founder, and Tobbie Jones, Jr., assistant director, conspired to collect illegally almost a half million dollars. The agency, which derived almost all its funds from Medicare and Medicaid, submitted phony home care claims for real patients. Had Charles Drew clients reviewed their Medicare statement (even though they did not have to pay for care out of pocket), they might have spotted the phony claims.

As in other cases of known home care fraud, there was no evidence that these crimes hurt home care clients directly. However, such fraud hurts us all. Added costs further undermine Medicare's crumbling financial base, thereby promoting reduced health care benefits for the elderly and increased rates for all taxpayers.

If you receive home care through Medicare, Medicaid, or other public funds, keep records and review all copies of claims submitted for your care. If you spot errors, notify the appropriate agencies, as discussed in the next chapter.

Home care fraud may also involve kickbacks. These are fees, gifts, or other payoffs given to health personnel in return for referring Medicare "customers" to home care providers, usually durable medical equipment suppliers. Calvin Anderson explains: "Usually a hospital therapist, social worker, or other employee who has access to, and has excellent rapport with, patients may tell them, 'I know of a good company where you can get . . .'"

It's certainly okay for doctors, hospital, or home care personnel to refer patients to services. After all, given the large number of companies competing for business, most consumers are bewildered and grateful for recommendations about honest, reliable service. But problems arise when personnel push a particular provider and profit from doing so.

Anderson reports: "Sometimes employees may get $10 a head for referrals or in some cases they may own or have an interest in a medical equipment company to which patients are referred." The recommended company may give good service, but it may also be more costly than others the consumer might choose.

When you need help, personnel normally should recommend several providers and let you decide. You can and should ask if personnel prefer one provider versus another. If they do, always ask why. Check all recommendations yourself, then choose the provider that is best for you.

If you have good reason to suspect a kickback, do your part. Alert government officials. Under a new federal anti-kickback law, offenders are subject to stiff penalties.

HOME CARE ABUSE

Abuse does not mean your average, run-of-the-mill, home care problems or disputes that may be at best annoying and at worst unpleasant. These instances do not involve misconduct with the intent and/or the result of victimizing or endangering home care clients. Abuse is theft, outright physical or verbal assault, or mental terrorism in your own home. It is also poor, substandard care that harms or endangers health or life, or greedily exhausts precious finances, leaving you broke, or without care, or both.

Abuse can, and does, often occur in do-it-yourself situations or when agencies fail to follow strict professional standards for screening, supervision, and care. Problems abound with the fly-by-nighters and those would-be "professional agencies" whose advertising is good, but whose services fall short. Almost *every* case of abuse involves a high-risk home care situation. The person needing help is usually elderly, sick, or frail, and lives alone. Caring friends or relatives may live nearby, but unless they monitor the home care situation closely, abuse can occur. Here are some reported examples of agency abuse:

- An agency provided an elderly woman with round-the-clock care, despite her doctor's prescription for part-time assistance. After her money was exhausted, she was "dumped" into a nursing home on Medicaid for further care. The agency got away with this because, once hired, neither the agency nor anyone on the client's behalf ever contacted the doctor again.
- In her elderly client's home, an agency aide regularly entertained her boyfriend, stole food, and did her laundry. She also failed to keep her client clean and groomed. In-home supervision of the aide was not provided. The

agency also ignored reports by other personnel that misconduct was occurring.

- An agency sent a licensed practical nurse as a temporary live-in for a 72-year-old woman while the family vacationed. The nurse drove drunk twice with the client in the car, the second time getting into an accident. Luckily the elderly client was not hurt. The agency later learned that the nurse had a drunk-driving record.
- A licensed practical nurse, sent to care for an 89-year-old woman, overdosed on drugs while at the client's home. Again the client was not hurt, but the nurse required hospitalization. In nearly five months of work, the agency had only supervised the nurse once on the job. All other contact with the nurse was by phone.
- An agency aide put her elderly client into the bathtub to soak, then cleaned out the client's apartment. The agency, which hadn't checked the aide's references, found out, after the fact, that the aide had given a phony name and address.

Additional horror stories could be cited, but dwelling on them distorts the noteworthy picture of professional home care. Don't let these cases dissuade you from getting needed help, but read the messages they send loud and clear. Choose a professional agency, and take the time to do so. Be more cautious in high-risk situations, and involve an advocate in your care. Whenever there is a hint of a problem, take it to the agency right away. If the agency is indifferent or does not respond immediately, change agencies. There are professional agencies that can and will do the job well.

HOME CARE MALPRACTICE

Malpractice fever has hit health care. Doctors and hospitals charge that the ever-growing number of malpractice lawsuits has helped drive up the cost of care. Malpractice lawyers counter that these claims are a smokescreen to divert attention from the real issue—justified compensation for consumers who suffer because of substandard care.

Though there are few reported cases of home care malpractice, home care agencies are also concerned about potential lawsuits, especially with the advent of high-tech home care. Most home care agencies carry malpractice or professional liability insurance that covers the actions of their employees. In some cases, employees themselves carry these insurances. However, should problems occur, don't regard a malpractice suit as an opportunity to get rich quick. As one lawyer wryly commented, "The lawyer never loses." But consumers often do. Despite the headlines of huge settlements for medical malpractice, the majority of cases are lost by those suing.

Malpractice is a murky area of the law. To win a malpractice suit, the lawyer must first prove "fault"—that is, that "negligence" or "liability" exists. Second, the lawyer must prove that as a result of fault, damages or injuries have occurred. Near misses do not count. This is like stopping your car for a light and being hit from the rear. If you are not injured, even though the other driver is at fault, no suit exists.

Should injury or ill health occur during a home care situation, home care agencies (and their personnel) bear the same responsibility for patient care as do hospitals. Therefore, just because you are getting your care at home, don't blame yourself or assume it is "one of those things" if something serious goes wrong. The agency and/or its personnel may be at fault.

Attorney Elliot Ozment of Good Samaritan Home Health in Tennessee, who counsels home care agencies on how to avoid malpractice suits, points out that juries are more sympathetic to cases involving children and the elderly, or to someone who is mentally impaired. "Therefore," he cautions, "agencies should exercise even higher standards." On the other hand, consumers in these groups should exercise higher caution too.

As with patient malpractice suits of any kind, the fault is seldom obvious and clear-cut. An agency or personnel may be liable regardless of any waiver of liability you may have signed as part of your service agreement. Mr. Ozment advises that agencies may be liable if, for example, they fail to:

- Hire qualified staff and check references
- Provide in-service training so staff skills are maintained
- Provide good instruction for equipment supplied by the agency, or check any in-home equipment for obvious defects or malfunctions
- Do an adequate assessment of the home environment in order to prevent accidents or injuries

Home care personnel may also be liable if they fail to perform their duties within the accepted scope of the profession. For example, a nurse may be liable if the wrong drug or dosage is administered, or if patient care is not properly monitored and if the doctor is not informed when problems occur.

Don't seek a malpractice suit frivolously. But if serious harm occurs, you may want to seek sound legal advice for any remedies open to you.

—24—

Consumer Clout

Consumers cannot rely on federal or state regulations or voluntary standards alone to ensure quality in home care services. To be effective, these must be enforced; but often there are too few personnel to tackle this job adequately. In many states, agencies or services are not subject to any controls other than those of the free enterprise system.

When you are dissatisfied with service or encounter serious troubles, you may solve your problem by switching agencies, by firing, and hiring, another self-employed worker, or if necessary, by seeking police or legal action. But don't stop there; also make your complaints a matter of record. Use your consumer clout to help improve home care quality for other consumers in your community.

HOW TO COMPLAIN

A complaint is usually more effective if you put it in writing. Do so if you switch agencies or when you notify other organizations about your problem. Your letter does not have to be elaborate. It need only summarize the key facts:

- Who is involved? Cite the agency, dealer, and so on, and name of the person with whom you dealt. Include the agency mailing address. Give your name, address, and phone number (optional).
- What happened? Be brief and specific. Outline the nature of the problem, the results, any action you took.
- When and where did it happen? Give the date(s) and pinpoint the location of the incident (as best you can).
- Why did it happen (if known)?

Along with your complaint, enclose anything that supports the complaint, such as a *copy* of a bill or any letters sent about the problem. If you wish, file complaints with several organizations simultaneously. This can often be more effective than relying on just one organization for action. If you would rather phone your complaint, make sure you note the time, the date, and the person with whom you registered your problem.

What type of results can you expect? That largely depends on the organization's jurisdiction and the nature of the infractions. Within a two- to three-week period, you should receive a written response to your complaint outlining the next step. Clearly, before any serious action is taken against an agency or worker, a full investigation of all charges will be required. However, generally all complaints are noted and a history of even minor complaints may alert an organization to take a more serious look at the agency's operations.

WHERE TO COMPLAIN— REFERRAL SOURCES

Did your doctor or the hospital discharge planner refer you to the agency or the dealer that you're dissatisfied with? By all means, let professionals or whoever referred you know. If you keep them in the dark, they will go on referring, thinking their recommendations were sound.

In this competitive home care area, this is one of the surest and quickest ways to blacklist a substandard agency. This is also one time you needn't wait to put it in writing. Give the person who advised you a call.

Office of the Inspector General (OIG)

If you know of, or suspect, Medicare or Medicaid waste, fraud, or abuse of any kind, home care or not, lodge your complaint here. This office is charged by law with preventing the misuse of any funds budgeted to the U.S. Department of Health and Human Services (DHHS).

OIG maintains a toll-free telephone hotline to take consumer complaints. The hotline operates from 8:30 to 5:00 on all federal workdays. The nationwide number is (800) 368–5779. Maryland residents should call (800) 638–3986. Spanish-speaking personnel are available, if needed, to take complaints.

A hotline operator will take your complaint over the phone, but hotline director Anderson recommends that you put any serious complaints in writing as well. When you contact OIG, Anderson advises: "Be prepared to give pertinent details—the who, what, why, where, and how."

Your complaint will be forwarded to the proper office within the Health Care Financing Administration (HCFA), the agency that oversees Medicare and Medicaid programs. All complaints are investigated and are referred, when appropriate, to proper state agencies.

The Business Community

While home care is a special kind of health care, it is also a consumer service. In this sense, home care agencies, as well as equipment dealers, are part of the business community. When you cannot resolve a problem or dispute satisfactorily, make it known to business leadership.

If the agency in question is a local branch of a national or regional firm and you have not otherwise been able to resolve your problem locally, let top management know. Conscientious firms have a reputation they want to maintain. Make sure to enclose copies of your original complaint, as well as any supporting correspondence sent to other government agencies or community organizations.

The Better Business Bureau has an established reputation for helping consumers through education about fair business practices and by providing information, when requested, about an individual business's track record in the community. What many consumers do not realize is that the BBB also helps mediate complaints. Before you take a dispute to court, you can use the BBB's arbitration program. Its decisions are legally binding on all parties. But don't expect BBB to provide legal advice about a home care dispute. Nor will it judge the quality of services or equipment you received.

Most BBBs will require that you file a written complaint. (Some have developed their own forms for this purpose.) They will then send your complaint to the agency involved for a reply and hopefully a satisfactory resolution. If not, mediation and arbitration are next steps. Nonresolved complaints become part of the BBB file on the agency.

National and State Home Care Associations

"We're definitely interested in hearing from consumers," says National Association for Home Care (NAHC) president Val Halamandaris. The association is unusual. It is a trade association composed of members who provide home care services, yet it advocates for the clients home care serves as well.

This strange duality undoubtedly stems from president Halamandaris's background. While serving on Senate and House staffs, Mr. Halamandaris championed the rights of the elderly, leading a hard-hitting congressional investigation into nursing home abuses, medical quackery, and other scams victimizing the elderly.

"We make no bones about the fact we don't want people in our association who are on the wrong side of the law or that take shortcuts in home care," he firmly states.

The NAHC Code of Ethics addresses quality of patient care and ethical financial practices. It's likely that any serious consumer problem would qualify as a code violation. The NAHC code also provides that consumers "aggrieved by agency action" receive a fair hearing if needed in order to resolve problems, including the denial, reduction, or termination of services. NAHC warns members that "failure to comply will result in expulsion from membership in the association in addition to other penalties prescribed by law." NAHC is leading efforts to assure consumers quality in home care and to improve home care benefits through Medicare and other programs as well.

In addition to NAHC, the state home care associations, which are also listed in the Resource Guide, want to know about professional member misconduct or local consumer problems in home care. These agencies cannot resolve your problems, but they are involved in legislative and other activity aimed at improving home care quality in their areas.

Funding Sources

Community-funded home care services must continuously compete for dollars with other community agencies. When you voice your complaints to funding sources, you strike at the agency's lifeblood. The Area Agencies on Aging, United Way, philanthropic foundations, corporate giving programs, and other such funding sources do not like to hear that the agencies they support or may consider funding are doing consumers a disservice. If funding sources receive several complaints, you can be sure that serious questions will be raised regarding any funding or contracts for that agency.

Licensing, Certification, Accrediting Bodies

If the agency or the home care worker at fault is "credentialed"—that is, licensed, certified, accredited, or registered by a governmental office or voluntary organization, as described in Chapter 3—register your complaint there. These groups have the clout to suspend or rescind professional credentials, which can have a devastating effect on the party in question. Without the necessary credentials, agencies or home care personnel may not be able to provide home care services to the public until such time as the penalty is served and the party proves trustworthy again.

Fiscal Intermediaries

If the agency is Medicare-certified, it has a fiscal intermediary that serves as a government-agency payment go-between. Under government contract, FIs review all agency claims and records and issue Medicare payments to agencies within their geographic area. FIs are also supposed to stay alert to any signs that may mean questionable quality of care or business practices.

If you run into trouble with a Medicare-certified agency, the FIs would definitely like to hear from you. You can reach FIs through their mailing address, listed in the Medicare handbook for beneficiaries, or your social security office can direct you.

Federal Trade Commission (FTC)

If your complaint deals with fraud, price-fixing, or deceptive advertising, contact the FTC. The FTC is also interested in anticompetitive practices—for example, if you felt you had no choice but to use a certain home care agency or equipment dealer as a precondition for continuing hospital or physician services.

The FTC serves all consumers, but has special interest in the elderly, who are more often the victims of such activities. In a statement to the Senate Special Committee on Aging, FTC Commissioner James C. Miller notes: "Because many persons over 65 live on fixed incomes, Commission activities aimed at preventing anti-competitive conduct in the health care industry [are] of substantial benefit to them. The purpose of our efforts in this area is to stimulate and strengthen competitive forces, thereby decreasing the need for government regulation, increasing consumer choice among providers of health care services, and lowering their costs." Contact the FTC by phone or mail:

FTC, Correspondence Branch
Pennsylvania Ave at 6th St NW
Washington, DC 20580
(202) 523–3567

Other Suggestions

Don't overlook consumer watchdog organizations, whether public or private.

Many states maintain hotlines to report cases of child or

elder abuse, regardless of whether abuse occurs at home or in an institution. The state Department of Social Services or Aging, or the home care or long-term care division within the state Department of Health, may run or fund these programs or may investigate home care complaints independently of licensing duties.

If your city or county has a consumer affairs office, register the problem there. The state attorney general's office is also charged with consumer protection against fraud and abuse. Many local health planning councils or health systems agencies (HSAs) are concerned with consumer affairs. If possible, phone the agency first in order to identify the correct department or individual before writing. If the telephone operator is not familiar with home care (and most aren't), speak to someone involved with nursing homes or long-term care, who should be.

If the agency receives public funds, complain to elected officials. Health care, particularly Medicare and Medicaid, has become prime political fodder. Legislation that benefits senior citizens often grows out of greater awareness of their consumer problems. Most elected officials maintain offices geared to helping consumers resolve problems, and an inquiry from a congressional office, for example, is bound to get an agency's attention.

VI

ALTERNATIVES TO HOME CARE

—25—

Adult Day Care and Foster Care

ADULT DAY CARE

After Mrs. C., age 76, had a stroke, she was left severely disabled. Home care helped her daughter Mary care for Mrs. C. at the home they shared together; but Mrs. C. needed long-term help, the kind of assistance Medicare would not pay for. The daughter, who worked, could no longer take time from her job. The doctor suggested a nursing home; the home care agency suggested adult day care.

Over 1,000 adult day care centers exist nationwide, and the number is growing rapidly. Day care serves a variety of needs. Like home care, centers help frail or health-impaired adults like Mrs. C. maintain independence at home and provide family caregivers like Mary respite from daily care and the opportunity to work worry-free.

Day care's relatively low cost makes it attractive too. According to the National Institute on Adult Daycare (NIAD), in 1984 the average daily costs nationwide for day care ranged from $20 to $24, although individual rates may be higher. This figure compares well with usually more expensive options, such as all-day companion or home health aide services or institutional care. In many cases, adult day care supplements home care a few times a week, rather than totally substituting for it.

Most day care centers operate Monday through Friday

during standard work hours. However, centers differ in the services they provide. Centers may offer services in an intensive, highly individualized program geared to rehabilitation, or in a maintenance program aimed at sustaining physical and mental health or both. In some areas, specialized day care programs exist to help those suffering with certain problems, such as Alzheimer's disease or "developmental disabilities" (cerebral palsy, mental retardation, autism).

ADULTS SERVED BY DAY CARE

As a movement, day care centers (sometimes called day treatment, day health care, psychiatric day treatment, and day hospital care) provide help to adults, age 18 and over, who have a wide variety of problems.

They may be adults who have physical, emotional, or mental problems and need assistance and supervision. These could include an older person who requires help with basic activities of daily living, or someone who has suffered a critical memory loss that prevents normal self-care, or perhaps someone with a physical problem that requires ongoing monitoring and nursing supervision. Day care can also work wonders with those who are declining because of lack of stimulation and loss of interest in life.

Day care also serves adults who need rehabilitation-type services to reach their best ability to function. This group includes recently discharged patients who may have suffered a stroke or a broken limb, or those with chronic conditions whose life could be improved through therapy and new self-care skills. Some younger disabled adults may need help making the changeover from group care to independent living. Here again, day care can help.

Essentially, day care tries to help bridge the gap between long-term institutional care and home independence.

DAY CARE SERVICES

Services may include:

- Health monitoring*
- Medical supervision
- Dentistry
- Therapy (physical, occupational, speech, respiratory, art, music, or dance)
- Audiology
- Skilled nursing
- Social services, including case management, information, and referral
- Shopping escort
- Personal care*
- Social, physical, and recreational activities geared to improving physical and mental well-being*
- Psychological and psychiatric services
- Podiatry
- Protective services
- Nutritional counseling
- One or more nutritious meals, including snacks, beverages, and special diets*
- Health education, including self-care
- Spiritual counseling
- Life skills counseling (how to cope, use community resources, problem-solving)*
- Vision care
- Transportation to and from center, and center-sponsored outings*

The asterisked services are considered the essentials of any sound day care center. The additional services provided by a given center may be more social or health-oriented, depending on how the day care center is funded. But to assist properly its ailing clientele, who are often seniors, most centers offer a variety of both social *and* health services.

Though services are provided outside the home, day care centers are vitally concerned with the home situation. Center personnel often make home visits to better assess a participant's day-to-day functioning, as well as to meet any other family members. Center staff members frequently work with families on an ongoing basis to ease the pressures of difficult care situations.

DAY CARE VERSUS HOME CARE

Day and home care share many services in common. However, day care has one special advantage. It provides the kind of social support and interaction that home care usually cannot. At the center, participants have an opportunity to develop friendships with other community residents and to participate in individual group activities that improve self-image and self-esteem.

For many senior participants, day care days are eagerly anticipated each week. Day care helps reduce the awful social isolation many elderly or disabled people experience when they do not go out into the community.

Services for the withdrawn or confused elderly often focus on remotivating seniors to take an interest in life and helping them orient themselves to their environment. Such help is often the key to preventing institutionalization.

Day care also brings another dimension to care—fun! Even treatment and rehabilitation-oriented programs provide plenty of opportunity for participants to relax and enjoy life.

ADULT DAY CARE
VERSUS SENIOR CENTERS

Should you look for an adult day care center, don't confuse it with a senior center. *Senior centers* are multipurpose activity centers that only occasionally include a day care program.

Unlike day care centers, senior centers typically serve a generally healthy senior population, providing educational, recreational, and social activities. Many include general health activities, such as exercise or fitness classes or health screenings for high blood pressure or hearing and vision problems. Senior centers are also a good source of community information. Staff can probably direct you to any existing adult day care programs within your community.

OBTAINING DAY CARE

You're most likely to find adult day care available in larger urban and suburban areas. Look for centers sponsored by reliable public or private community groups. Centers are often affiliated with hospitals, nursing homes, rehabilitation, or multiservice geriatric centers.

Avoid any so-called private day care centers which may operate in individual private homes. While there are no solid statistics to document the extent of "cottage" day care, Betty Ransom, coordinator of NIAD, a division of the National Council on Aging, reports that she frequently gets calls from homeowners seeking to open an adult day care center in their own homes. "From these conversations," Ms. Ransom reports, "I gather their intention is to give seniors a meal and have them watch T.V. That's not day care," she declared emphatically. "That's babysitting!"

Community referral sources, or your closest Area Agency on Aging, can help you identify reliable programs that may be available locally. The National Institute on Adult Daycare can also refer you to centers nationwide.

Admission requirements vary widely among centers. All require some degree of incapacity. Other requirements may be tied to income, where you live, and the availability of space in the program.

Most centers charge a flat daily rate for care regardless of the services received. Medicare and other insurance seldom pay for long-term adult day care. Insurance may reimburse you for the cost of certain day care services, such as physical therapy, provided you are eligible for and would otherwise be covered for therapy received at any qualifying outpatient facility.

Many centers do receive funds from government and public or private philanthropic sources that help underwrite the center's total costs. Such centers often scale their fees according to income level, so a financial assessment may also be part of a preadmission review. The average client at such centers pays less than the full day rate, and some receive free care. The only practical way you can determine what your out-of-pocket costs for day care may be is to discuss payment in advance with appropriate center staff.

EVALUATING THE CENTER

Before enrolling, visit the center so you can see the facility, meet staff, and get an overall impression of daily operation. Ms. Ransom advises, "Because adult day care is a young field, still looking for direction, the quality of day care programs varies."

As of 1984, 34 states had developed some standards for care, but these range from sound to very superficial. In order to provide national direction, the National Institute on Adult Daycare has developed basic uniform standards for quality care.

Consumer Guidelines

NIAD guidelines of interest to consumers include these:

- *Adequate staff.* When you visit the center, notice what the patients are doing. Ms. Ransom counsels, "If you walk into a room of 30 patients and some are sitting off in the corner doing nothing, this is one tip-off that there isn't enough staff to meet patient needs." Generally you should expect at least one staff person for every eight day care attendees.
- *Assessment and a plan of care.* As with home care, when you enroll in a day care program, a professional should conduct an initial assessment of your health and social needs. This should be followed by the development, with your participation, of a plan of day care with established goals. Your doctor should also be consulted about your medical needs. Assessment may be made during a center interview, but an in-home visit is highly recommended.
- *Termination.* As a participant or family caregiver, you should receive no less than two weeks' notice of termination or discharge from the program for any reason

other than the sudden worsening of a health condition.

- *Emergency services.* You and the center should have a written agreement regarding emergency care, including ambulance service. At least one person on staff should be trained in first aid and cardiopulmonary resuscitation (CPR).
- *Scope of activities.* Look for a balance of activities geared to physical, social, emotional, cultural, and economic needs. Activities should give you the opportunity for individual activities as well as small and large group activities, participant or spectator. Many centers sponsor intergenerational activities, or activities involved in community events.
- *Coordination with other services.* The day care staff should coordinate your planning care with help provided by other local organizations, including home care agencies. When such services are coordinated, your overall care improves. For example, a day care physical therapist should coordinate his or her plan with that of the home care agency therapist.

When you visit the center, talk to participants. Ask staff for a copy of the monthly calendar of activities and menus. Daily activities should be posted.

Note whether surroundings are clean, comfortable, well-lit, hazard-free, and pleasing to the eye. The center should also be barrier-free, with toilet and doorways accessible to wheelchairs. There should be a small personal locker available to store personal garments. A rest area should be available, as well as enough space to ensure privacy if needed.

Participants' Rights

As a day care participant, NIAD stresses that you have inpatient rights. Foremost among these is the right to be treated as an adult, with respect and dignity. NIAD's Statement of Rights also emphasizes participation in services that will encourage learning, growth, and awareness, but also the right to decide whether or not you wish to participate in any given activity.

Consumer Follow-up

If you want more information on adult day care, including standards, or to locate the state day care association, contact:

National Institute on Adult Daycare
600 Maryland Ave SW, West Wing 100
Washington, DC 20024
(202) 479–1200

ADULT FOSTER CARE

For those who live alone or with someone unable to provide enough care, even with home care support, sometimes independent living may not be possible. This was the case for Martha L., age 56, following a disabling stroke. Her mind, which wandered at times, was generally good, good enough to know that she did not want to enter a nursing home for the expected long months of therapy and recovery ahead. For her, adult foster care was a much-welcomed option. It provided home care, although not in her own home. She was placed in a home where the two children soon called her "Grandma," and she adjusted and improved under adult foster care.

Adult foster care places adults in need of assistance into a warm family environment. The program essentially is similar to foster care programs traditionally provided for children. Families are carefully prescreened and receive a stipend of upwards of $400 a month to provide care. The stipend may be scaled according to the adult's disability level and need for care. Family caregivers normally undergo special training in basic home nursing, problems of the elderly, and rehabilitation before an adult is placed in the home. Nurses and other home care personnel are assigned when skilled professional services are needed.

Most programs, which are usually hospital-sponsored or operated by a state department of social services, limit participation to adults in need of skilled care who would otherwise require nursing home placement. In some cases, the adult may contribute toward the family's stipend. In such programs, a social worker works closely with the adult and the family to ensure that the arrangement is satisfactory and the treatment goals are met.

Placement may be short term, as was Martha's case, or permanent. Foster care programs have been slowly growing as the value of this option is realized. Johns Hopkins University Hospital in Baltimore and Massachusetts General Hospital in Boston have operated programs since 1978. Queen's Medical Center in Honolulu started its program in 1979. To locate any available programs in your area, contact the local department of social services or department of community or family medicine if you have a teaching hospital nearby.

—26—

Life Care Communities

When Senator John Heinz opened a 1983 hearing on life care communities before the Senate Special Committee on Aging, he characterized *life care communities* as the "fast-growing and increasingly important housing and health care alternative for Older Americans."

Indeed, growth over the last few years has been fast-paced, with the industry doubling in size. Estimates vary on the number of such communities, from between 300 to 500, housing more than 100,000 seniors and taking in an excess of $1 billion annually. As our population continues to age, the number of life care communities is expected to expand more rapidly.

THE LIFE CARE CONCEPT

Robert W. Marans, director of the Urban Environmental Research Program at the University of Michigan, Ann Arbor, who studies life care and retirement communities, reports that most older people he talks to consider this sort of life style.

What's the attraction? These retirement communities—sometimes referred to as *continuing care residential communities (CCRC)*—combine lifetime housing with the promise of nursing care when needed. They also provide the usual variety of retirement-community social activities and other amenities, such as transportation and beauty shop or barber services.

It is the health care dimension, however, that principally

distinguishes these communities from the garden-variety retirement housing development. This is also the feature that evokes so much interest among seniors.

With payment of a lump-sum entrance fee, residents enter a bona fide life care community with a " 'til death do us part" contract that provides lifetime housing (not ownership) and guaranteed nursing care, exclusive of hospitalization.

Life care is supposed to free residents from the grim specter of illness depleting their life savings for nursing home care. In effect, seniors buying into a life care community "purchase" a prepaid insurance policy that does not give them home equity, but provides nursing care should they need it. If they don't ever need nursing care, they will have paid a premium for this protection. But most residents consider the fees affordable and the security of lifetime care well worth the investment.

Community Life and Fees

At first glance, you might mistake the average life care community for a college campus or condominium complex. Architecturally, they often comprise a complex of low or high-rise residential units in a scenic setting, frequently with separate facilities for recreation, nursing care, or other services. Individual residential units are usually available as studios, or one- or two-bedroom apartments. In some cases, three-bedroom units or even small separate homes or townhouses are offered.

Most units provide modern conveniences such as central air conditioning, and often include basic household accessories such as carpeting and drapes. Furnishings may or may not be provided. Units are often equipped with bathroom grab bars and other safety features and designed with extra-wide doorways for wheelchair access. Many newer communities feature built-in emergency response devices, often connected to the community's 24-hour health facility. Weekly maid and/or linen service is usually provided, plus one or more communal meals daily. In brief, the communities are designed to enhance independent living.

All this, including health care and social activities, doesn't come cheaply. Typically these communities charge a hefty entrance or "endowment" or "founder's" fee, which varies based on the residential unit that is selected. Fees range from $20,000 to $100,000. A study of 85 life care communities by the accounting firm of Laventhal & Horwath found that the median entrance fee for a one-bedroom apartment was about $45,000 in 1983. In lieu of an endowment fee, a few communities require that incoming residents sign over all capital assets as a precondition for acceptance.

On top of the entrance fee, residents almost always pay a monthly service fee ranging from several hundred dollars to more than a thousand dollars. Monthly fees generally vary with the selected unit and the number of occupants. The additional fee required for the second occupant is usually lower and generally runs about 40 to 60 percent less than the single rate. The Laventhal & Horwath study reported that the 1983 median monthly fee for a one-bedroom apartment was $630 for one occupant, $885 for two.

Promises and Problems

Most seniors who consider this option are described as middle-class Americans, comfortable but by no means rich. Many who eventually opt for life care finance the initial entrance fee through the profits realized on the sale of their principal asset—their home. Thus, for many investing in life care means investing most of their life savings, so the risk is high. Unfortunately, in many cases a commitment to life care has brought disappointment and even destitution. Senator Heinz noted that "the promise of life care has too often been thwarted by inept management, mismanagement, and outright fraud." As a result, in recent years scores of life care facilities have been forced to declare bankruptcy.

Despite these serious problems, a life care community can be a sound alternative for many older Americans. Residents in solidly managed facilities usually express a high level of satisfaction.

Speaking before the Senate committee, Doris Schwartz, a

faculty member of the University of Pennsylvania School of Nursing and a resident of the Foulkeways Life Care Community, Gwynedd, Pennsylvania, summed up her experience: "It is a lifestyle for alert, active people who are 65 and over, and it provides lifetime security, independence, dignity and privacy. If long-term care is required, the move, complete with selected pieces of one's own furniture, is likely to be a short distance on already familiar grounds, to a setting where one remains ensconced among one's former friends and neighbors in a community where the resident has already put down roots. I like my apartment and grounds very much. Everything is close and living there is convenient."

Lack of Consumer Safeguards

Whether life care proves one of the best or worst experiences of a lifetime largely depends on how carefully consumers evaluate such communities *before* residency. Seniors considering life care should be aware that they are in a "buyer beware" situation.

As of 1984, there were no federal regulations governing the life care industry, and only 11 states (Arizona, California, Colorado, Florida, Illinois, Indiana, Maryland, Michigan, Minnesota, Missouri, Oregon) regulate life care operations in any way. However, such regulations are no guarantee of consumer protection.

Ten years after regulations were in effect in California, the first state to enact life care laws, one of the worst life care failures occurred. Pacific Homes, a life care community related to the Methodist Church, which had been in operation for 25 years, went bankrupt, resulting in financial losses for thousands of residents and leaving many homeless. In its report pursuant to the California Bankruptcy Act, the trustee of Pacific Homes directly traced its final collapse to "gross mismanagement over an extended period of time" and charged that the state "ignored its mandatory duty."

The moral of the story is, don't rely on state regulations as a safeguard. If you (or someone you know) are considering life care, approach this option with your eyes open. Don't be charmed by the glossy brochures or a professional sales pitch. Ask questions.

Lloyd Lewis, executive director of Kendal Crosslands, a nationally recognized model life care community in Kennet Square, Pennsylvania, reports that few consumers do. He advised the Senate committee: "Rarely am I asked penetrating questions about our finances, non-profit status, or overall approach to the subject of aging. Even more rarely am I asked searching questions about our health care facilities and programs. We are only occasionally asked questions about our most intimate and important services."

In many cases, consumers probably do not ask because they simply do not know what to ask and what to look for when they evaluate a life care community. Some basic pointers follow. Also the following organizations have useful, low-cost consumer booklets available that can help you evaluate life care.

National Consumers League
600 Maryland Ave SW, Suite 202, West Wing
Washington, DC 20024
(202) 554–1600

American Association of Homes for the Aging
1050 17th St NW, Suite 770
Washington, DC 20036
(202) 296–5960

HOW TO EVALUATE LIFE CARE

Finances

Consider all the financial aspects to life care first. No matter how appealing a life care community and its contract may appear, if the community is not on solid financial ground, you face serious potential risk. The financial side to life care is one of the most difficult areas to evaluate. With life care, you cannot use longevity as a sign that a community is financially sound. As the Pacific Homes case illustrated, established communities may go bankrupt unless they have been managed properly through the years.

Keep in mind too that you should consider the financial picture far into the future. Seniors over age 85 represent the fastest-growing segment of our population. If you enter a life care community at age 65, you may live there more than twenty years. The community that does not plan for the extended future could fail at a time when you most need help.

Conduct your own financial analysis of the community first. Then, if the figures seem economically sound, have a professional with actuarial experience, if possible, review them. This review will be well worth the additional cost. Your study should examine the following factors.

Entrance and Monthly Fees

Most consumers want to know about these costs first. But a dollar amount alone tells you little. You should consider more than what size unit and services these figures provide.

One critical factor that determines a community's financial stability is *how* these funds are used on a larger scale. The entrance fee is supposed to cover your allocation for expected nursing care, and major repairs, maintenance, and improvements. The monthly fee covers all basic services, such as meals, maid service, and so on, plus your prorated portion of the community's overall debt. Faulty practices include using entrance fees to cover initial construction costs or to expand facilities. Some communities keep the monthly fee low so they can attract residents. They then use the entrance fee to subsidize monthly service fees. Such practices can spell future financial ruin.

Writing in *Modern Healthcare,* Richard Cole, of Blyth Eastman Paine Webber Health Care Funding, New York, who rescues failing retirement communities, notes that this "life care syndrome" has occurred repeatedly in the communities he works with. According to Mr. Cole, these practices can exhaust the entrance fee fund within a six- to ten-year period, unless there is enough resident turnover. Therefore, without additional entrance fees from new residents coming in, the monthly fees collected cannot meet the basic service costs. Then, typically, mortgage payments on the facilities are missed and bills to service suppliers go unpaid. The community teeters on the brink of financial disaster.

One tipoff to such fiscal distress is a "deferred residence" sales campaign. Potential residents are encouraged to pay now in full but move in later, thereby ensuring themselves against any future hikes in the endowment fee. Funds raised this way can then be used immediately to pay off creditors.

In a financially sound community, monthly fees are set high enough so that the community is self-supporting and does not have to depend on a constant flow of new resident endowments. Therefore current fees may be higher than current expenses in order to provide properly for the future.

You must expect eventual increases in monthly fees. Check the basis for increasing monthly fees. Many communities have automatic built-in cost-of-living escalation clauses in their contracts. It is also common practice for contracts to limit the number of annual increases and/or annual percentage increases in fees. Be careful when the increases allowed may be less than the inflation rate. At face value this practice attracts incoming residents; but the fact remains that unless the monthly fee structure has been planned to meet rising costs over the long haul, the community is headed for problems.

Reserve Funds

Whether a community is old or new, to avoid the life care syndrome described earlier, sufficient money from the entrance fee fund should be held in reserve or placed in escrow. Check the stated purpose of the reserve fund and any limitations placed on its use. The reserve fund's purpose is to tide the community over those periods when nursing care use may be high and resident turnover low. It is also for prudent future capital expenses. In some cases, reserve funds have been established to protect the mortgage lender's interest, not those of the residents.

Just how much money should be placed in reserve depends

on the size and the age of the community. (This is where actuarial advice is valuable.) Clearly any community that doesn't have a healthy reserve fund is risky.

Sponsorship, Ownership, and Management

Whether the community is owned or sponsored by a nonprofit or profit-making enterprise does not indicate its financial reliability.

Traditionally, life care communities were sponsored by nonprofit altruistic groups, often church-related. More recently, entrepreneurs, some unscrupulous, have entered the field. In some instances, hospitals and nursing homes and even universities looking for additional funds are turning to life care as a potential investment venture.

Look carefully at who *actually* sponsors, owns, and manages the community, and what legal and financial obligations that entity maintains. Many communities maintain close affiliations with groups that assert a "moral" responsibility. But morality does not mean *financial* responsibility or consumer protection.

In the Pacific Homes scandal, many residents had joined believing that the Methodist Church would fully protect them against default; yet this was not the case. In another instance, a Federal Trade Commission investigation found that Christian Services Incorporated (CSI), a proprietary corporation that developed, marketed, and operated some 200 nonprofit life care communities across the United States, had engaged in deceptive sales practices. Though CSI communities were in no way affiliated with the Presbyterian Church, many of these communities were (and still are) promoted and managed under the name "John Knox Village," John Knox being the founder of the Presbyterian Church.

Sound professional management is critical. Some communities are self-managed, while others contract with proprietary management firms for this service. In some cases where outside contractors have been used, this arrangement has led to "sweetheart" deals that bilked community funds. On behalf of the community, these contractors purchased goods and services at inflated prices from subsidiary contractor-owned businesses, instead of using competitive bidding. If the community is self-managed, find out whether it has professional expertise. Many communities have failed in the past because of inept management, not deliberate wrongdoing. The board of directors should have business and financial experience, not just good intentions.

When you study sponsorship, ownership, and management, don't forget to check reliability with your basic consumer references, such as the state attorney general's office. Ask about and investigate past performance in similar or other financial ventures.

Your Personal Finances

When you consider the financial side to life care, analyze your own finances carefully too. Some communities require a financial statement prior to enrollment and deny admittance if finances appear inadequate. Compare your present budget against that projected for lifetime life care residency. Entrance fee aside, can you meet the monthly fee today and in the future?

In a statement prepared for the Senate committee, Robert Ball, former long-time commissioner of social security, noted that couples who received near maximum social security benefits would probably be able to meet the monthly fee in many life care communities, even assuming modest raises, since social security benefits provide cost-of-living increases. For those below the highest social security rates, he stated: "Income from non-social-security sources probably needs to be at least twice the current monthly fee in order to meet present and future monthly payments over the resident's lifetime."

When you figure your cost of life care, take into account that certain items you would normally pay for, such as daily meals, linen service, and recreation, may be covered under the life care contract. Budget for Medicare or other insurance costs and medical expenses, as outlined in the next section.

Consider taxes. Under IRS regulations, you can include as part of your medical expenses that portion of the entrance fee or monthly fee that is allocated for medical care. However, to be deductible a specific amount or percentage must be designated for care in your contract. Also, the contract must state that it requires a "lump-sum or advance payment" for the community's promise to provide lifetime medical care.

Health Care

Prior to the rapid rise of health care costs, most communities provided the long-term health care benefits traditionally associated with life care. These included the kind of ongoing health services and care normally provided by nursing homes. Such care was usually rendered at an on-site nursing facility and was provided when needed for as long as needed, at little or no additional increase in the monthly fee.

Not so today. Health benefits vary widely among individual communities from those just described to little or no free nursing care. In order to assess any potential advantage of life care, you must analyze all the issues related to health care. Then carefully compare the cost and convenience of life care against your health care options in another retirement life style.

Health-Related Admission Requirements

Some communities deny admission to persons who are not in reasonably good health *at the time of initial occupancy.* Good health is often defined as the ability to live independently, to shop for oneself, or the ability to walk unassisted to communal dining facilities.

If a community has a long waiting list, you may find yourself out of luck by the time your name comes up, as happened to one elderly woman. At age 72, Mrs. C. was ablebodied but arthritic when she applied and was placed on the waiting list of a California life care community. But some four years later, when housing was available, her condition had deteriorated to the point where she needed a walker for assistance. Though she was financially independent, in good health otherwise, and mentally alert, she was turned down.

Scrutinize the health requirements and contract language. Should you have a preexisting condition such as cancer which can seriously affect health but may not always impair mobility, make sure you are still eligible for life care health benefits. Some contracts may permit communities to "evict" residents or revoke health benefits on the basis of misrepresentation of health status.

Also note whether you are required to maintain Medicare, Parts A and B, or other health insurance, in order to be accepted. Most communities *require* that you carry some health insurance. Generally the services that communities do provide pick up only where insurance ends. Even if insurance is not required, you would be wise to maintain your coverage. Few communities provide all the common insurance benefits, such as hospitalization, outpatient therapies, or medical equipment.

Contracted Health Benefits and Extra Costs

Refer *only* to the contract as the basis for this information. When you do, distinguish carefully between those benefits which are *included* versus those which are merely *available* or *accessible* to residents.

Look for specific exclusions of benefits. Most communities do not provide routine preventive care, dental care, psychiatric, podiatric, and eye care, drugs, eyeglasses, and hearing aids.

Review all included benefits, but focus primarily on the long-term care benefits that are offered. These benefits are not generally provided by Medicare or other insurance and therefore represent the true value of a life care commitment. Many communities no longer provide unlimited nursing care. Some allow only a certain number of "free" days, often thirty to sixty. After that, you are charged full nursing rates.

Note if communities charge a substantially higher monthly fee to residents when they must occupy the community nursing facility. Compare these increased monthly fees with the rates for care charged by local nursing homes. When life care charges approximate or exceed local nursing home rates, as they often do, ask yourself: "What benefits am I really getting in return for that hefty entrance fee without home equity?" To help quantify the answer, weigh the dollar value of any "free" nursing care days offered against the entrance fee.

Consider that the average nursing home patient is in residence for more than a year. How would such fees affect your finances over a long period? Check any special eligibility requirements for inpatient nursing care. For example, must you exhaust all Medicare nursing home benefits first? Unless the community's facility is Medicare-certified, this may mean placement in another facility first, perhaps far away, and additional out-of-pocket costs.

Learn what provisions will be made if you need an inpatient service that is unavailable or more skilled care than the nursing facility provides. What happens if you need a bed, but the nursing facility is fully occupied?

Home Care Benefits

Note carefully whether the community's contract provides for home care services in addition to Medicare home care benefits. Be wary when the community does not provide any in-home assistance with personal care or other basic services. Medicare does not provide these services, yet they are so often needed to remain independent at home. If a community does not provide home care, you could find yourself placed prematurely into the community nursing facility. (This would free a housing unit for a new resident and another entrance fee.) Ideally, communities should provide a continuum of care and use inpatient nursing care only as a last resort.

If the community provides such help, who actually gives assistance? What is their training? Is there an extra cost? Personnel who provide such care and the overall care given should meet the home care standards already described.

The Nursing Home Facilities and Care

Nursing facilities must be state licensed or certified as skilled nursing facilities (SNFs) or as intermediate care facilities that provide less intensive care. Most life care nursing facilities are *not* certified for Medicare and/or Medicaid participation.

The few communities with certified facilities provide some consumer advantages.

If Medicare-certified, you may be able to combine your Medicare and life care benefits to extend any free care days and reduce out-of-pocket costs. If the facility is Medicaid-certified, you would have the security of receiving uninterrupted care at the same location if your financial resources should ever become exhausted.

You should look carefully at the nursing care provided. State-certified or licensed facilities are reviewed periodically for *minimum* standards of care. A copy of the most recent review should be available. Realize that the problems that exist in regular nursing homes also can happen here. One consumer wrote me: "If patients are 'troublesome' in any way, minor or major, they are sedated to the point where they can't do anything. A friend's father was so far gone, he seemed to have lost his mind. The friend visited him every day for two weeks. He was soon making macrame projects. We concluded that when the family was present daily, they took him off of sedatives and he returned to normal. He stopped sleeping most of the day and became active." Use published consumer guidelines for nursing homes as an indication of quality care.

Where physician's care is included, such care should be provided by physicians trained in appropriate specialty areas, such as internal medicine, family practice, or geriatric care.

Check whether the facility is located on or very near the community grounds. If it is not, you may become socially isolated from important community ties. Also, check the accommodations in individual nursing units. Are they all semi-private, or are private rooms available too? Find out if you can partially furnish the nursing unit with any of your personal belongings. Are nursing units strictly segregated by sex, or can provisions be made for couples to share accommodations when both parties require care?

Compare the number of nursing beds available to the number of community residents. A ratio of better than 1:5 may mean long waiting lists for admission. Ask about nonresident use of facilities. Some communities use this practice in order to keep nursing beds full. This gives the community additional money to operate, but may also increase waiting time for bona fide life care residents.

Your Consumer Rights

Before signing the contract, know your consumer rights. Many states that do not specifically regulate life care communities provide some consumer protection through general contract laws.

Check the refund policy carefully for both the lump sum entrance fee and any application fee. Note the amount and conditions of refund and whether refunds can be made to your estate in the event of death.

Most life care contracts grant you an *occupancy* license. Make sure your rights under this arrangement are clearly spelled out for every possible personal contingency. For example, what happens in the case of death of a spouse and/ or subsequent remarriage? Or in the event of financial setback and inability to pay monthly fees as a regular or nursing care resident?

Also review the contract to determine your rights in the event that the community fails financially. Because of past problems, some contracts now provide a *small* return to residents of record should failure actually occur.

Reviewing the contract will take time. Take the contract home and read it. Question the motives of any community that will not give you this opportunity. During a National Consumers League (NCL) study of life care, administrators at one life care community would not permit the NCL staff to examine their contract outside the administrative office. Though the community seemingly had nothing to hide, one can only wonder why a request to review the contract independently would be denied.

GENERAL ADVICE

Life care is usually a lifetime commitment, so proceed slowly and with care. "Consumers are very vulnerable when they look at life care," says NCL executive director Barbara Warden. "It's the psychological factor. People want to believe they will be protected for life." Get all the printed material available, including price lists, in advance. Then read this information at your leisure. Take notes and prepare your questions. Consider and evaluate several communities, not just one. There will be differences. The American Association of Homes for the Aging publishes a directory that profiles about 400 life care communities and includes information on services and fees.

Don't rely on the testimonials in the advertising brochures. Be prepared to visit the community in person. This is the only practical way to evaluate a community and to get a feel for what day-to-day living there would be like.

Look at all the facilities, including the health care units. Talk to several current residents, including those in the nursing units, about their experiences. Sit in on recreational or social activities. Talk to and observe the attitude of the life care staff. Meet with the medical and nursing directors.

One common complaint about communities is the food. If possible, dine at the residential facility; otherwise just observe the quality of the food. Review a copy of the week's menus.

If you can, visit the community more than once, if your first impression is favorable. Become familiar with the general geographic area if it is new to you. One allergy-ridden life care resident found out too late that the community she chose was situated in the hay fever belt. Consider the availability of shopping areas, cultural activities, and nearby transportation.

Be wary of any sales attempts to have you make a fast decision. One-day discounts, warnings that there are few units left, or similar tactics may be used by unreliable developers to pressure you into a quick commitment.

If you decide in favor of life care, seek professional advice. Have an independent financial advisor—an accountant or banker for example—review the financial details. Consult a lawyer about your contract; don't automatically sign.

—27—

Board and Care Facilities

Group homes, community or residential care homes, adult congregate living facilities, domiciliary care facilities, and enriched or sheltered housing are among the names used to describe *board and care facilities*. These facilities offer the elderly and disabled an option to traditional housing and certain home care services. They might be viewed as "halfway houses" between one's own home and a nursing home environment.

SERVICES AND FEES

Unlike life care communities, these facilities do not require any entrance fee. They operate on a strictly weekly or monthly payment, like that of old-fashioned boarding homes or standard apartment rentals. However, they provide not only housing, but housekeeping, meals, personal care assistance, and often recreational activities too. In some cases, if state laws permit, self-administered medication may be dispensed to residents, but the extent of health-related services usually stops there. Normally board and care residents cannot be bedridden and must be able to leave their homes by foot or wheelchair.

Nationally, well over 30,000 such facilities exist, with the number increasing substantially each year. This continued growth has been fueled by the large demand for noninstitutional care. The accommodations available and their costs run the gamut from high-priced ($1,000+ per month), professionally managed retirement apartment buildings with hundreds of units to tiny, private home "mom and pop" operations with as few as two to four beds, room-sharing, and welfare rates of $200 to $400 per month. In Florida's Pinellas County, monthly board and care rates averaged $625 in 1984. Most facilities operate as for-profit enterprises.

CONSUMERS BEWARE

Past abuses in many board and care homes have been glaring. Outright physical abuse and neglect of residents, bilking of funds, and deaths due to absence of basic fire or safety devices made headlines during the mid-seventies. Such public scandals finally prompted some states to initiate regulatory action.

Where licensing and regulation exist, this responsibility usually falls under the jurisdiction of one or more of the following state departments: Social or Human Services, Human Resources, Health and Public Health, Public Welfare, Aging or Community Affairs. To further curb abuses, most states encourage the reporting of any endangerment of resident health and safety or infringement of basic rights via the ombudsman hotlines set up for nursing homes or other long-term-care housing.

In many states, existing board and care regulations are weak. The state standards for operating these facilities often focus primarily on fire and safety measures and certain administrative procedures. Too often little real attention is given to standards relating to actual services and the care that may be provided. Even when stiffer state regulations exist, enforcement can be a problem. The size of enforcement staffs has not kept pace with the rapid board and care growth. With too many facilities and too little staff, pen and paper surveys often replace periodic on-site inspections.

Therefore you cannot rely on state authorities to monitor board and care facilities adequately. If you are considering a board and care facility yourself or assisting someone else, investigate all angles of the arrangement beforehand. Make sure that you have explored the many home care services now available before you turn to board and care.

If you enter or place a loved one in a board and care facility, make sure that interested "others"—family members, friends, religious or community social services personnel— visit regularly to ensure that a satisfactory quality of life is being maintained.

CONSUMER GUIDELINES

Before you investigate the facility itself, find out whether board and care facilities must be licensed in your state in order to operate, and if so, which state agency has this responsibility. Local senior citizen organizations, health planning councils, or nursing home ombudsmen programs can generally help you identify the appropriate state agency if state licensing exists.

Contact the state agency or its local branch and learn the general licensing requirements insofar as resident health, safety, personal care, and consumer protection are concerned. If your state has a resident Bill of Rights (for board and care or nursing homes), obtain a copy and use it as a guide for the minimum living standards you should look for and expect. Also check with the agency and learn if the facility in question is properly licensed and if there are any complaints on file.

When you contact the facility, ask about:

- *References.* Is the facility recommended by local community health or social service personnel or senior or disabled advocate groups? Get specific names and follow up with phone calls.
- *Services.* What basic services are included in the standard fee? What optional services are available?

Consider your current needs for assistance as well as services you may need in the future. Make sure you get specific answers on services; if not, ask specific questions. For example, with respect to meals: How many meals a day are provided? Are snacks provided? Where are meals served? Is in-room meal service available if needed or requested? What provisions are made for special diets for medical or religious reasons?

For personal care, ask whether facility staff will assist with daily activities such as medications, toileting, shaving, dressing, bathing, feeding, and so on if need be.

Facilities typically provide housekeeping. Does this mean that they will change the bed linens at least weekly? Clean your room? Do personal laundry? Assist with shopping? What social or recreational activities are provided or available? Are transportation services provided?

- *Accommodations.* How many residents does the facility house? Are rooms private or shared? If shared, how are roommates matched? What happens should personalities prove incompatible? Can spouses or other companion couples share a room? Can you furnish your room yourself in whole or part? What bathroom facilities are there? Must you provide your own phone, or is there telephone access? If access is provided, during what hours are incoming and outgoing calls permitted? What access can you have to common living areas? During what hours? Are visitors permitted? (They should be.) During what hours? What about overnight guests? Are kitchen privileges available? Are pets allowed?
- *Costs and payment.* What is the basic charge for daily, weekly, or monthly residence? What services cost extra, and what is the charge? Is there a "security" charge? If so, how much? When is payment due, and how must it be made? What penalties are there for late payment? What is the policy on refunds? Are any discounts available; and if so, under what conditions? For example, what if you go on vacation and therefore do not need meals? On what basis are fees increased? How often have increases occurred in the past? How large were the increases? When was the last increase?
- *Security.* What provisions have been made to ensure safety, such as the installation of safety devices? Can you have a key to your room, or is a locked area provided

for important personal items? What measures have been made to ensure that the facility itself is secure from intruders?

- *Facility ownership and personnel.* Who actually owns the facility? (Frequent changeovers are not uncommon.) What is the background of the owners and service personnel? Apply the guidelines used for home care agencies. Also note the ratio of service staff to residents; higher ratios are better.
- *Grievance and resident participation policies.* How are problems and complaints resolved? What input do residents have in the day-to-day operations that directly affect them; for example, meal planning, recreational activities, visitor hours?
- *Termination policies and follow-up assistance.* In some states, these policies are regulated by law or administrative codes. Florida, for example, requires that residents receive a 30-day notice of relocation or termination of residency *in writing.* It does not require that the facility provide any help in relocation, nor does it regulate the conditions under which the owner can terminate residents. Florida also requires that residents be relocated should they become bedridden for longer than seven days. This stipulation stands even if residents can arrange for appropriate home care services at the residence.

Clearly, termination policies are critical for any potential resident and should be checked. Ask what happens should you become unable to meet the facility's full charge. Or if your health status (mental or physical) seriously declines. How long will your room be held in case of hospitalization or temporary nursing home care? If you become bedridden, how long can you remain in the facility? Must you personally make additional provisions for care there? What kind of assistance does the facility provide in relocation or in obtaining additional care if needed?

Answers to these questions can be provided over the phone. If satisfactory, follow up with a visit to the facility itself.

WHEN YOU VISIT

Look beyond basic cleanliness and the amenities. Observe the physical environment from a health and safety view. Note whether there are obvious safety hazards, such as scatter rugs, shaky stair railings, or dimly lit, cluttered stairs. Are there safety grab bars in bathroom(s), outdoor wheelchair ramps, smoke detectors on every floor? Consider your own mobility and proximity to bathrooms and dining areas. Ask to see copies of the latest fire and health inspection reports. Note whether any state-mandated Bill of Rights is posted. Talk to the staff about the facility's philosophy and the general life style.

Large and small facilities may have individual pluses or minuses. Diana Cruz, a specialist in Florida's Office of Licensure and Certification, regularly visits facilities of all sizes. She notes that "smaller facilities often tend to do too much for residents if the owners or staff have no experience in gerontology (care of the aged). They may mean well, but they don't give residents an opportunity to do for themselves." On the plus side, however, "some small homes have children or pets. They may allow residents to get involved in normal daily living activities like filling a dishwasher. This wouldn't happen in larger facilities."

The familylike atmosphere of some small facilities can have a very positive effect on the health of residents.

In larger facilities, many organized social activities are frequently available. While this can be a plus for many seniors, it can be a drawback too. Larger facilities can be impersonal, despite the outward trappings of color-coordinated rooms and activity areas. It is easy for the mildly confused or less socially inclined senior to become forgotten amid a large resident population. Unless staff is truly concerned, such residents often become more isolated and withdrawn, making their mental and physical decline more likely.

Check the facility's accessibility to shopping, to the community in general, and to health care. Also consider whether the overall makeup of the resident population suits you.

Some facilities have mostly senior citizens, while others mix adults of all age groups.

Talk to other residents privately about their living conditions. If possible, spend a day or at least several hours at the facility to get a better sense of what daily living there might be like. Many legitimate complaints of today's board and care residences do not involve direct abuse. Rather, residents complain about indifferent care, poor meals, and infringements, sometimes subtle, on their privacy, dignity, right to make their own decisions, go where and when they want, manage their money, and practice their religion.

If you sense any reluctance on the part of residents to discuss life there freely, this is a sign that something is amiss.

When you visit a facility, drop in unannounced if possible. Or if you must prearrange a visit, follow this up with an unexpected call. This strategy has helped many consumers get a true picture of nursing home life, and it applies equally to board and care facilities.

If you decide on a board and care facility, review carefully any contract or agreement you may be asked to sign, and of course get a copy. All facilities, even the smallest, should have written statements outlining services, costs, and mutual obligations.

As with other care options, compare several facilities and have a backup plan ready should the arrangement fail to work out.

—28—

Shared Housing

The newspaper ad placed by the New York Foundation for Senior Citizens read: "We match and place persons in need of housing in the apartments and homes of senior citizens, thus helping to solve the problems of both individuals: financial hardship, loneliness and isolation." What the ad didn't mention was that this arrangement—home sharing—also provides for many seniors, or others who need some assistance, an alternative to home care services such as homemaking or companion services.

The home sharing option, sometimes referred to as joint households, is slowly growing into a more organized movement. While exact figures are not available, the National Shared Housing Resource Center (NSHRC) estimates that 300 organizations or projects exist nationwide to help match consumers with one or more unrelated persons to share a common household.

Often the homeowner or apartment lessee is a senior citizen. About one-half million seniors now share their households. Financial hardship is not always a prerequisite for such programs. Many programs require only that a human need exist, such as security, companionship, and the need for helpful services. A senior is matched with a compatible roommate(s) in need of housing.

Each match is different. The financial arrangements between the two parties involved in home sharing may be based on a straight 50–50 split; others may trade services for a lesser household share or even a rent-free situation. The program benefits both parties. Some people who have chosen to share explain.

"I have outlived my family," said one woman, "and faced the dilemma of having to choose either to maintain my home alone or move into an institution. I choose instead to share my house with others and it has been a wonderful experience."

Said a roommate of his experience, "I was 64 when I moved in here, and I didn't know if I could learn to share a kitchen, having only lived in a nuclear family.... After a while, it's the differences that intrigue you. You want stimulation. That's why we're here instead of sitting alone somewhere.... It doesn't matter how old you are, as long as you keep growing."

Group residence shared housing programs also exist. In such arrangements, a home is purchased or leased, usually by a nonprofit community organization, to provide a shared home for four or more residents in a familylike setting. Groups normally range between 6 and 15 residents.

NSHRC reports that about half of all programs mix residents of all ages.

IF YOU ARE INTERESTED

Anyone interested in this option should first contact a local home sharing program if available.

When people handle their own home sharing arrangements they often experience problems, some serious, unless careful screening of potential home sharers has been done. The most common problems are the everyday ones of unrealistic expectations and troubles in adjusting and getting along together. An organization geared to matching couples professionally can help you avoid these difficulties. If no program exists in your area, NSHRC has a useful self-help guide that will steer you clear of major problems and show you step-by-step how to proceed.

You should also get advice on any tax consequences such an arrangement may have or how it might affect any social security income (SSI) supplements, Medicaid, or other public benefit programs which you may be receiving.

To locate such organizations, contact the appropriate resources listed in Chapter 5. These include I&Rs, 3As, and local social service or community organizations, particularly those that deal with services for seniors. Social work staffs at a community-based home care agency such as a visiting nurse association are also likely to know about any local community matching programs. Often organizations that assist in home sharing arrangements provide many other services and are not engaged in home sharing alone. Steer clear of any organization that matches people for a healthy fee. Most community service organizations provide assistance on a free or very low fee basis. Some organizations serve only residents living within specified geographic areas or may limit services according to age or income, so check any requirements in advance.

Programs operate differently, but in general, whether you have a home to share or are seeking a home with another, you should expect to provide plenty of information about yourself regarding your health, your personal habits, your preferences for a housemate, your finances, and details of your current housing arrangement. All such information is strictly confidential, and only very general information is revealed to a potential home sharing partner. You will be interviewed by a trained staff person. Then there is generally a waiting period until a potentially suitable partner is found.

Staff provide each potential partner with some background information about the other person and if both parties agree, an informal get-acquainted meeting is arranged. Normally the first meeting takes place on "neutral" ground, rather than in the home that will be shared. After the meeting, both parties talk privately to staff about their impressions. If favorable, subsequent meetings are arranged in the home in question; if not, then on to the next potential match.

Throughout the matching process, staff acts as a buffer and intermediary to help negotiate the living and financial arrangements and help both parties satisfactorily adjust to the new situation before and after home sharing begins.

To make a proper match usually takes time, so don't delay

if you seriously want to participate in such a program. For more information, contact:

The National Shared Housing Resource Center
6344 Greene St
Philadelphia, PA 19144
(215) 848–1220

VII

RESOURCE GUIDE TO HOME CARE

Self-Assessment Checklist for Home Care Services

Check all items. Home health aides, homemakers, and companions help with these activities to varying degrees. Anyone experiencing moderate difficulties in carrying out these tasks due to chronic illness, advancing age, or disability should consider seeking advice from an occupational therapist. This may decrease the need to rely on others for help. Remember too that some community organizations provide certain services, such as transportation, meals, companionship.

ACTIVITIES OF DAILY LIVING

	Help Needed?		Who Will Provide?			
	No	Yes	Family/ Friend	No. of Days/ Week	Agency/ Hiree	No. of Days/ Week
Bathing	☐	☐	☐	☐	☐	☐
Toileting	☐	☐	☐	☐	☐	☐
Transfer in/out bed	☐	☐	☐	☐	☐	☐
Walking	☐	☐	☐	☐	☐	☐
Teeth and/or mouth/denture care	☐	☐	☐	☐	☐	☐
Shaving	☐	☐	☐	☐	☐	☐
Comb hair	☐	☐	☐	☐	☐	☐
Wash hair	☐	☐	☐	☐	☐	☐
Nail care:	☐	☐	☐	☐	☐	☐
· Hands	☐	☐	☐	☐	☐	☐
· Feet	☐	☐	☐	☐	☐	☐
Dressing	☐	☐	☐	☐	☐	☐
Eating	☐	☐	☐	☐	☐	☐
Meal preparation:	☐	☐	☐	☐	☐	☐
· Regular diet	☐	☐	☐	☐	☐	☐
· Special diet	☐	☐	☐	☐	☐	☐
Tidy:						
· Bedroom	☐	☐	☐	☐	☐	☐
· Living room	☐	☐	☐	☐	☐	☐
· Bathroom	☐	☐	☐	☐	☐	☐
· Kitchen	☐	☐	☐	☐	☐	☐
Wash dishes	☐	☐	☐	☐	☐	☐
Laundry:	☐	☐	☐	☐	☐	☐
· Personal	☐	☐	☐	☐	☐	☐
· Linens	☐	☐	☐	☐	☐	☐
Change bed(s)	☐	☐	☐	☐	☐	☐
Telephoning	☐	☐	☐	☐	☐	☐
Letter writing	☐	☐	☐	☐	☐	☐
Recreation/social activities	☐	☐	☐	☐	☐	☐
Shopping:						
· Personal	☐	☐	☐	☐	☐	☐
· Food	☐	☐	☐	☐	☐	☐
List needed household supplies	☐	☐	☐	☐	☐	☐
Banking	☐	☐	☐	☐	☐	☐
Pay bills	☐	☐	☐	☐	☐	☐
Other errands _____	☐	☐	☐	☐	☐	☐
Transportation escort:						
· Doctor/medical care	☐	☐	☐	☐	☐	☐
· Community recreation	☐	☐	☐	☐	☐	☐
· Other _____	☐	☐	☐	☐	☐	☐

BASIC NURSING

	Help Needed?		Who Will Provide?			
	No	Yes	Family/ Friend	No. of Days/ Week	Agency/ Hiree	No. of Days/ Week
Temperature/pulse respiration	☐	☐	☐	☐	☐	☐
Exercises as prescribed	☐	☐	☐	☐	☐	☐
Assist with self-administered medications	☐	☐	☐	☐	☐	☐
Measure intake and output	☐	☐	☐	☐	☐	☐
Keep basic patient records	☐	☐	☐	☐	☐	☐
*Irrigate Foley catheter	☐	☐	☐	☐	☐	☐
*Change/reinforce nonsterile dressing	☐	☐	☐	☐	☐	☐
*Assist with skin care	☐	☐	☐	☐	☐	☐
*Apply cold or heat	☐	☐	☐	☐	☐	☐
Collect urine specimen	☐	☐	☐	☐	☐	☐
*Urine test for sugar, etc.	☐	☐	☐	☐	☐	☐
*Colostomy bag change	☐	☐	☐	☐	☐	☐

Note: Basic nursing tasks are usually carried out by home health aides or by LPNs and RNs when skilled nursing is also needed. (*) activities require an aide with advanced training and skills.

SKILLED NURSING

	Help Needed?		Who Will Provide?			
	No	Yes	Family/ Friend	No. of Days/ Week	Agency/ Hiree	No. of Days/ Week
Monitor health status	☐	☐	☐	☐	☐	☐
Change sterile dressing	☐	☐	☐	☐	☐	☐
Bowel and bladder training	☐	☐	☐	☐	☐	☐
Enema	☐	☐	☐	☐	☐	☐
Catheter insertion and care	☐	☐	☐	☐	☐	☐
Give injections or drugs	☐	☐	☐	☐	☐	☐
Ostomy care	☐	☐	☐	☐	☐	☐
Suctioning	☐	☐	☐	☐	☐	☐
Administer oxygen	☐	☐	☐	☐	☐	☐
Other physician-prescribed treatment ..	☐	☐	☐	☐	☐	☐
Draw blood for testing	☐	☐	☐	☐	☐	☐
Assist with:						
· Rehabilitation (basic)	☐	☐	☐	☐	☐	☐
· Rehabilitation (intensive)	☐	☐	☐	☐	☐	☐
· Dialysis	☐	☐	☐	☐	☐	☐
· Hyperalimentation	☐	☐	☐	☐	☐	☐
· IV therapy	☐	☐	☐	☐	☐	☐
· Ventilator care	☐	☐	☐	☐	☐	☐
Teach self-care skills	☐	☐	☐	☐	☐	☐
Teach equipment use	☐	☐	☐	☐	☐	☐
Inhalation treatment	☐	☐	☐	☐	☐	☐
Bedsore (decubitus) care	☐	☐	☐	☐	☐	☐

SOCIAL SERVICES

Note: If you answer yes to any of the items below, consult a social worker.

	Yes	No
Need information on community services?		
· Meals-on-Wheels	☐	☐
· Day care	☐	☐
· Hospice	☐	☐
· Friendly visiting	☐	☐
· Community companion service	☐	☐
· Telephone reassurance	☐	☐
· Respite care	☐	☐
· Chore services	☐	☐
· Transportation service	☐	☐
· Escort service	☐	☐
· Support groups	☐	☐
· Adult protective services	☐	☐
· Adult foster care	☐	☐
· Housing options (shared housing/board and care)	☐	☐
Need information/application assistance?		
· Medicare	☐	☐
· Health insurance coverage	☐	☐
· Veterans benefits	☐	☐
· Home equity	☐	☐
· Workers compensation	☐	☐
· Disability insurance	☐	☐
· Medicaid/Medi-Cal	☐	☐
· Supplemental social security (SSI)	☐	☐
· Food stamps	☐	☐
· Public assistance	☐	☐
Anxious, angry or depressed or guilty about failing health or disability?	☐	☐
Dislike self following body-changing surgery?	☐	☐
Frequent mood changes?	☐	☐
Frequently angry at others?	☐	☐
Little interest in daily life or in caring for self?	☐	☐
Overwhelmed by illness or disability?	☐	☐
Frequent family quarrels?	☐	☐
Worried about maintaining normal family role (husband, wife, breadwinner, parent)?	☐	☐
Trouble following prescribed treatment, drugs, exercise, etc.?	☐	☐
Abnormal eating, sleeping, or other personal habits?	☐	☐
Depend on others for help with tasks that could be self-performed?	☐	☐

Checklist for Choosing a Home Care Agency

Check or fill in information where needed

PART 1: QUALITY ISSUES

The Agency's Résumé	Agency A			Agency B		
	Yes	No	Notes	Yes	No	Notes
Professional references available?	☐	☐		☐	☐	
State licensed?	☐	☐		☐	☐	
Medicare/Medicaid certified?	☐	☐		☐	☐	
Accredited?	☐	☐		☐	☐	
Fully insured?						
· Malpractice	☐	☐		☐	☐	
· Liability	☐	☐		☐	☐	
· Bonding	☐	☐		☐	☐	
Office in business over 1 yr?	☐	☐		☐	☐	
Management qualifications:						
· Health degree?	☐	☐		☐	☐	
· Prior home care experience?	☐	☐		☐	☐	
· Other related education/experience?	☐	☐		☐	☐	

PART 1: QUALITY ISSUES (continued)

Services Offered	Agency A			Agency B		
	Yes	No	Notes	Yes	No	Notes
Member NAHC?	☐	☐		☐	☐	
Member state home care association?	☐	☐		☐	☐	
Professional or community advisory committee?	☐	☐		☐	☐	
Annual report available?	☐	☐		☐	☐	
Rates in writing?	☐	☐		☐	☐	
Written personnel and care procedures?	☐	☐		☐	☐	
Provides in-service education?	☐	☐		☐	☐	

Professional References

Agency A

1. _____ _____ _____
   Name of professional   Affiliation   Phone

2. _____ _____ _____
   Name of professional   Affiliation   Phone

Agency B

1. _____ _____ _____
   Name of professional   Affiliation   Phone

2. _____ _____ _____
   Name of professional   Affiliation   Phone

☐	☐	☐	☐	☐	☐	☐	☐	☐	☐	☐	☐	☐	☐	☐		☐
☐	☐	☐	☐	☐	☐	☐	☐	☐	☐	☐	☐	☐	☐	☐		☐

☐	☐	☐	☐	☐	☐	☐	☐	☐	☐	☐	☐	☐	☐	☐		☐
☐	☐	☐	☐	☐	☐	☐	☐	☐	☐	☐	☐	☐	☐	☐		☐

Skilled nursing?

Physical therapy?

Occupational therapy?

Speech therapy?

Social services?

Respiratory therapy?

Dietitian services?

Home health aides (HHA)?

Homemakers?

Companions?

Live-In?

Chore services?

Sells/rents DME/supplies?

Coordinates DME supplies?

Equipment loan closet?

Transportation (ambulette, etc)?

Emergency response system?

Coordinates community services, Meals-on-Wheels, transportation, etc)?

PART 1: QUALITY ISSUES (continued)

Assessment/Care Plan	Agency A			Agency B		
	Yes	No	Notes	Yes	No	Notes
Special Services						
Doctor's services?	☐	☐		☐	☐	
Dental care?	☐	☐		☐	☐	
Hyperalimentation?	☐	☐		☐	☐	
Dialysis?	☐	☐		☐	☐	
Respiratory-ventilator support?	☐	☐		☐	☐	
IV therapy?	☐	☐		☐	☐	
Intensive rehabilitation (trauma, burn, etc)?	☐	☐		☐	☐	
Air ambulance?	☐	☐		☐	☐	
Other?	☐	☐		☐	☐	
Service Availability						
24-hour?	☐	☐		☐	☐	
Daytime only (hours)?	☐	☐		☐	☐	
Evening-partial (hours)?	☐	☐		☐	☐	
Seven days/week?	☐	☐		☐	☐	
Weekdays only?	☐	☐		☐	☐	
Holidays?	☐	☐		☐	☐	
Personnel placement within 48–72 hours?	☐	☐		☐	☐	
Therapy within 48 hours if needed?	☐	☐		☐	☐	

	☐ ☐	☐ ☐
In-home assessment before care?	☐ ☐	☐ ☐
Conducted by professional?	☐ ☐	☐ ☐
Evaluates:		
• Ability to perform daily living tasks?	☐	☐
• State of health, "hands-on exam," if indicated?	☐	☐
• Social support?	☐	☐
• Home environment?	☐	☐
• Finances?	☐	☐
Consult your doctor?	☐	☐
Consult other organizations involved?	☐	☐
Care plan:		
• Written out?	☐	☐
• Lists problems, services, & goals for health care?	☐	☐
• Copy given to you or left in the home?	☐	☐

PART 1: QUALITY ISSUES (continued)

Personnel Policies (Paraprofessionals)	Agency A			Agency B		
	Yes	No	Notes	Yes	No	Notes
Supervision						
In-home?	☐	☐		☐	☐	
Frequency						
• Every two weeks?	☐	☐		☐	☐	
• Once a month?	☐	☐		☐	☐	
• Other? _____	☐	☐		☐	☐	
Telephone						
• Daily?	☐	☐		☐	☐	
• Weekly?	☐	☐		☐	☐	
• Other? _____	☐	☐		☐	☐	
Supervisor's qualifications						
• RN?	☐	☐		☐	☐	
• Public health or community experience?	☐	☐		☐	☐	
• Social worker (BSW/MSW)?	☐	☐		☐	☐	
• Other _____	☐	☐		☐	☐	
Supervisor availability						
• During working hrs?	☐	☐		☐	☐	
• On call 24 hrs?	☐	☐		☐	☐	

Employed directly by agency?

Training required? Amount?

· Home health aides?

· Homemakers?

· Companions?

Employer references checked?

Personal interview?

Skills tested? How?

Personnel Policies (Professionals)

Experience required? Amount?

Additional education? (specify): _____

Employer references checked?

Current licenses checked?

Skills inventory?

PART 1: QUALITY ISSUES (continued)

Potential Problems

1. What method(s) does the agency employ to prevent problems?

A. _____

B. _____

2. What happens in cases of theft? Property loss or damage?

A. _____

B. _____

3. Does the agency have a grievance procedure for problems? What is it?

A. _____

B. _____

PART II: COST ISSUES

Basic Policies	Agency A			Agency B		
	Yes	No	Notes	Yes	No	Notes
Fee flexibility if needed?	☐	☐		☐	☐	
Any minimum service charge for:						
• Hours/day?	☐	☐		☐	☐	
• Days/week?	☐	☐		☐	☐	
• Hours/week?	☐	☐		☐	☐	
Any charge for:						
• Assessment?	☐	☐		☐	☐	
• Supervision?	☐	☐		☐	☐	
• Professional consultation?	☐	☐		☐	☐	
• Team conferences?	☐	☐		☐	☐	
• Social work information and referral?	☐	☐		☐	☐	
• Written reports to doctors?	☐	☐		☐	☐	
• Written reports to family?	☐	☐		☐	☐	
• Completing and filing insurance forms?	☐	☐		☐	☐	
• Copies of records for tax purposes?	☐	☐		☐	☐	

PART II: COST ISSUES (continued)

Basic Policies	Agency A			Agency B		
	Yes	No	Notes	Yes	No	Notes
• Employee transportation?	☐	☐		☐	☐	
• Travel time?	☐	☐		☐	☐	
Accepts credit card? Which?	☐	☐		☐	☐	
Flexible billing?	☐	☐		☐	☐	
If insurance benefits run out or payment difficulties arise, the agency will:						
1.						
2.						
Insurance Policies						
Investigates your insurance coverage?	☐	☐		☐	☐	
Your insurance covers the service of this agency?	☐	☐		☐	☐	
Limits fees to customary and reasonable?	☐	☐		☐	☐	
Accepts insurance assignment?	☐	☐		☐	☐	

PART II: COST ISSUES (continued)

Rates for Service	Agency A		Agency B	
	Per Visit	Per Hour	Per Visit	Per Hour
Physician				
Registered nurse				
Licensed practical nurse				
Physical therapist				
Occupational therapist				
Speech therapist				
Dietitian				
Respiratory therapist				
Home health aide				
Homemaker				
Companion				
Chore service				
Live-in:				
• RN				
• LPN				
• HHA				
• Companion/homemaker				
Hyperalimentation				
Dialysis				
IV therapy				
Respiratory—ventilator support				
Special rehabilitation				
Bed/bath service				

Insurance Worksheet for Home Care/Hospice Coverage

Will your insurer pay for home care or hospice? Consult your policy, then complete or check items that apply. Complete a separate worksheet if you are covered under another insurance plan (as dependent on spouse's plan) so you can coordinate benefits. If you are not sure about an item, ask your insurer or benefits claims representative.

1. Insurance carrier:

Policy or group no. _____

Submit claims to: _____

Local contact for insurance information: _____
(Name)

_____
(Phone)

2. Specific coverage available:

	Home Care	Hospice
No specific benefits provided? (If not skip to #6)	_____	_____
Benefits provided—hospital insurance	_____	_____
Benefits provided—medical insurance	_____	_____
Maternity benefits	_____	(N/A)

3. Eligibility for coverage:

Hospitalization *not* required ....

Prior hospital stay required ....

First visit provided no later than (state # of days after discharge) _____

Other requirements (e.g., precertification): _____

4. Benefits limits:

Deductible required (state $ amt or none): _____

Co-payment (state $ amt, % or none): _____

Maximum dollar coverage (state $ amt or none): _____

Maximum visits allowed (state # or none): _____

Other limits: _____

5. Covered home care expenses

Ambulance services ....

Doctor visits ....

Registered nurse ....

Licensed practical nurse ....

Occupational therapy ....

Physical therapy ....

INSURANCE WORKSHEET (continued)

	Home Care	Hospice
Speech therapy		
Dietitian		
Medical social services		
Respiratory therapy		
Home health aide		
Homemaker		
Drugs		
EKG		
Home improvements (catastrophic illness or injury)		
Laboratory		
Medical equipment		
Medical supplies		
Oxygen		
X rays		

6. **Coverage available under other policy provisions**

Private duty: RN ....

Private duty: LPN ....

Outpatient: ....

    Laboratory ....

    Physical therapy ....

    Occupational therapy ....

    Speech therapy ....

    Oxygen ....

    X rays ....

Medical social services (check counselling/mental health clauses) _____

Other: (check disability clauses) _____

Checklist for Choosing a Medical Equipment Dealer

Check or fill in information where needed

Customer Service	Dealer A			Dealer B		
	Yes	No	Notes	Yes	No	Notes
Medicare-certified?	☐	☐		☐	☐	
Handles all types of equipment?	☐	☐		☐	☐	
How soon delivers?						
24-hour, seven-day-a-week service available for:						
· Repair/maintenance?	☐	☐		☐	☐	
· Delivery of supplies or equipment replacement?	☐	☐		☐	☐	
Helps with inventory control of oxygen, supplies, etc.?	☐	☐		☐	☐	
Can provide needed supplies if you travel?	☐	☐		☐	☐	
Replaces or loans equipment free when your regular equipment needs repair?	☐	☐		☐	☐	
Does own repairs and maintenance?	☐	☐		☐	☐	
Service available after warranty expires?	☐	☐		☐	☐	
In-home visit prior to equipment selection?	☐	☐		☐	☐	
Follows up all customers to ensure satisfaction?	☐	☐		☐	☐	
References available?						
Professionals	☐	☐		☐	☐	
Consumers	☐	☐		☐	☐	

Checklist for Choosing a Medical Equipment Dealer (continued)

	Dealer A			Dealer B		
	Yes	No	Notes	Yes	No	Notes
Dealer Personnel						
Service workers well trained?	☐	☐		☐	☐	
Professionals credentialled?	☐	☐		☐	☐	
Some full-time service staff?	☐	☐		☐	☐	
Some full-time professional staff?	☐	☐		☐	☐	
Cost/Payment Terms						
Any extra charge for:						
Delivery?	☐	☐		☐	☐	
Repair?	☐	☐		☐	☐	
Maintenance?	☐	☐		☐	☐	
After-hours call?	☐	☐		☐	☐	
In-home evaluation visits?	☐	☐		☐	☐	
Setup/installation?	☐	☐		☐	☐	
Training in equipment use?	☐	☐		☐	☐	
or consultation?	☐	☐		☐	☐	

Payment due on delivery? .... ☐ ☐

Will bill later? .... ☐ ☐

Credit cards accepted? Which one(s)? .... ☐ ☐

Charges interest on overdue payments? ☐ ☐

Fully itemizes all bills? ☐ ☐

Full credit or exchange for returned equipment? ☐ ☐

Free equipment trial period? ☐ ☐

Accepts assignment of insurance benefits? ☐ ☐

References

A. _____ (Name) _____ (Phone)

_____ (Name) _____ (Phone)

B. _____ (Name) _____ (Phone)

_____ (Name) _____ (Phone)

Home Care Tax Deductions

This list is based on IRS publications *and* various tax rulings. For more information, contact an experienced tax advisor (accountant, attorney). Do not rely on the IRS advisory service. Consumer studies confirm that, with the exception of very basic questions, taxpayers often receive incomplete, incorrect, or misleading information.

Ambulance/ambulette service
Antiseptic solutions*
Attendant services*
Autoette
Blood transfusions
Canes
Catheters
Colostomy supplies
Crutches
Dietitian fees
Doctor fees
Drugs, physician-prescribed
EKG at home
Emergency response systems*
Employer expenses for self-hired home care personnel
Glucose tests (self-administered) if physician prescribes
Health insurance premiums including Medicare, HMO fees

Home health aide fees*
Home improvements*
Homemaker fees*
Hyperalimentation products/equipment
Ileostomy supplies
Incontinent products*
Insulin
Irrigating solutions*
Laboratory tests including medically prescribed self-administered tests
Meals for medically necessary personnel
Medical equipment
    Purchase or rental fees
    Maintenance
    Repair
    Replacement parts
Medical social service fees
Medical supplies*
Medicine, over-the-counter, if physician-prescribed*

Minerals, physician-prescribed*
Nursing fees (RNs, LPNs, aides)*
Ostomy supplies
Oxygen equipment/supplies
Personal care fees*
Prescription drugs
Prosthetic devices
Refrigerator*
Respiratory equipment
Special diets, food and drink*
Syringes
Therapy fees
Transportation, all medically necessary
Urine tests (self-administered) if physician-prescribed
Utilities*
Vitamins, physician-prescribed*
Walkers
Wheelchairs
Wigs*
X rays

* Certain conditions apply; see Chapter 12.

National Home Care Related Organizations

This list is selective. Many other organizations which serve older or disabled persons or consumers with health problems or other special interests or needs are also involved in home care (see Chapter 5). The organizations noted below (✓) provide free or low-cost consumer publications. For more information, contact them directly.

American Affiliation of Visiting Nurse
    Associations and Services
21 Maryland Plaza, Suite 300
St. Louis, MO 63108
(314) 367-7744

American Association for Continuity of Care
1101 Connecticut Ave NW, Suite 700
Washington, DC 20036
(202) 857-1194

American Federation of Home Health Agencies
429 N St SW, Suite S-605
Washington, DC 20024
(202) 554-0526

American Hospital Association (✓)
Division of Ambulatory Care
840 N Lake Shore Dr
Chicago, IL 60611
(312) 280-6216

American Medical Association (✓)
535 N Dearborn St
Chicago, IL 60610
(312) 645-5000

American Society for Parenteral and Enteral
    Nutrition
1025 Vermont Ave NW, Suite 810
Washington, DC 20005
(205) 638-5881

Council on Accreditation of Services for
    Families and Children
67 Irving Pl
New York, NY 10003
(212) 254-9330

Family Service America
44 E 23 St
New York, NY 10010
(212) 674-6100

Health Insurance Association of America (✓)
1850 K St NW
Washington, DC 2006-2284
(202) 331-1336

Home Health Care Medical Directors
    Association
PO Box 16626
Mobile, AL 36616
(205) 476-0192

Home Health Services & Staffing Association
2101 L St NW, Suite 800
Washington, DC 20037
(202) 775-4707

Joint Commission on Accreditation of Hospitals
875 N Michigan Ave
Chicago, IL 60611
(312) 642-6061

National Association for Home Care (✓)
519 C St NE
Washington, DC 20002
(202) 547-7424

National Association of Meal Programs
Box 6344
604 W North Ave
Pittsburgh, PA 15212

National Citizens' Coalition for Nursing Home
    Reform (✓)
1825 Connecticut Ave NW, Suite 417
Washington, DC 20009
(202) 797-0657

National Foundation of Dentistry for the
    Handicapped
1250 14th St, Suite 610
Denver, CO 80202
(303) 573-0264

National HomeCaring Council (✓)
235 Park Ave S, 11th floor
New York, NY 10003
(212) 674-4990

National Hospice Organization (✓)
1901 N Fort Myer Dr
Arlington, VA 22209
(703) 243-5900

National Institute on Adult Daycare (✓)
600 Maryland Ave SW, West Wing 100
Washington, DC 20024
(202) 479-1200

National League for Nursing
10 Columbus Circle
New York, NY 10019
(212) 582-1022

U.S. Department of Health and Human
  Services (✓)
Administration on Aging
330 Independence Ave SW
Washington, DC 20201
(202) 245-0724

U.S. Department of Health and Human Services
Health Care Financing Administration
310G Humphrey Bldg
200 Independence Ave SW
Washington, DC 20201
(202) 245-6726

U.S. Department of Health and Human Services
Public Health Service
716G Humphrey Bldg
200 Independence Ave SW
Washington, DC 20201
(202) 245-7694

U.S. Federal Trade Commission (✓)
Correspondence Branch
Pennsylvania Ave at 6th St NW
Washington, DC 20580
(202) 523-3567

U.S. Veterans Administration
Department of Medicine and Surgery
810 Vermont Ave NW
Washington, DC 20420
(202) 389-2596

State Home Care Associations

This list includes only those state associations that have permanent mailing addresses.
For information on unlisted states, contact the National Association for Home Care.

ARIZONA

Arizona Association for Home Care
3602 E Campbell
Phoenix, AZ 85018
(602) 957-0773

ARKANSAS

Arkansas Association for Home Health Agencies
1501 N University, Suite 400
Little Rock, AR 72207
(501) 664-7870

CALIFORNIA

California Association for Health Services at
  Home (CAHSAH)
660 J St, Suite 290
Sacramento, CA 95814
(916) 443-8055

COLORADO

Colorado Association of Home Health Agencies
7235 S Newport Way
Englewood, CO 80122
(303) 694-4728

CONNECTICUT

Connecticut Association for Home Care
110 Barnes Rd
PO Box 90
Wallingford, CT 06492
(203) 265-8931

DISTRICT OF COLUMBIA

Capitol Home Health Association
PO Box 70407
Washington, DC 20088
(202) 547-7424

FLORIDA

Florida Association of Home Health Agencies
201 S Monroe St, Suite 201
Tallahassee, FL 32301
(904) 224-4226

GEORGIA

Georgia Association of Home Health Agencies
1260 S Omni International
Atlanta, GA 30303
(404) 577-9144

ILLINOIS

Illinois Council of Home Health Services
1619 Ashland Ave
Evanston, IL 60201
(312) 328–6654

INDIANA

Indiana Association of Home Health Agencies
PO Box 1457
Carmel, IN 46032
(317) 848–2942

IOWA

Iowa Assembly of Home Health Agencies
3000 SW 40 St
Des Moines, IA 50321
(515) 282–6498

KANSAS

Kansas Association of Home Health Agencies
1526 N Market St
Wichita, KS 67214
(316) 265–5888

KENTUCKY

Kentucky Home Health Association
1804 Darien Dr
Lexington, KY 40504
(606) 277–7983

MAINE

Maine Community Health Association
71 Sewall St
Augusta, ME 04330
(207) 622–3276

MARYLAND

Maryland Association of Home Health Agencies
PO Box 1307
Columbia, MD 21044
(301) 964–9698

MASSACHUSETTS

Massachusetts Association of Community
Health Agencies
6 Beacon St, Suite 915
Boston, MA 02108
(617) 893–4792

MICHIGAN

Michigan Home Health Association
Seymour Ave, Suite 22079
Lansing, MI 48933
(513) 372–6143

MINNESOTA

Minnesota Assembly of Home and Community
Health Nursing Agencies
PO Box 300110
Minneapolis, MN 55403
(612) 374–5404

MISSISSIPPI

Mississippi Home Health Association
455 N Lamar St, Suite 410
Jackson, MS 39202
(601) 353–0015

MISSOURI

Missouri Association of Home Health Agencies
101 Madison St
Jefferson City, MO 65101
(314) 634–7772

NEW HAMPSHIRE

Community Health Care Association of New
Hampshire
117 Manchester St
Concord, NH 03301
(603) 225–5597

NEW JERSEY

Home Health Agency Assembly of New Jersey
760 Alexander Rd, CN-1
Princeton, NJ 08540
(609) 452–9280

NEW YORK

Home Care Association of New York State
840 James St
Syracuse, NY 13203
(315) 475–7229

NORTH CAROLINA

North Carolina Association for Home Care
714 W Johnson St
Raleigh, NC 27603
(919) 821–3575

NORTH DAKOTA

North Dakota Nurse Corps, P.C.
212 N 4th Greentree Sq
Bismarck, ND 58501
(701) 223–1385

OHIO

Ohio Council of Home Health Agencies
175 S Third St, Suite 925
Columbus, OH 43215
(614) 461–1960

OREGON

Oregon Association for Home Care
Box 510
Salem, OR 97308
(503) 399-9395

PENNSYLVANIA

Pennsylvania Association of Home Health
  Agencies
1200 Camp Hill By-pass
PO Box 608
Camp Hill, PA 17011
(717) 763-7053

RHODE ISLAND

Association of Home Health Agencies of Rhode
  Island
2845 Post Rd
Warwick, RI 02886
(401) 738-8280

TENNESSEE

Tennessee Association for Home Health
4711 Trousdale Dr
Nashville, TN 37220
(615) 331-0463

Tennessee Council for Home Care Service
394 W Main St
Hendersonville, TN 37075
(615) 822-3094

TEXAS

Texas Association of Home Health Agencies
One La Costa Office Bldg
1016 La Posada Dr, Suite 296
Austin, TX 78752
(512) 459-4303

VERMONT

Vermont Assembly of Home Health Agencies
148 Main St
Montpelier, VT 05602
(802) 229-0579

WASHINGTON

Home Care Association of Washington
PO Box 55967
Seattle, WA 98155
(206) 363-3801

WEST VIRGINIA

West Virginia Council of Home Health Agencies
PO Box 4227
Star City, WV 26504-4227
(304) 599-9583

WISCONSIN

Wisconsin Homecare Organization
330 E Lakeside St
Madison, WI 53715
(608) 257-6781

State Units on Aging

ALABAMA

Commission on Aging
State Capitol
Montgomery, AL 36130
(205) 261-5743

ALASKA

Older Alaskans Commission
Department of Administration
Pouch C-Mail Station 0209
Juneau, AK 99811
(907) 465-3250

ARIZONA

Aging and Adult Administration
Department of Economic Security
1400 W Washington St
Phoenix, AZ 85007
(602) 255-4446

ARKANSAS

Office of Aging and Adult Services
Department of Social and Rehabilitative
  Services
Donaghey Bldg, Suite 1428
7th and Main St
Little Rock, AR 72201
(501) 371-2441

CALIFORNIA

Department of Aging
1020 19 St
Sacramento, CA 95814
(916) 322-5290

COLORADO

Aging and Adult Services Division
Department of Social Services
1575 Sherman St, Room 503
Denver, CO 80203
(303) 866-3672

CONNECTICUT

Department on Aging
175 Main St
Hartford, CT 06106
(203) 566-3238

DELAWARE

Division on Aging
Department of Health and Social Services
1901 N DuPont Highway
New Castle, DE 19720
(302) 421-6791

DISTRICT OF COLUMBIA

Office on Aging
1424 K St NW, 2nd floor
Washington, DC 20005
(202) 724-5622

FLORIDA

Program Office of Aging and Adult Services
Department of Health and Rehabilitation
    Services
1317 Winewood Blvd
Tallahassee, FL 32301
(904) 488-8922

GEORGIA

Office of Aging
878 Peachtree St NE, Room 632
Atlanta, GA 30309
(404) 894-5333

HAWAII

Executive Office on Aging
Office of the Governor
1149 Bethel St, Room 307
Honolulu, HI 96813
(808) 548-2593

IDAHO

Office on Aging
Room 114—Statehouse
Boise, ID 83720
(208) 334-3833

ILLINOIS

Department on Aging
421 East Capitol Avenue
Springfield, IL 62706
(217) 785-3356

INDIANA

Department of Aging and Community Services
115 N Pennsylvania St
Suite 1350 Consolidated Bldg
Indianapolis, IN 46204
(317) 232-7006

IOWA

Commission on Aging
Suite 236, Jewett Bldg
914 Grand Ave
Des Moines, IA 50319
(515) 281-5187

KANSAS

Department on Aging
610 W Tenth
Topeka, KS 66612
(913) 296-4986

KENTUCKY

Division for Aging Services
Department of Human Resources
DHR Bldg—6th floor
275 E Main St
Frankfort, KY 40601
(502) 564-6930

LOUISIANA

Office of Elderly Affairs
PO Box 80374
Baton Rouge, LA 70898
(504) 925-1700

MAINE

Bureau of Maine's Elderly
Department of Human Services
State House—Station #11
Augusta, ME 04333
(207) 289-2561

MARYLAND

Office on Aging
State Office Building
301 W Preston St
Baltimore, MD 21201
(301) 383-5064

MASSACHUSETTS

Department of Elder Affairs
38 Chauncy St
Boston, MA 02111
(617) 727-7750

MICHIGAN

Office of Services to the Aging
PO Box 30026
Lansing, MI 48909
(517) 373-8230

MINNESOTA

Board on Aging
Metro Square Bldg, Room 204
Seventh and Robert St
St. Paul, MN 55101
(612) 296-2544

MISSISSIPPI

Council on Aging
802 N State St
Executive Bldg, Suite 301
Jackson, MS 39201
(601) 354-6590

MISSOURI

Division on Aging
Department of Social Services
Broadway State Office—PO Box 570
Jefferson City, MO 65101
(314) 751-3082

MONTANA

Community Services Division
PO Box 4210
Helena, MT 59604
(406) 444-3865

NEBRASKA

Department on Aging
PO Box 95044
301 Centennial Mall—South
Lincoln, NE 68509
(402) 471-2306

NEVADA

Division on Aging
Department of Human Resources
505 E King St
Kinkead Bldg, Room 101
Carson City, NV 89710
(702) 885-4210

NEW HAMPSHIRE

Council on Aging
14 Depot St
Concord, NH 03301
(603) 271-2751

NEW JERSEY

Division on Aging
Department of Community Affairs
PO Box 2768
363 W State St
Trenton, NJ 08625
(609) 292-4833

NEW MEXICO

State Agency on Aging
224 E Palace Ave, 4th Floor
La Villa Rivera Bldg
Santa Fe, NM 87501
(505) 827-7640

NEW YORK

Office for the Aging
New York State Plaza
Agency Building #2
Albany, NY 12223
(518) 474-5731

NORTH CAROLINA

Division on Aging
708 Hillsborough St., Suite 200
Raleigh, NC 27603
(919) 733-3983

NORTH DAKOTA

Aging Services
Department of Human Services
State Capitol Bldg
Bismarck, ND 58505
(701) 224-2577

OHIO

Commission on Aging
50 W Broad St, 9th floor
Columbus, OH 43215
(614) 466-5500

OKLAHOMA

Special Unit on Aging
Department of Human Services
PO Box 25352
Oklahoma City, OK 73125
(405) 521-2281

OREGON

Senior Services Division
313 Public Service Bldg
Salem, OR 97310
(503) 378-4728

PENNSYLVANIA

Department of Aging
231 State St
Harrisburg, PA 17101-1195
(717) 783-1550

RHODE ISLAND

Department of Elderly Affairs
79 Washington St
Providence, RI 02903
(401) 277-2858

SOUTH CAROLINA

Commission on Aging
915 Main St
Columbia, SC 29201
(803) 758-2576

SOUTH DAKOTA

Office of Adult Services and Aging
700 N Illinois St
Kneip Bldg
Pierre, SD 57501
(605) 773-3656

TENNESSEE

Commission on Aging
703 Tennessee Bldg
535 Church St
Nashville, TN 37219
(615) 741-2056

TEXAS

Department on Aging
210 Barton Springs Rd, 5th floor
PO Box 12768 Capitol Station
Austin, TX 78704
(512) 475-2717

UTAH

Division of Aging and Adult Services
Department of Social Services
150 W North Temple
Box 2500
Salt Lake City, UT 84102
(801) 533-6422

VERMONT

Office on Aging
103 S Main St
Waterbury, VT 05676
(802) 241-2400

VIRGINIA

Department on Aging
101 N 14th St, 18th floor
James Monroe Bldg
Richmond, VA 23219
(804) 225-2271

WASHINGTON

Bureau of Aging and Adult Services
Department of Social and Health Services
   OB-43G
Olympia, WA 98504
(206) 753-2502

WEST VIRGINIA

Commission on Aging
Holly Grove—State Capitol
Charleston, WV 25305
(304) 348-3317

WISCONSIN

Bureau of Aging
Division of Community Services
One W Wilson St
Madison, WI 53702
(608) 266-2536

WYOMING

Commission on Aging
401 W 19 St
Cheyenne, WY 82002
(307) 777-7986

State Hospice Organizations

***Denotes no existing state organization

ALABAMA

Alabama State Hospice Organization
Janice Quick, President
701 Princeton Ave SW
Birmingham, AL 35211
(205) 592-1738

ALASKA

Hospice of Juneau
Mary Tonsmeire, Coordinator
419-6th St
Juneau, AK 99802
(907) 586-3414

ARIZONA

Arizona State Hospice Organization
Sue Vandenbroeck
St. Mary's Hospice
1601 West St Mary's Rd
Tucson, AZ 85705
(602) 622-5833

ARKANSAS

Arkansas State Hospice Organization
Elizabeth F. King, President
PO Box 725
Jonesboro, AR 72401
(501) 972-6270

CALIFORNIA

Hospice Organization of Southern California
Joyce Green, President
637 S Lucas
Los Angeles, CA 90017
(818) 788-3295

Northern California Hospice Association
Sarah Gorodezky
703 Market St, Suite 550
San Francisco, CA 94103
(415) 543-9393

COLORADO

Colorado Hospice Coalition
Susan Langsraff
3534 Kirkwood Pl
Boulder, CO 80302
(303) 449-7740

CONNECTICUT

Hospice Council of Connecticut
Janice Casey, Home Care Coordinator
461 Atlantic St
Stamford, CT 06901
(203) 324-2592

DELAWARE

Delaware Hospices, Inc.***
A. Murray Goodwin, Executive Director
3509 Silvergate Rd, Suite 109 Talley Bldg
Wilmington, DE 19810
(302) 478-5707

DISTRICT OF COLUMBIA

Hospice Care of the DC***
Anne Towne, Executive Director
1749 St. Matthews Court, NW
Washington, DC 20036
(202) 347-1700

FLORIDA

Florida Hospices, Inc.
Becky McDonald, President
Hospice of Volusia
PO Box 1990
Daytona Beach, FL 32724
(904) 254-4237

GEORGIA

Georgia Hospice Organization
Nancy Paris, President
Hospice of the Golden Isles
1326 Union St
Brunswick, GA 31520
(215) 265-4735

HAWAII

St. Francis Hospital***
Maureen Keleher
2230 Liliha St
Honolulu, HI 96817
(808) 845-1727

IDAHO

Council of Idaho Hospice Organizations
Betty L. Johnson, President
Hospice Mercy Medical Center
1512 12th Ave
Nampa, ID 83651
(208) 467-1171, ext. 174

ILLINOIS

Illinois State Hospice Organization
Anne Rooney, President
Hospice of Proviso-Leÿden
330 Eastern Ave
Bellwood, IL 60104
(312) 547-8282

INDIANA

Indiana Association of Hospices
Stephen G. Arter, President
2200 Randalea Dr
Fort Wayne, IN 46805
(219) 484-6636, ext. 4183

IOWA

Iowa Hospice Organization
Marilyn Story, President
205 Loma St
Waterloo, IA 50701
(319) 273-2702 or 273-2814

KANSAS

Association of Kansas Hospices
Nancy Solscheid, President
7540 Aberdeen
Prairie Village, KS 66208
(913) 341-5476

KENTUCKY

Kentucky Association of Hospices
Gretchen Brown, President
1105 Nicholasville Rd
Lexington, KY 40503
(606) 252-2308

LOUISIANA

Richard N. Murphy Hospice***
Lou Bordelon, RN
PO Box 111
Hammond, LA 70404
(504) 386-6130

MAINE

Coalition of Maine Hospices
Ellen Rogers, President
32 Thomas St
Portland, ME 04102
(207) 774-4417

MARYLAND

Maryland State Hospice Network
Susan Riggs, Co-Chairman
Sinai Hospital Home Care/Hospice
2401 Belvedere Ave
Baltimore, MD 21215
(301) 587-5600

MASSACHUSETTS

Hospice of Lynn
Carol Holden, President
VNA of Lynn
196 Ocean Ave
Lynn, MA 01902
(617) 598-2454

MICHIGAN

Michigan Hospice Organization
Karl Zeigler, President
1825 Watson Rd
Hemlock, MI 48626
(517) 642-8121

MINNESOTA

Minnesota Hospice Organization
Anne O'Brien, President
Metro Medical Center
900 S 8 St
Minneapolis, MN 55404
(612) 347-4377

MISSISSIPPI

South Mississippi Home Health***
Annette Drennan
PO Box 888
Hattiesburg, MS 39401
(601) 268-1842

MISSOURI

Missouri Hospice Organization
Karen Beckman, President
527 W 39 St
Kansas City, MO 64111
(816) 531-1200

MONTANA

Montana Hospice Exchange Council
St. Joseph's Mission Mountain Hospice
Sheila Gapay
PO Box 1010
Polson, MT 59860
(406) 883-5377

NEBRASKA

Nebraska Hospice Association, Inc.
M. Thomas Perkins, President
1010 E 35 St
Scotts Bluff, NE 69361
(308) 635-3171 or 632-5549

NEVADA

Nathan Adelson Hospice***
Linda Lehman
4141 S Swenson
Las Vegas, NV 89109
(702) 733-0320

NEW HAMPSHIRE

Hospice Affiliates of New Hampshire
Lutie K. Piper, Executive Director
Concord Regional VNA
8 Loudoun Rd
Concord, NH 03301
(603) 224-4093

NEW JERSEY

New Jersey Hospice Organization
Shelley Van Kempen, President
760 Alexander Rd
Princeton, NJ 08540
(609) 452-9280

NEW MEXICO

Visiting Nurse Services Hospice***
Bette Betts, Administrative Coordinator
PO Box 1951
Santa Fe, NM 87501
(505) 471-9201

NEW YORK

New York State Hospice Association, Inc.
Carole Selinske, Executive Director
468 Rosedale Ave
White Plains, NY 10605
(914) 946-7699

NORTH CAROLINA

Hospice of North Carolina, Inc.
Judi Lund, Executive Director
800 St. Mary's St, Suite 401
Raleigh, NC 27605
(919) 829-9588

NORTH DAKOTA

St. Joseph's Hospice
Patricia F. Drake, Coordinator
7th Ave, W
Dickinson, ND 58601
(701) 225-7200

OHIO

Ohio Hospice Organization, Inc.
Betty Schmoll, President
2181 Embury Park Rd
Dayton, OH 45414
(513) 278-0060

OKLAHOMA

Oklahoma Hospice Organization
James A. Eselin, Executive Director
Hospice of Central Oklahoma
4500 N Lincoln
Oklahoma City, OK 73105
(405) 424-7263

OREGON

Oregon Council of Hospices
Maryanne Memorial Hospice
Valarie Ivey, President
PO Box 191
Forest Grove, OR 97116
(503) 640-2737

PENNSYLVANIA

Pennsylvania Hospice Network
Francis Cohen, President
South Hills Family Hospice
1000 Bower Hill Rd
Pittsburgh, PA 15243
(412) 561-4900

RHODE ISLAND

Hospice Care of Rhode Island***
Robert J. Canny, Executive Director
1400 Pawtucket Ave
Rumford, RI 02916
(401) 434-4740

SOUTH CAROLINA

Hospice of Charleston, Inc.***
Roberta H. Frank, Executive Director
PO Box 1125
Charleston, SC 29402
(803) 577-0186

TENNESSEE

Hospice of Tennessee
Iris A. Kozil
Alive—Hospice of Nashville
1908 21 Ave, S
Nashville, TN 37212
(615) 298-3351

TEXAS

Texas Hospice Organization, Inc.
Jo Edmundson, Coordinator
2525 Wallingwood #104
Austin, TX 78746
(512) 327-9149

UTAH

Utah Hospice Organization, Inc.
Helen Rollings, President
1370 South West Temple
Salt Lake City, UT 84115
(801) 627-2504

VERMONT

Vermont Ecumenical Council
Patricia Healy Sullivan, President
Visiting Nurse Association, Inc.
260 College St
Burlington, VT 15401
(802) 658-1900

VIRGINIA

Virginia Association of Hospices
Jacke White
Hospice of N Virginia
316 Main St
Arlington, VA
(804) 525-7070

WASHINGTON

Washington Hospice Organization
Elaine McIntosh, President
7814 Greenwood Ave, N
Seattle, WA 98103
(206) 784-9221

WEST VIRGINIA

Hospice Council of West Virginia
Morgantown Hospice, Inc.
PO Box 4222
Morgantown, WV 26505
(304) 598-3424

WISCONSIN

Milwaukee Hospice Home Care
Jim Ewens
1022 N Ninth St
Milwaukee, WI 53233
(414) 271-3686

WYOMING

Sheridan County Hospice, Inc.***
William J. Browning, MD
2000 Suite 515
Sheridan, WY 82801
(307) 672-3473

Self-Help Clearinghouses

NATIONAL

National Self-Help Clearinghouse
Graduate School and University Center/CUNY
33 W 42 St
New York, NY 10036
(212) 840-7606

CANADA

Self-Help Clearinghouse
CAMAC, Inc.
14 Aberdeen
Montreal, Quebec, Canada J4P 1R3
(514) 937-5621

CALIFORNIA

Self-Help and Mutual Aid Association (SHAMA)
% Alfred Katz
UCLA School of Public Health
405 Hilgard Ave
Los Angeles, CA 90024
(213) 825-5418

San Diego Self-Help Clearinghouse
1172 Morena Blvd, PO Box 86246
San Diego, CA 92138
(619) 275-2344

San Francisco Self-Help Clearinghouse
Mental Health Assn. of San Francisco
2398 Fine St
San Francisco, CA 94115
(415) 921-4401

CONNECTICUT

Hamden Mental Health Center
300 Dixwell Ave
Hamden, CT 06514
(203) 789-7645

Connecticut Self-Help Mutual Support Network
19 Howe St
New Haven, CT 06511
(800) 842-1501 or (203) 789-7645

ILLINOIS

Self-Help Center
1600 Dodge Center, Suite S-122
Evanston, IL 60201
(312) 328-0470

MICHIGAN

Berrien County Self-Help Clearinghouse
Riverwood Community Mental Health Center
2681 Morton Ave
St. Joseph, MI 49085
(616) 983-7781

MINNESOTA

Community Care Unit
Wilder Center
919 Lafond Ave
St. Paul, MN 55104
(612) 642-4060

NEBRASKA

Self-Help Information Services
1601 Euclid Ave
Lincoln, NE 68502
(402) 476-9668

NEW JERSEY

Self-Help Clearinghouse of New Jersey
St. Clare's Hospital
Pocono Rd
Denville, NJ 07834
(800) 452-9790 or (201) 625-6395

NEW YORK

New York City Self-Help Clearinghouse, Inc.
186 Joralemon St
Brooklyn, NY 11201
(718) 852-4291

Long Island Self-Help Clearinghouse
New York Institute of Technology
6350 Jericho Turnpike
Commack, NY 11725
(516) 499-8800 or 686-7505

Orange County Department of Mental Health
Consultation and Education Department
Harriman Dr, Drawer 471
Goshen, NY 10925
(914) 294-6185

New York City Self-Help Clearinghouse
Graduate School and University Center/CUNY
33 West 42 Street
New York, NY 10036
(212) 840-7606

Rockland County CMHC
Sanitorium Road
Pomona, NY 10970
(914) 354-0200, ext. 2237

Westchester Self-Help Clearinghouse
Westchester Community College
Academic Arts Building
75 Grasslands Road
Valhalla, NY 10595
(914) 347-3620

OREGON

Portland Self-Help Information Service
Regional Research Institute
Portland State University
1912 Southwest Sixth
Portland, OR 97207
(503) 222-5555 or 229-4040

PENNSYLVANIA

Philadelphia Self-Help Clearinghouse
John F. Kennedy, CMHC/MR
112 N. Ercad St, 5th floor
Philadelphia, PA 19102
(215) 568-0860, ext. 276

Self-Help Information Network Exchange
Voluntary Action Center
200 Adams Ave, Room 317
Scranton, PA 18503
(717) 961-1234

TENNESSEE

Overlook Mental Health Center
6906 Kingston Pike
Knoxville, TN 36919
(615) 588-9747

TEXAS

Dallas County Self-Help Clearinghouse
Dallas County Mental Health Assn.
2500 Maple Ave
Dallas, TX 75206
(214) 748-7825

Tarrant County Self-Help Clearinghouse
Tarrant County Mental Health Assn.
804 W 7 St
Fort Worth, TX 76102
(817) 335-5405

WASHINGTON, DC

Greater Washington Self-Help Coalition
Mental Health Association of Northern Virginia
100 North Washington St, Suite 232
Falls Church, VA 22046
(703) 536-4100

WISCONSIN

Continuing Education in Mental Health
University of Wisconsin Extension
414 Lowell Hall
610 Langden St
Madison, WI 53706
(608) 263-4432

Mutual Aid Self-Help Association (MASHA)
PO Box 09304
Milwaukee, WI 53209
(414) 461-1466

INDEX